MITLA
PASS

LEON URIS

NEW YORK   LONDON   TORONTO   SYDNEY   AUCKLAND

MITLA PASS

Doubleday

Published by Doubleday, a division of Bantam Doubleday Dell Publishing Group, Inc., 666 Fifth Avenue, New York, New York 10103

Doubleday and the portrayal of an anchor with a dolphin are trademarks of Doubleday, a division of Bantam Doubleday Dell Publishing Group, Inc.

This book is dedicated
to my beloved sister
ESSIE

ACKNOWLEDGMENT

This book required extraordinary research, and an extraordinary researcher. Clarifying confusing military history and accounts of battles plus running down a thousand and one little sticklers was a gigantic job, beautifully done. I would like to thank and acknowledge Priscilla Higham for her tremendous skill and ingenuity, for her complete devotion to this project, and mainly for her friendship, particularly when the waters got rough.

And to my wife Jill. God bless the writer's wife.

PART ONE

GERONIMO!

TEL AVIV

October 20, 1956

D DAY MINUS NINE

THE PRIME MINISTER'S COTTAGE, a remnant of the former German colony, sat unobtrusively in the midst of the outsized defense complex on the northern end of Tel Aviv. Midnight had come and gone. The stream of callers faded to a trickle, then halted.

For the moment David Ben-Gurion sat alone, his first opportunity all day for solitary contemplation. He was behind a desk that looked down a long conference table which was covered with green felt. Dead cigarette butts spilled over their ashtrays. The fruit baskets held spoiling apple and pear cores, grape seeds, banana skins, and peach pits, their fruit devoured. Half-empty soda bottles had lost their fizz and others, tipped over in disarray, appeared like a platoon of soldiers caught in a cross fire.

The cleanup crew of soldiers, two young men and two young women wearing top-security clearance badges, tiptoed in and attacked the mess.

"Can I get you anything—some tea?" one of the girls asked.

Ben-Gurion shook his head. It was a great head that seemed even greater perched on his short dumpling body. It was bald on top with an angry white mane flaring out in every which direction. The cherub face remained deceptively peaceful.

"Where are you from?" he asked.

"Morocco," one of the girls said.

"Romania. I live at Moshav Mikhmoret."

"South Africa. My family is in Haifa," the second girl said.

"I am a sabra, Kibbutz Ginnosar."

"Yigal Allon's kibbutz," Ben-Gurion said.

"Yes," the soldier boy answered proudly.

Ben-Gurion's head tilted and his eyes blinked. He was a past master at grabbing forty winks, a skill honed at a hundred Zionist conferences. When the crew departed it was nearly two o'clock in the morning.

The Old Man's eyes fluttered open and became fixed on a single paged document awaiting his signature, the approval of a plan, Operation Kadesh, that would commit his young nation to war. Only eight years earlier he had signed another document, a proud document that declared statehood. Would there even be a ninth birthday, or would it all end in horror like a biblical siege with a final ghastly scene of a national massacre?

The past three weeks had been nightmarish in the speed and intensity of events: the secret meetings in Paris with the French and later the British and the clandestine agreement to go to war together . . . the return of Israeli officers who had been training in military academies and army specialty schools around the world . . . the call-up of reserves . . . the near-disastrous raid on Kalkilia to make the world believe that Jordan, not Egypt, was the enemy of record . . . French equipment arriving without spare parts . . . pressure from Eisenhower and the Americans mounting daily . . . dire threats from the Russians . . .

Operation Kadesh. How esoteric, Ben-Gurion thought. The biblical site in the Sinai where the Jews dwelled for a time during their wanderings with Moses.

Operation Kadesh needed a series of miracles to succeed. Every assessment was frightfully the same: *Israel must win the war in the first four days. A prolonged conflict in which every Arab nation would join would be disastrous.*

No small country goes to war without the support of a major power, yet David Ben-Gurion felt, in the depths of his being, that Israel's partners, England and France, would falter, leaving her alone, outmanned and outgunned.

Israel must win the war in the first four days!

All sorts of things were going wrong as D day approached. The ordinance reports all but crushed the spirit: no spare steel matting to roll vehicles over the sucking sands of the desert . . . aged tanks being cannibalized, further reducing their already inferior armored force . . . rifles from Belgium not up to spec . . . no filters for the tracked vehicles to keep them from choking in the desert . . . a shortage of tank tracks, chains, pulleys, winches, flatbeds, four-wheel-drive trucks, repair stations, batteries, belts . . . an obsolete air force of World War II piston planes to face double the number of the latest MiGs owned by the Egyptians . . . no aircraft batteries to defend the cities against Egyptian bombers flown by "volunteers" from Poland and Czechoslovakia.

The orders to the brigade commanders were desperately simple. They said, in effect, "You have an objective. You must reach the Suez Canal in three days despite the resistance. You will not ask for reinforcements or further supplies for there are none available."

Worse was the constant gnawing conviction that the British and French would quit. This would release divisions of fresh Egyptian troops to reinforce the Sinai. If France and England failed to bomb out the Egyptian airfields, Nasser could put his Russian-made bombers to work on Israel's cities.

We must win the war in four days!

Two of the brigades must traverse over a hundred miles of semicharted wilderness . . .

. . . and the 7th Battalion, the Lion's Battalion, must be dropped deep into the Sinai behind enemy lines, exposed to a disaster, a sacrificial force. The Old Man had argued for hours with the Defense Chief of Staff, Moshe Dayan, to try to dissuade him from parachuting the Lion's Battalion near Mitla Pass. Dayan was adamant. It was the linchpin of the entire operation, a maneuver to initially confuse the enemy, then stop Egyptian reinforcements. When the brigade linked up with the battalion, the combined force would wheel south to free the blockaded passage to the Red Sea. Yes, there was great risk—but try to engage in a war without risk.

Jacob Herzog, B.G.'s confidant and closest adviser on the campaign, entered the room with Natasha Solomon. Herzog was pale, in a scholarly way; an Irish Jew, the son of the chief Ashkenazi rabbi, with a magnificent religious and legal mind. He put all the late communications and a day's summary before the Old Man.

Natasha Solomon set a batch of papers on the desk, translations of messages from the French. Even at this hour Natasha was a warming sight. She was one of those women who gained an extra dimension of beauty through weariness, a certain sensuality in the black rings of fatigue forming beneath her eyes, as if from exhaustion at the end of a day of lovemaking. She was softness itself, different from many of the roughhewn sabra and kibbutz women, groomed in a Middle European way that made the silk of her blouse float over her terrain and shout "female!" even at two in the morning. An all but forgotten memory flitted through the Old Man's mind . . . a girl, long ago. Such a thing to remember at a time like this.

Ben-Gurion picked up the summary but his eyes were fatigued. He handed the papers to Natasha and waved her into a seat, then took up a pad and pen to jot notes as she read.

The British were being very cautious, very cagey, deepening B.G.'s distrust. Herzog tried to tidy up the day's events, but new events were already overtaking them.

Both the Soviet Union and America were bogged down in their own problems. An American presidential election was to take place in a few days, and traditionally it was a good time to catch Washington off guard.

Revolts against the Russians were brewing in Poland and Hungary. The students in Budapest had rioted and the unrest was growing. Israeli intelligence estimated a Russian tank force would enter Budapest in a matter of days.

Herzog reckoned these events could give Israel a slight advantage. Russia and America might be slow to react to the Israeli attack on Egypt. If Israel could stall diplomatically for three days, her forces might reach the Canal and Israel's part of the war would be over.

But America was certain to be outraged that her two closest allies, England and France, would initiate military action without advising them. As for the Soviets, they had to put on a barking show for their Egyptian clients.

"Is there anything at all we haven't covered, Yakov? Anything . . . anything . . ."

Herzog pointed to the document setting Operation Kadesh into motion.

"Your signature," he said.

Ben-Gurion would not quit, gleaning for the stray, minute detail that might have been overlooked. It all boiled down to the same thing. Gamal Abdel Nasser, the Egyptian president, was on a heady binge. He had seized the Suez Canal and evicted the British and French. He had closed the Strait of Tiran, at the tip of the Sinai Peninsula, to Israeli shipping. He had turned the Gaza Strip into one enormous terrorist base which violated the Israeli border hourly. He had massed a huge army in the Sinai armed with a larder filled with Russian weapons. The bottom line was that Israel had no choice other than military action—with or without the British and French.

He scribbled his name on the paper. His nation was at war!

"Anything else?" he asked.

Herzog put before him a memo requiring initialing.

"What is this?"

"A small piece of business. Permission for Gideon Zadok to go into the Sinai with a forward unit. He has had a standing request that if there was ever to be a major action, to be allowed to join it as an observer. Research for his book."

"Am I mistaken, or didn't he go on the Kalkilia raid?"

"He did," Herzog answered. "Both Zechariah and Ben Asher told me he conducted himself very well under fire."

"How is his intelligence clearance?" B.G. asked.

"Early during his trip here, we realized he was in a position to gain very valuable information to pass to the Americans. Both Beham and Pearlman fed him false intelligence on the Ramon Rocket and the atomic project at the Haifa North Plant. The kind of data we gave him would be easy to trace if he had turned it over to the Americans. Our boys have no qualms about him as a security risk and I personally give him my vote, but I believe Natasha is in the best position to judge."

"Natasha?"

"Gideon Zadok is family," she said. "He's been on five or six border and desert patrols with units of the Lion's Battalion. They swear by him, as well."

"So, why not," Ben-Gurion said. "He's a good boy. I like him. He has funny ideas about not settling in Israel. I'll change his mind about that. But . . . who knows, he might write us an important book." The Old Man scribbled his initials on the memo. "Who are you assigning him to?"

I believe," Natasha said, "if Gideon knew about the plans, he'd choose to be dropped with the Lions at Mitla Pass."

"That's one part of this I don't like," Herzog interjected. "He is an American, after all. If we sent him back to Eisenhower in a wooden box it could create an ugly incident."

B.G. pondered. "We are entitled to a poor man's Hemingway. Send him with the Lions. He's a writer. He should be in the action. God knows he doesn't write like Hemingway, but I hear he drinks as well."

"I can vouch for that," Natasha said.

"Don't get yourself broken up with this boy," the Old Man said.

"I already have," she answered.

GIDEON

HERZLIA, ISRAEL
October 29, 1956
D DAY, H HOUR MINUS NINE

I COULD NOT MOVE. My feet felt as though they were encased in cement. My brain was whirling with a mishmash of bloated, horrifying images. Weird-shaped airplanes fell out of the sky . . . distorted, terrorized faces of my daughters screamed for help . . . Valerie was humping some faceless bastard and screeching venomously and laughing at me . . . a band of headless musicians played a military march. . . . Shit, what was all this about? Baby waves breaking on a beach . . . hush . . . hush . . . hush . . .

I blinked my eyes open.

Hush . . . hush . . . hush . . .

Where the hell am I? My mouth was filled with sand. I strained to move. Trapped! Dammit! I can't move!

I jerked hard and inched up on my elbows. The beach was empty. My face dropped to the sand again. Get it together, Gideon. Think, man. All right, I know. I . . . I . . . left the hotel and . . . uh . . . I left the hotel and took a walk on the beach to clear my head. Let me think, now. I must have stopped at the water's edge and . . . I guess I passed out from exhaustion. Where is the hotel? Dammit, I can't see too well . . . sand.

Think. The tide has washed over me. My legs and feet are sunk in the wet sand. I worked my feet and legs loose and wobbled upright, then staggered to the water and plunged my face into an oncoming little wave. Shit! Sand washed out of my face, ears, mouth, nostrils, hair. My eyes stung from the salt water. I plunged in, took a mouthful, rinsed it, spit it out. Phew!

I looked about. Not a soul, not even a bird. Nothing more empty than an empty beach.

Oh, Jesus! The past twenty-four hours flooded in. The evacuation and watching Valerie and the girls fly off. How'd I get here? I remember now. I went home but couldn't stay there alone, so I went to the hotel. It was deserted.

Our dog, Grover! Come on, Gideon, get a handle on it. I went home, decided to go to my office in the hotel. Grover had a fever. I took him with me and had to carry him up four flights to my room. The hotel was dark and empty, scary.

Where was Grover? Yeah, okay, that's it. I put him into the car to wait for me. I was going to take him into Tel Aviv to the vet. Then I took a walk on the beach to try to clear my head. I sat down for a rest and must have dropped off. Lucky I didn't drown myself.

Oh, dear Lord, where were Val and the girls now? What a mess I've made! I began once more to replay the evacuation scene. Blow the trumpets. Gideon has just made a triumphal entry into shit city.

"Gideon!" a voice called from the distance. "Gideon!"

Now I'm hearing things.

"Gideon!" it repeated.

If that voice isn't real, I'm in big trouble.

"Gideon!"

I squinted, tried to clear the sting from my eyes, and brought into focus the figure of a woman standing on the bluff near the hotel, shouting and waving.

"Natasha!"

I sprinted down the beach along the waterline, where the sand was hard, stopped and caught my breath, then cut over the soft sand toward the hotel. A path led up to the bluff. I grunted and growled as sharp little pebbles and shells nipped hard at the soles of my feet, and then I stood before her nearly doubled up.

Natasha clawed so hard at my back I felt and heard my shirt rip. She bit at my shoulders, weeping crazily. She pulled at my wet, salty, sandy hair and I came back at her squeezing the breath from her with my embrace.

After a time we stood holding each other up like a pair of fighters who have punched themselves out and are clinched and staggering. Our bodies became still, only wavering a bit as we fought to control our breathing. A puff of wind blew her hair into her face where it joined her tears. I pushed free and hobbled off the path to where the sand was soft in a patch surrounded by high spiky tufts of dune grass.

"They're gone," I managed to blurt.

"I was with B.G. all day," she rasped. "I heard about the evacuation, but didn't dare try to telephone out. Everything goes through the switchboard. I was crazy out of my mind. I thought—I thought you had left with them."

I flopped my arms.

"You wanted to go with them, didn't you?"

"I'm here, aren't I?"

"But you wanted to go."

Her eyes mirrored her hurt.

"I'm here."

"Why?"

"I guess I was more scared of evacuating than I was of staying. I wanted to stick around for the raid, or the battle, or the war . . . whatever the hell is coming."

She turned acid. Unmistakable, vintage Natasha.

"You stayed because you weren't going to show yourself to be a coward in front of the whole country. After all, everyone knows what a tough Marine you are. Your blessed novel is the bible of the army of Israel. Prophets don't flee."

"Come on, get off it. I'm here." I reached out and touched that fine silky red hair of hers and brought her against me, this time softly. "Maybe I stayed for you."

"For me? Why? I'm poison. You've told me I'm poison a dozen times." She turned sharply out of my grasp and walked away, off the little path and into a wave of small dunes that formed part of the bluff. She relented for a moment as I put my arm around her shoulder and we stared at the unearthly emptiness below.

"So quiet around here now," I said. "You okay?"

She sighed and leaned against me. "My head is spinning like crazy. It's been chaos. Everything is crazy. Ben-Gurion fell sick last night. He got up out of his chair and just collapsed. Jackie Herzog set up a hospital room for him right in the cottage. It's got twenty guards around it."

"What's the matter with him?"

"I don't know. He's running a high fever. Two hundred people are trying to get to see him. He's—he's—throwing up. He's sick like a dog. We're spreading the story that he's out of the country on a secret meeting. I've only got a few hours. I've got to get back."

She suddenly shivered and walked away from me. Natasha could play deadpan for everyone but me. The color left her face and she bit nervously at her lip.

"Are we at war?" I asked.

Her lack of a reply was answer enough.

"When?"

"Tonight," she managed shakily. "You can still leave. There's an American destroyer heading for Haifa."

I had known it was coming. Everyone had known it was coming. Yet it jolted me. That flash of fear that sends tingles throughout the body. You can't divide fear up into halves and quarters, but I knew I was more afraid for Israel than for myself . . . or Val . . . or the girls. I was very afraid for Natasha.

"I want to go out with the troops," I said.

"It's been arranged," she managed. "The Old Man himself gave approval."

"Who am I going with?"

"The Lions. Your lucky outfit."

"Where?"

"I shouldn't say any more."

"Okay, I'll find out when I find out." My mind checked out a number of possibilities over the Jordanian border. Maybe it was going to be a push to capture the West Bank and straighten out the borders along the Jordan River. Maybe Israel would try to capture East Jerusalem. That would be a dream.

"You're going to make a drop in the Sinai," she said abruptly.

"The Sinai! Are you sure?"

"I'm sure."

"Mother of God, are you sure?"

"Yes, it's the Sinai. All this rumbling and the threats against Jordan have been a decoy. Egypt has been the real target all along."

"French and British involved in this?"

"Draw your own conclusions."

The ramifications were staggering. These audacious Israelis were going to take the Sinai Peninsula while the Anglo-French snatched the Canal back. This was the whole ball of wax . . . major, major.

"Where are we going to be dropped?"

"A place called Mitla Pass."

I sat in the sand and with my finger drew a map. The Sinai was fairly clear in my mind. "Mitla . . . Mitla . . ." It was somewhere quite close to the Canal and, I think, near the Gulf of Suez as well. Something else occurred to me.

"Shit! I've never jumped out of an airplane."

Her white teeth showed. "That's very funny," she said. "No matter. A lot of people here are convinced that nothing is too tough for you."

"I jumped from a practice tower once. Scared the hell out of me."

"Oh, I don't worry about you, *chéri*. You'll bounce right up like a ball. Shlomo says it's easy, like pie. He'll be right in back of you to push you out of the plane."

"Jesus," I said and dropped my head onto my knees. "It isn't funny." Natasha stood over me—back to bitch again, the master of Hungarian mood swings.

"You wouldn't back out, Gideon," she said sarcastically. "After all, war is where little boys go to prove they are big boys. You wouldn't miss this for the world."

She was right. She generally was. I realized my posturing had convinced the Israelis that I was rattlesnake-mean. I'd sold them a real sackful of B.S. Out of an airplane, huh? Well, I hoped I wouldn't make an ass of myself. I didn't make an ass of myself that one time, long ago . . . I almost did . . . I almost broke with fear, but I held on—barely.

We were coming into the beach at Tarawa. My boat was in the first wave and I was up front, right next to the ramp. We were hitting one of the smaller islands on the atoll and not expecting much opposition. We'd been circling around for hours and most of us were pretty nauseated as the line of landing craft straightened out and moved for the beach. Just then, Japanese machine-gun fire opened up and raked us. The bullets hit the armor plating on the ramp and their impact nearly shook us out of the water like a wounded sailfish. In a matter of a few seconds the ramp would be lowered and I'd be the first out, into the water. All I could think about clearly was that I couldn't disgrace myself because I was a Jew. I almost fainted with fright. I managed to dare a peek back into the boat. Almost half of the guys, including the major, were puking out of sheer fear. Pedro, the toughest guy I ever knew, was on his knees praying to Jesus, Mary, and an assortment of Mexican saints. And just like that, a miracle happened. I was no longer afraid. The ramp lowered and bashed the water and I leaped in without hesitation. We were pretty near chest high and being fired at as, grunting, we waded forward. Funny part of it is how other things take over. I had a lot of work to do when we hit the beach—set up a radio and contact our command ship. Then my mind went to Ser-

geant Bleaker in back of me. He was the tallest guy in the company so we all gave him our cigarettes to keep dry inside his helmet. . . .

So, them were the apples. I was going to jump out of an airplane and I couldn't dream or wish it away. Thirteen years had passed since Tarawa, with a lot of fat living in between. I put my face in my hands and sighed away my trepidations.

Natasha stood over me, her hands on her hips and her legs apart provocatively. Natasha did not assume that stance accidentally.

"What are you thinking about?" she said.

"It's been a real shit night," I said.

"The first destination of your family was to be Athens. They cleared our airspace without any problems. Your wife is probably enjoying an ouzo . . ."

So, finish your fucking sentence . . . with some nice, handsome, young officer from the embassy. . . .

Hungarian bitch!

"You love me now or you hate me now?" she persisted.

"Bitch!"

I lifted my head, the same instant her skirt fell to the ground and she stepped out of it. Her blouse and bra followed.

"Come on, Natasha, only a rat could make love at a time like this."

"That's right," she answered, "we're rats, both of us, so let's do a little rat fucking."

She hurled herself atop me, grabbed two handfuls of sand, and ran them up and down my back, hard.

"I make it raw. I want to see blood from you. I want it to hurt so bad that when you jump out of the airplane your shirt will stick to you from blood and you'll be thinking of Natasha!"

Natasha did have a nice way of getting your mind off your troubles.

If you considered things from Natasha's point of view, she'd been waiting for a long time to make tartare out of my back. For the better part of six months I'd been chastising her.

"For Christ sake, stop wearing perfume!"

"Look what you've done. I've got a bite mark on me."

"Easy with the fingernails."

Those times we soared, and they were often, restraint was not one of Natasha's commendable qualities. From time to time she'd deliberately leave a calling card in the form of a high-visibility mark, a bite bruise, scratches, which obviously didn't come from wrestling with the family dog. ("The platoon was scaling some rocks and I slipped and tore the hell out of my back.")

Valerie's response was always double-edged. ("Poor baby. These Israeli rocks *do* have teeth in them.")

Now the family was gone, and Natasha jumped me in the sand dunes. She had me as she used to have me, before Val came to Israel. Natasha went ape. She was the only woman who could make love while cursing you in seven languages.

An hour or so later we went to my hotel room to survey the damage. Natasha was filled with remorse. Scrubbing very gingerly, it took over a half an hour to get the sand cleaned out of a lot of unlikely places. As she examined my back, she chastised herself but reckoned I could get by without stitches.

In the shower, she started up again. Natasha adored making love in the shower . . . or out of the shower . . . or in bed . . . or locked in a public rest room . . . or on the desk in the Prime Minister's office after he had gone for the day.

"Oh, poor baby, look at what I've done. Natasha, you are an animal," she said of herself.

There was a Swedish mouthwash in my cabinet that could peel the paint off a battleship or make a leper aseptic. The tenderness with which she dabbed it on my wounds was the flip side to her character.

From the rape in the sand dunes, one would hardly get the notion that Natasha Solomon was also the most gentle, patient woman and lover I had ever known. She could play with my eyelashes for an hour with her whisper touch and lips and make every moment of it new.

She cried as she patched me up. All I could manage was to hang on to the bedposts, clench my teeth, and fight off the tears.

The alarm clock woke us up a bit later. She went out onto the balcony as I dressed and she read my new pages. I couldn't help myself, but it felt good—damned good, wonderful—as I laced up my old Marine boots and strapped a .45 pistol on my belt. I wondered why it should be feeling good . . . khaki shirt and trousers . . . fatigue jacket with an IDF logo . . .

I came out to the balcony. Her white knuckles gave her away as she gripped the railing like a vise. I put my arm about her shoulder as she slowly calmed, and we watched the sea as we had watched it from there in fifty stolen rendezvous.

"You're writing beautifully," she said.

"I wonder how it sounds in Hungarian."

"Don't worry about the dog," she said. "I'll take him to Dr. Klement. Grover will keep me company. Put him in my car. I parked right next to you."

"Natasha . . ."

She broke. Seeing someone off always terrified her . . . since she had seen her mother sent to the gas chambers at Auschwitz . . . God almighty!

"See you around," I said.

SLOW TRANSPORTS ALWAYS "lumber." Our formation of twenty Dakotas lumbered over the Negev Desert toward the Sinai Peninsula. The twilight was fading fast. This military version of the DC-3, the famed Gooney Bird, was built for neither speed nor comfort. Twenty-five of us were crammed into miserable bucket seats along either bulkhead.

First time I flew in a Gooney Bird was to cross the States returning from furlough. The trip from Philly to L.A. took almost twenty hours. I had to transfer to four different airlines. From L.A. it was a train to San Diego, because there was no air service.

On the other hand, there was something comforting about the Gooney Bird. I used to read a bedtime storybook to the girls called *The Little Engine That Could.* This little engine was a small-time train and found itself in a rough situation. It had to huff and puff its tiny heart out to make it over a mountain, in order to take candy and toys and food to the kids on the other side. I acted out the story with nail-biting suspense a hundred and one times, but in the end the little engine always made it. So did the Gooney Bird. Sometimes it landed with one engine out, or half the tail assembly shot off. But the Gooney Bird was the mainstay of the lift over the Hump, the Himalayas, and it carried the Berlin Air Lift.

During the briefing earlier today, we had been told that at the same moment, a pair of World War II F-51 fighter planes were crisscrossing over the Sinai Peninsula, cutting the telephone lines with their propellers. For that dandy little maneuver, the pilots had to fly ten feet off the ground. Amen!

We had been sequestered in a hangar on the military side of Lydda Airport. Colonel Zechariah, the founder and commander of the Paratroop Brigade, briefed us. Zechariah was a comforting sight, a sort of Hebrew-speaking Marine-type commander, working diligently on becoming a living legend.

The plan was simple enough. The Lion's Battalion—four hundred paratroopers under the command of Major Ben Asher—had been given the "honor" of dropping deep into the Sinai Peninsula to open Operation Kadesh.

The actual site was called the Parker Monument, a marker in honor of a former British military governor. From the Parker Monument to Egypt proper, on the other side of the Suez Canal, was a distance of thirty miles. Sixteen or seventeen of those miles was Mitla Pass—a treacherous, narrow defile of mountain, rock, and cliff. An Egyptian force of unknown size was inside the Pass in fortified positions. Fortunately, we would not have to go in and try to take the Pass itself.

The Lions were to seal the eastern end of Mitla to stop reinforcements from getting through to the Sinai. Meanwhile, the balance of the Para Brigade under Zechariah would cross a hundred and fifty miles of desert track, capture three fortified positions, and link up with us sometime around D day plus two.

There were a thousand *What ifs* in my mind. I'm certain Dayan and the Old Man and Jackie Herzog and the rest of them had already *What if*'d themselves to death.

Israel wasn't going to initiate a war unless she was forced. She was undermanned and underarmed against Egypt alone. *What if* we were jumped by Jordan, Syria, and Iraq as well?

And *What if* the Egyptian Air Force caught us in the open . . .

And *What if* Zechariah didn't link up with us . . .

And *What if*—forget it, Gideon.

The nonchalance, the downright boredom of the Lions had to be partly playacting. We did it in the Marines before battle. In fact, my dog Grover was probably the best in the world at fake macho.

The Lions were sprawled about, seemingly oblivious of the bouncing and rolling. The sergeant major checked his Uzi gun as though it were a sweetheart he never got tired of caressing.

Shlomo Bar Adon, my assistant, who had been lent to me by the Foreign Ministry, was dead asleep, his bearded angry-looking head bobbing on my shoulder, unresponsive to my elbow whacks into his ribs. I don't know whether I could have gone through a parachute jump without Shlomo. I loved him like a brother most of the time and some of the time hated him twice as much.

I didn't want to think about Val and the girls right at that moment. If a writer can't block his family out of his thoughts, he can't go to war. During years of long research trips I had mastered the art of not thinking about them. I'd get maudlin . . . I'd cry at bars . . . I'd never get my work done if I couldn't get my family out of my mind. Or so I made myself believe. Val says writers are the total masters at suffering. She says everyone suffers just as much, but writers can say it better.

For a time I thought my decision to bring my family to Israel was going to work. I'd been there four months when they arrived, and was already heavily involved with Natasha. All three of my girls adapted and seemed happy. We lived in a lovely neighborhood near the sea and I had an extra hotel room a few miles away to work in. Our neighbors were mostly affluent South Africans who were bedrock Zionists and had come to settle.

Life wasn't easy in Israel in 1956, but what was lacking in comforts was more than made up by an explosion of spirit and a lust for life and a purpose for living and a feeling of brotherly love that I never would have believed could exist in an entire people. For me, being here was reaching nirvana.

The government had shown a lot of confidence in me, and the armed forces loved my early novel on the Marines. I had finished most of the research on my new book. Writing was going extremely well. To be the first Jew in centuries to write about Jews as warriors was more than an obsession, it was life itself.

Even the madness of my affair with Natasha was controllable. Or so I led myself to believe. She was by far the cleverest person I'd ever met. Far too clever to cross that final bit of no-man's-land and force me into a decision between her and my family.

So I'd go to my room at the Accadia Hotel every day and write and make believe that Natasha really wasn't going to be a problem. And I had reckoned that by the time I finished the novel and was ready to return to the States, Natasha and I would have burned the affair out—past history. Everything would resolve itself like magic . . . yeah, sure, man. Gideon, you are one stupid Jew.

An abrupt downdraft got me in the pit of the stomach. A few of the Lions were annoyed enough to shift positions, grunt, and continue to snore.

So, Gideon, the best-laid plans of mice and men . . . I was an idiot to think I could tightrope between two warring females.

I did manage to hold everything together and move the book along well and keep our heads above water financially. Then came the border raids, the sudden, swift escalation, and the inevitable conflict. Things started to really become unhinged with the Kalkilia raid. Good Lord, it was only seventeen days ago.

Major Ben Asher opened the door from the cockpit. This woke everyone up in a hurry.

"One hour to drop," he bellowed over the engines. "We'll be going down to five hundred feet to get under their radar."

. . . The Kalkilia raid . . . only nineteen days ago . . .

HERZLIA, ISRAEL
October 9, 1956

IT WAS COMING up to six o'clock, time for the English-language news. Gideon never missed the news; he should be back. The whole country stopped every hour, on the hour. Good news was scarce these days.

The sun played out its daily ritual, drifting downward toward a sea that was mirror-smooth tonight. From the kitchen window Valerie could just about make them out coming up from the beach. She shaded her eyes and squinted toward the path, then wiped her hands at the sink and stepped out onto the rear veranda and waved.

Penelope enjoyed her royal seat on Daddy's shoulders, while Roxanne walked ahead of them swinging a bucket.

Val never failed to react every time she caught sight of him. Gideon was on the slight side, but most people thought of him as being larger. It was his bearing, a determined manner of stride, hunched forward, pondering. Val loved his looks. Feisty little bastard. Gideon had overpowering eyes that could express a full range of emotions with a glance, and when his look was for you and filled with lust, it always brought on shivers.

The first time she ever saw him was on a USO dance floor. He was in Marine uniform and she was a student at Mills College, a few miles away from the Oak Knoll Naval Hospital. Gideon just moved right in— cut in and whisked her away from her partner. He was pure driving male.

And cocky! "You'd better put in your dibs for me now, Val, because I'm going to be a great writer." Hell, he was only nineteen years old when he told her that, two nights after they met.

"Here's a pair of tickets for a play at the hospital next week." Gideon was a patient. He was also the playwright, director, producer, and star of the show.

It was frightening meeting someone so strong that early in life, but Lord, he was magic.

Grover Vandover, their golden retriever, a lollipop of a family dog, flopped up the path alongside them. Roxanne broke away, running toward the house, and opened the back gate onto a lawn of coarse grass.

"Mommy! Look! Coins!" She opened her palm revealing three bits of irregularly shaped metal, blackened by time, with the image and lettering no longer visible.

"Daddy says they may be Roman, even Israelite."

What Roxy didn't know was that when Professor Ben Zohar had been over the night before, he had slipped the coins to Gideon who had planted them at the tel earlier in the day. The Professor was their self-appointed Hebrew teacher and he kept an eye on their school progress. The only English-language school was run by Franciscan Brothers in Jaffa, too far for them to travel. It fell on Val to see to the girls' studies.

Gideon lowered Penelope from his shoulders and she ran to embrace her mother. She still had a slight limp from the accident three years earlier. It had happened in the blink of an eye. Val had turned her back for only a few seconds when Penelope ran into the street as a bus came roaring through the intersection and sideswiped her . . . fractured skull . . . broken ribs . . . wrecked knee.

It took over two years for Penny to heal. Val, with great compassion and support from Gideon, learned to manage her guilt but would take some of it with her to her grave.

They looked at her and smiled and said silent "thank Gods." They always did.

Val ordered the girls to strip and they squealed under the outdoor shower. She rubbed them dry with big towels, dressed them in muumuus, and sent them to their room to do their lessons.

In the kitchen, Gideon reached under Val's muumuu and caressed her backside. Most of the Jewish men she had met since Gideon often as not had their hands on their women. A lovely horny breed.

"What's for dinner?"

"Surprise. We've got prime rib."

Gideon peeked into the oven. "Chicken," he grumbled. Gideon hungered for a thick, juicy slab of prime rib. His visions of food, which grew daily, always ended up at Lawry's Restaurant. He'd get off the plane at L.A. International and all the customs officers would have been alerted to pass him through without formalities. A helicopter would be waiting to fly him directly to the Lawry parking lot. The big silver cart would be rolled up to his table, the lid would be opened, and there would be . . . one entire steer. He wouldn't get up from the table until he was so bloated that a pair of waiters would have to pack him out on a hand-cart. . . . Well, anyhow, the fruits and vegetables were outstanding in Israel.

Gideon seated himself at the kitchen table and snapped on the radio. His hand snaked over to the fruit bowl as he checked the mail.

Oh, thank God, a letter from F. Todd Wallace, his literary agent! Gideon had bombarded Wallace with letters pleading with him to find some writing assignments—a magazine article, a guest column, anything to augment the foundering bank account.

Val watched Gideon's anxiety turn to deflation and then to anger. "Incompetent, lazy son of a bitch. All that mother knows how to do is collect commissions like a hungry landlord. The whole God-damned Middle East is about to blow up, he's got a writer in place, and he can't get me a nickel's worth of work!"

"Why don't you just replace him?"

"He's got me tied up on this book and there's no way he's going to give it up. You remember how it was? We were in a real mess with J. III and Reaves Brothers Publishers and in comes Wallace, Princeton charm in Brooks Brothers' uniform. We thought we were lucky to have him at the time."

"Honey, don't get yourself all churned up."

"Depend on that literary pimp to pull you through and you're dead, man, dead. You've got to lay a winner in that sucker's lap. Give him any God-damned task requiring creative selling and you might as well be represented by the seals at Sea World."

"Listen, we can only eat two chickens a day. We'll get through."

Gideon was pacing, throwing his middle finger up. "F. Todd Wallace and his God-damned club. Harvard and Yalie blimps with rigor mortis, in their overstuffed chairs, sneering down on Fifth Avenue. That crowd is drunk by noon. Can you believe it? God, I hate that crowd. Hey, Wallace, how'd they let me in? Do they know I'm a Jew?"

"Calm down, Junior, *gor nisht helfen*," Val said, once again butchering an attempt at Yiddish.

Gideon jammed his hands into his pockets and continued his monologue. "If worse comes to worst I can always do a doctoring job on a screenplay. That'll set the novel back three months. I'd better write and see what's doing at the studios. There's always a script in trouble."

He flopped back down. Val had taken one of the letters and put it in her apron pocket. A letter from Nathan, Gideon's father.

"Might as well let me have it," he said.

"Maybe you ought to save it till after dinner."

He took the envelope from her pocket and held it as one would handle a box with an unexploded bomb inside, sighed, and tore it open.

"Want me to read it?" she asked.

"Yeah."

My Dear Son,

I am still trying to get used to being deprived of your weekly letter, which I came to depend on when you were home in California. Now I come home to the usually empty mailbox. Am I to blame for having the blues?

Val sighed. "Honey, you really don't need this," she said.

"Go on, finish it."

"As you wish. Let's see . . . 'blame for having the blues?' "

Son! I am getting nasty letters from the relatives in Israel that you are boycotting their homes. I am having terrible difficulty to convince them that Gideon is not a snob. Son, I beg of you. It wouldn't hurt a thing to drop in for a meal once in a while. You still like gefilte fish! Even though Valerie doesn't know how to make such dishes and seems reluctant to learn.

However, that is not the point. Especially you should every so often see my brother, Mordechai, who suffered so brutally at the hands of the Nazis. He pleads with me for you to read his essays, which are world-famous in some circles, a highly respected scholar. You could easily, with a letter or two to your famous friends, get him published in America. It would do miracles for his health (ruined by the Nazis) if you could accomplish this small favor. Or maybe I'm asking too much.

Also, to visit my sister (your aunt) Rifka, who sits in a dark room all day grieving for my beloved mother (your grandmother), who was murdered at Treblinka. She is not a well person, mentally speaking, and it is my firm belief and honest opinion that a visit from you would make her well. Thank you, son, for not ignoring the relatives.

How are Valerie and my beautiful *eynikles? Ah laben auf dier kups.* I love them all! I embrace them. I kiss them. Perhaps you could convince Valerie to drop the old man a few sentences, a post card. It would be nice to get from her regular mail IF IT'S NOT TOO PAINFUL FOR HER. Also, is there a reason that Roxanne and Penny should be ashamed of their *zayde?* I have for each of them a little Channukah *gelt* in exchange for a letter. Please, so they shouldn't forget, have them write regularly. It would also alleviate my loneliness.

Now, let me address you on a very serious matter. I am not no literary expert, although I have read all the classics in a number of languages. I am only a humble worker, but you must listen to what I have to tell you. Menachem Begin and his crowd are nothing but fascists. Don't let them convince you they are Hollywood heroes. The Jewish people will never forgive you if you glorify, in your book, these thugs and hoodlums. God forbid I should tell you what to write. I am only offering a suggestion that should be carefully followed, FOR YOUR SAKE.

I miss you. I long to see you. I embrace you. I plead with you, don't take chances and also MOST IMPORTANTLY to write. Lena sends love.

Your loving,
Dad
P.S. We are okay for old folks. Nothing happens new in Philly except to wait to die.

The letter sent Gideon directly to the liquor cupboard over the sink. "He gets better with age," Val said.

"Shit!" They had finished up the Scotch last night. Gideon took down a bottle of Israeli brandy and glared at it as though it were an adversary. A few ice cubes, without integrity, were scraped from the tray. He poured a brandy and diluted it with soda water. The ice cubes vanished on contact. The first swallow was the worst.

Kol Israel radio beeped out its signal. Gideon turned up the sound. Syria and Jordan were meeting with Egypt to form a joint military command. Val watched her husband tense up. His back and neck would be as hard as a billiard table tonight.

More news. A fedayeen raid from Jordan. The marauders caught a girl from the kibbutz, raped her, and stabbed her to death. The Arab Legion fired into West Jerusalem from the walls of the Old City.

Well, at least the sunset was reliable. Gideon repaired to a tiny porch on a flat part of the cottage roof that afforded almost a full-circle panorama.

Between their cottage and the sea was a smattering of cottages and small villas, randomly scattered in the dunes and anchored by a pair of hotels, the Accadia and the Sharon, on the beach about a mile apart.

Before Val and the girls arrived, Gideon had lived at the Accadia.

Now they gave him a room to write in and the family was able to use the hotel switchboard for phone messages.

In the opposite direction lay the Plain of Sharon, now glistening from the sprays of overhead sprinklers. Jordan was only ten miles away. Gideon was certain there would have to be a major reprisal against the Jordanians. Something big, a real *klop* to sober up Hussein and stop him from joining up with Nasser and the Egyptians.

His thoughts were interrupted as Val brought up a second drink. If you survived the first one, the second one was almost palatable.

They were invaded by squadrons of fighter-plane gnats followed by squadrons of bomber mosquitoes.

"Where's the bug spray, baby?" he asked.

"The store was out. The store was out of everything."

"Except chickens with pinfeathers. I'll get some bug spray in Tel Aviv tomorrow," he said, dipping his finger into his drink and rubbing the brandy on his cheeks, ankles, and exposed arms. No self-respecting mosquito would touch the stuff.

"Tel Aviv is out of just about everything as well," Val said. "I've got a long shopping list of things we're out of."

Val had that expression on her face that implied, "you *know* where you can get anything you want, if you really want to."

Gideon had managed to circumvent a quagmire of rules and regulations. He had hustled a full-time assistant, Shlomo Bar Adon, from the Foreign Ministry, commandeered the last electric typewriter in the Defense Ministry, borrowed a jeep from the Army, slid around a variety of currency laws, import regulations, and taxations. Customs was still trying to figure out how one G. Zadok managed to get a Ford through Haifa port with phony diplomatic plates. Gideon was a bulldog when it came to clearing himself a path and getting at his research. He was chutzpah personified.

"You know, honey," Val said, "if you really wanted to spare your family from all this privation, you could do it with an itty-bitty phone call to Rich Cromwell at the embassy. He's offered us use of the diplomatic commissary a half-dozen times."

Gideon's non-reply was definitive.

"Just think about it. Scotch, non-scratchy toilet paper, bacon, *prime rib.*"

Richard Cromwell, a purchasing agent in the American Embassy, was also the CIA station chief. Cromwell knew, of course, that Gideon was well connected in the high Israeli echelons. Rich had cultivated Gideon's friendship early on. From time to time Cromwell had dangled Pol-

ish hams, tobacco, booze, butter, and assorted other goodies before
Gideon's eyes, at wholesale prices. Gideon wasn't buying.

Val couldn't come to terms with her husband's being so sanctimo-
nious about using the commissary. After all, they *were* Americans, and
what would be the damned sin in slipping a little information to Cromwell now and then? Not that he knew any Israeli state secrets, and it
wasn't as though Israel and America were enemies. Gideon was wearing
his honorable jut-jawed boy scout expression. Honorable prick! She
dropped the subject.

"How about a walk on the beach after we put the girls down?" she
asked.

"We can't, honey. It's off limits after dark now. Being patrolled. Let's
get downstairs before these little bastards eat us up."

AFTER THE GIRLS' lessons and dinner, there was a family rough-
house. Gideon noted that it was becoming more difficult to wrestle with
Roxanne and get a decent grip on her these days. She was filling out
beautifully. Kisses and more kisses good night. Maybe a ride up to
Jerusalem in a few days.

Then came an awkward, uncomfortable moment. Gideon had new
pages. "I'd better get these into the hotel safe," he said. "I'll leave you
the carbons. Oh, incidentally, I asked Shlomo to meet me at the hotel
tonight. We've got to work out some appointments and next week's
travel plans."

Valerie used to be privy to all the plans, but Gideon seldom talked
them over with her anymore. Once upon a time, it had been a wonderful
nightly ritual for her to read the new pages back to him while he took
notes. She hadn't read to him for weeks.

The pleasure had faded. Val didn't laugh at his funny lines anymore,
only the mistakes. She would get combative and argue over meaningless
points. Val seemed very distant from what he was writing and trying to
say. Her barbs left him fuming. Little by little, the pages stopped coming to her on one pretense or another. He'd leave the carbon for her to
read on her own.

"I wouldn't mind reading to you, tonight." Val's expressed desire was
now a desperate attempt not to be shut out.

"Aw, hell. I've really got a ton of stuff to go over with Shlomo."

They exchanged cold kisses and a "See you later, honey . . . don't
wait up for me."

GIDEON WHEELED the jeep through the breezeway of the Accadia Hotel and spotted Shlomo Bar Adon. Shlomo was an unpolished gem, a native-born sabra who coordinated all of Gideon's interviews, travels, translations, and showed him every corner of the land. Shlomo knew Israel and taught it with the zeal of an ancient seer. For Gideon, Shlomo's rough edges were more than compensated for by the breadth of his knowledge.

Valerie barely tolerated him and Roxanne generally mirrored her mother. Val had eased Shlomo out of coming to their home, but he had become indispensable to Gideon. Perhaps she was even a bit jealous.

Shlomo indicated that they should get out of earshot, so they walked to the bluffs.

"We've been invited to join an operation," Shlomo said.

"When?"

"Tomorrow."

Gideon registered a flush of excitement. "Reprisal? Jordan?"

Shlomo shrugged that he didn't know.

Gideon had pestered, demanded, pleaded for a chance to go out on an action over the border. He knew there was something different about these soldiers, different from any others in the world. Their connection with the ancient biblical warriors intrigued him. The pieces of a six-thousand-year-old puzzle could not be found hidden away in an office drawer. He could only find them by going out and putting the puzzle together with his own hands.

Most of his prodding of the authorities had been done before Val and the girls arrived. They changed the picture. His embarking on such a risky adventure would be brutally unfair to them. But what the hell, writing is unfair. It takes from everyone—the writer, the wife, the children. Everyone's blood ends up hidden in the pages. Was this beyond reasonable unfairness?

"So, what do you think, Shlomo?"

"Val?"

"Val."

Shlomo's black beard and head rolled from side to side: maybe yes, maybe no. "There's going to be gunfire. People are going to get hurt . . . killed . . . maimed. You don't have to smell gunpowder to write about it. Something else pushing you to go out?"

"Maybe."

"What is it, Gideon?"

"I don't know. But I do know the only way I'm going to find out. I'm coming."

"We'll keep our asses down low."

"Your assignment with me doesn't call for this kind of crap. You don't have to come."

Shlomo puffed out his chest. An insult. "Be here at the hotel at five in the morning," he said. "I'll take you to the staging area."

VALERIE SAT cross-legged on the bed, her gown drawn up so that her thighs were bared. The international edition of *Time* was balanced between her legs as she wiped her reading glasses. She had hit the wastebasket with the Jerusalem *Post* and *Herald Trib*. Four points. Gideon's pages were on the bedstand to read last, for dessert.

Val turned to the *Time* book review. A full page in frothing lionization of a minor talent who couldn't sell twenty thousand books if they spotted him nineteen thousand.

"Pricks," she said, tossing the magazine. She picked up Gideon's pages, teased herself with them. She had looked forward to them voraciously.

Val read half a page, then lay back on the pillows with a thud and rubbed her eyes. My God, I'm finding fault. Nit-picking. I'm not reading what he's saying, but what I want it to say. I've become just like those God-damned critics I loathe. It's become insatiable. Why? To annoy him? Hell no, to hurt him. My head's not clear anymore. You just can't read with a hate bird sitting on your shoulder.

Val, damn you, you've got to be more supportive. Read what this guy is reaching for. He's good. He's ripping himself open to find meanings. That's when a writer can really be great, on a voyage of discovery.

What the hell, I came to Israel, didn't I? Isn't that being supportive enough? Did you come for Gideon or to save your own ass?

She heard Grover growl and the rubber flap of his dog door snap open and shut. Sounds disturbed her here, adding to the jittery feeling she always had when Gideon was away. Everything in this damned country ran on nerves and anxiety.

Val drew images of him whispering into the phone, calling that woman. Perhaps that woman was waiting for him at the hotel and they'd go at it desperately. If he smelled of a fresh shower, it was no doubt to get rid of her scent. He usually wore his guilt like a neon sign.

Lots of parties in Israel. Big social life. You know what it's like to feel every pair of eyes in the room glaring at you. That's the poor wife. Pity. No big deal in Israel, this bed-hopping: sophistication personified.

Natasha Solomon. She's a bloody charmer all right. So sweet to Penelope and Roxy at the Savyon Club.

"When you come up to Jerusalem, I'd love to take your daughters around."

And I'd like to bust you one in the mouth, lady!

Come on, Val, read the pages . . . no use. She flung them down rudely. Stinks! Oh God, it hurts!

There was that awful night, not long after I had arrived in Israel. Gideon was working late at the hotel. Or so I thought. I decided to drive over and surprise him and maybe talk him into a little romantic stroll on the beach.

When I parked the car in the front of the Accadia, I heard riotous laughter coming from the beach.

"What's going on down there?" I asked the doorman.

"A reunion of Hungarian survivors, from all over Israel," he answered.

I was magnetically drawn to the bluffs that ran along the rear of the hotel. The Hungarians were strung all up and down the beach; a crowd of them around a campfire were having a boisterous time. Some of the revelers began to shed their clothing, daring others to do the same. They plunged naked into the water and indulged in horseplay that bordered on the sexy. I felt like a bit of a peeping Tom, but it was so damned joyous down there I almost had the urge to join them. Good Lord, if anyone deserved happiness, they certainly did. Seeing their naked bodies, I shuddered for an instant . . . that was the way they were sent into the gas chambers.

And then it came back to me. The first time someone reached out to embrace me and I saw a number tattooed on her arm, I screamed and turned into Gideon's arms, weeping. I was shaken for days. So, I thought, have a good time, guys! Thank God for Israel.

I turned and retraced my steps from the bluff and glanced up to Gideon's window on the fourth floor. A large beach towel was draped over his balcony railing. Strange. Oh well, he must have taken a dip earlier—wait, what the hell's that? A woman darted out of Gideon's room, took the towel, and wrapped it about herself quickly.

I just stood there, stunned. From my vantage point I could see the door that led from the hotel to the beach. In a few moments the same woman emerged, ran across the beach, flung off the towel and joined the merrymaking in the sea. I looked up. Gideon was now on the balcony, watching her. I learned a short time later her name was Natasha Solomon. Apparently they had begun a not so discreet affair before my arrival.

Oh God, Gideon, God! Why! Why! Why! Oh God! She was wild and beautiful, an untamed bird. I almost went insane but I held my tongue. It hurt, it hurt, it hurt but I didn't face him with it. That was my damned fault . . . but . . . I guess . . . I wanted him, no matter what the price.

Suddenly Gideon's words captured her and she was at peace. It's beautiful stuff, she thought. I guess it must be worth the price we have to pay. One page, and another and another. I've got to tell him. I really do.

Grover barked and she heard the sound of Gideon's jeep. Pleasant surprise. There was an impulse to turn off the lights and feign sleep. That's childish, Val. Tell him what you think of the pages. Maybe he'll talk about what's coming up next, maybe we'll talk halfway through the night, the way we used to.

She pretended to read, but was now taken by his sounds, the door of the jeep slamming shut, his unmistakable gait, the jingling as he fumbled for the correct key, the careful closing of the front door, the click of the refrigerator door opening and closing, a stop at the girls' room and a final whispered word to Grover.

"Hi, you're home early," she said doffing her glasses. Gideon stared at her thighs from the doorway and watched her deliberately jiggle her breasts through the sheer gown. No matter how rotten things were, it could heat up between them in a hurry.

Why don't I just take it off and welcome him home? she thought. She remained formal, unconcerned at his stare.

"Your friends must all be up in Jerusalem tonight," she said. Why? I didn't mean to. It just came out.

Thanks, pal. You didn't disappoint me, he mused to himself.

"No phone calls?" Val went on.

Translation. No phone calls from *her?* Did you knock off a quickie with *her?* Say it, Val, God dammit. She has a name. Say it! I dare you.

"No phone calls," he said.

Val pulled down the gown covering her legs, set the pages aside without comment, lay back and drew the sheet over her. "God, I'm tired," she said.

Wacko! Bull's-eye! Whatever mellow mood he'd brought home was curdled.

"Let's knock off," he said. "I've got to get an early start tomorrow." There was a dreadful beat of silence. "I have to leave at four-thirty."

Val sat up slowly, afraid of the coming conversation. "Am I permitted to ask why?"

"I'm going out with the boys."

"The boys?"

"The troops."

"Good Lord, Gideon, you've been on two Negev patrols already this month. How many altogether—five? Seven?"

"Seven or eight, I don't know."

"What are you doing? Buying stock in the Lion's Battalion?"

"Val . . . Val . . . this isn't exactly a patrol."

Val became uneasy, frightened, not wanting to ask the next question. "Exactly what is it, then?" she asked tersely. No answer. "Well, do you care to tell me?"

"I've been invited to . . . join an action."

"Have you gone bonkers?" she shouted.

"Baby, you're going to wake up the kids. I've—I've been trying to get this arranged for months. If I pass on this one, I'll never get another chance."

"You're out of your God-damned mind!"

"Honey, the kids. I've got to get a night's sleep."

"Look at you, you bastard. You're in heaven, aren't you?"

"Val."

"Real bullets and everything this time. Old Marine blood all stirred up?"

"Shut up!" He was breathing hard now, teeth clenched. "I didn't come here to observe life from a sidewalk café on Dizengoff Street!"

"And I didn't come here to sit around and wait for you to be returned in a coffin. You're spoiling for it. I mean, really spoiling for it. You're not going to quit till you get your stupid head shot off!"

"Why is it! Why is it so difficult, so fucking impossible, for you to understand! Just once. Understand!"

"What is it you're after, boy? Tell me so I'll know what to tell the children."

He leaned over the bed, his hands like claws, tight, trembling. His voice became choked. "I want to feel it! I want to be scared shitless! I want to be exhausted! Feel it!"

"With your leg lying twenty yards away! You want to feel that too!" She stood in the bed and flung the pillow off. "How about us? Too bad you won't be around to watch us mourn. You don't have to do this!"

"No, I don't," he replied with menacing softness. "I can pack up tomorrow and hightail it back to Sherman Oaks and spend the rest of my life writing Doris Day comedies, or bowwow pictures at Disney. Hey, let's hire old Gideon Zadok, he's one of the best whores in town. Just wind him up and out comes dribble, dribble, dribble. Old Gideon won't give you any trouble. He's a pissant. Heard he wanted to be a real writer once. Can you imagine that? Shit, couldn't give up his monogrammed underwear. Not old Gideon."

"Isn't it about time for your zinger, that I wrecked your second novel because I wouldn't let you go live in the brothels of San Francisco?"

"No, no, no, honey, don't blame yourself. It's the tuition in those private schools that costs too much. Grover's got to see a psychiatrist. The Caddy has already got a thousand miles on it."

Val went to her knees, buried her face in her hands, and rocked back and forth, back and forth. She emitted a long, terrible sigh, lay down, turned her back to him, and drew the sheet over her. "Fuck off," she said.

"Baby," he cried, "please tell me you know what I'm trying to do. Please tell me."

She was calm now, deadly calm. "You're a war lover, Gideon. Even your jeep was making joyous sounds tonight when you pulled in."

Gideon was shattered. He fell back against the wall and hung his head. It was the damned truth. The thought of going on a raid had sent him into exaltation. How do you explain? How do you justify?

He knelt by the bed, reached out tentatively, and touched the rounded part of her hip. She was icy. "It's part of me, baby, I can't help myself. All right, I'm intoxicated by it. I've got to go for it, baby. I've got to reach for it. Don't make me go back . . . there . . . without going for it."

He waited but she did not stir. He came to his feet, rocky. "I'll go to the hotel," he said.

She reached behind her and pulled the sheet down for him to climb in. In a moment, he curled up tightly against her.

"Baby . . . baby . . ."

Val turned around, took his head, and held it on her breast.

"Try to sleep, Gideon. You'll need your strength."

"Take it off."

"You crazy fool. You're too much, Zadok. You horny Jew."

"This is what gives me strength," he said.

There was something incredible about the lovemaking, when it came on wings of such fury.

THERE HAD BEEN many other times I'd waited for Gideon with my
heart in my mouth. I always knew he'd find his way home. Not so, this
time. Val, I kept telling myself, it may be thirty-six hours before you get
any information. If I could only close my eyes and wake up tomorrow
with him standing over me. If I could only talk to someone about it!

All my options to kill time lost their appeal—reading a new book,
sewing a couple of dresses for the girls, giving them a heavy dose of
school lessons. I didn't seem to be able to concentrate.

Maybe jump into the car and take a trip up to Jerusalem, or go up to
the archaeological dig at Hazor. No, I didn't even want to take a long
walk on the beach. I should be on hand if a telephone message comes
through.

I found myself having tea with a couple of the neighbors. Nice girls,
South Africans. Part of their families stayed behind in Johannesburg to
operate the family businesses. Earnings were sent to Israel where the
other part of the family had immigrated and started up new enterprises.
Lifetime Zionists with clear-cut goals.

Where was Gideon now?

"Little more tea, Dara?"

"Thanks, Val. Little jumpy today?"

I didn't totally trust Dara Myerson. She was too gorgeous. They all
flirted with Gideon.

I almost lost it. I dropped the kettle and grabbed the sink for support.

"Val, you look the color of paste."

They helped me to the bedroom and Selma left to find Dr. Hartmann. Dara said she'd take the girls for the day and see to my meals.

"What's wrong, Mom?"

"Just a little dizzy spell."

"Are you starting your period? Is it premenstrual tension?" Roxy asked. Roxanne had become very worldly about menstruation. She was a lady-in-waiting, about to start up at any time. She carried a sanitary napkin around with her everyplace, in case the big event should occur.

Dr. Hartmann treated a lot of concentration camp survivors. His medical bag was full of goodies. The girls were gone and it became quite peaceful as the medication took hold . . . wheeeee . . . praise the Lord . . . baby's flying . . .

The fucking clock had barely moved. It was only eleven in the morning. "Oh, cripes." I breathed deeply. It hurt, bad. The only other time I remembered feeling this kind of pain was during those hours of waiting when Penelope's life hung in the balance.

I focused in on the photograph on the dresser. There he is, staring down at me. Rear Admiral Warren Ballard and Mother. Mom's big-brimmed hat was gushy with lace. Both of them had military stiff backs and white gloves. Their joint smiles registered .001 on the Richter scale. Bulldog Ballard.

San Francisco Bay Area, 1944–1953

HIS SOFTEST TOUCH felt like a blackjack. If it didn't cruise at twenty-five knots, or wasn't 90 proof, the Admiral usually wasn't interested, particularly if it was a voice that came from inside a little girl. We were commodities. Mother was a grade A commodity. Sweet Sister Ellen was a commodity, bless her pissant soul. Brother Tom was no commodity. He was a *male!*

But Tom let the old team down. Yea, Tom! Instead of following Bulldog Ballard into Annapolis, Tom was somewhere on a mountaintop in South America, teaching ungrateful Indians how to use fertilizer.

Anthropology! What the hell is anthropology! Married a God-damned Peruvian woman, half-Indian, that's what!

"Best not to mention Tom this Christmas," Mother had warned; "the Admiral's maudlin about it."

No such problems with Sweet Sister Ellen. Navy forever! Fred Barrington, now there's as fine a young officer as this man's navy has laid eyes on in ten years. That lad will be commanding a cruiser before he's thirty-five. Yoicks! A cruiser before thirty-five! Sweet Sister Ellen, who, in secret, could outdrink the Admiral and Fine Lad Fred, had delivered a little boy. He was a little shit, but at last the Admiral knew the old tradition would live on despite brother Tom's perfidy.

I was the baby. By the time it was my turn at bat, Sweet Sister Ellen had caved in and Brother Tom had waved his middle finger under the Admiral's nose and jumped ship to South America.

Mother usually came down on Father's side, so I spent my childhood learning the art of compromise and not rocking the boat. From the beginning, I was good in art—damned good, actually. My dreams of studying in Paris had to be set aside by the war. Besides, Mother and I hadn't totally convinced the Admiral. I was good enough for Paris, mind you, but not quite ready. The really fine art schools in L.A. and New York were also just out of reach. I decided to spend the war getting ready for Paris.

Mills College, a sort of West Coast Vassar with a fairly snooty all-girl campus near San Francisco, seemed to be a good compromise. Pleased the hell out of the Admiral and kept peace in the home.

Home, incidentally, was Coronado Island, a ferry-boat hop over the bay from San Diego. Ships here, ships there, ships everywhere. All Navy, a yard wide. A retirement community, where old salts got rigor mortis before the final sail to the great beyond. Six commanders and five captains per square block. Flag officers on Ocean Boulevard. That's where we lived, in a big old airy place with shiplap siding and the Fourth of July all year round.

At Mills I gloried in my first real taste of freedom. I studied art history (yawn), and studio art, and mostly boned up on my French so I could crack the Sorbonne after the war.

That's when I met him. Gideon Zadok, Private First Class, USMC and well-known entrepreneur.

Gideon was a patient at the Oak Knoll Naval Hospital, just a skip and a holler down the road from the Mills College campus. So many poor wounded Marines and sailors so far from home needing a lot of tender loving care, and several hundred girls just coming into heat . . . it was a lovely mutual arrangement. In those days old-fashioned chivalry still prevailed . . . a few fierce French kisses, maybe a little squeeze of the tits, but nothing we couldn't talk to Mother about. We just didn't sack out unless the situation had reached a very serious stage. Christ, the world was demure then. It was nice.

Gideon didn't talk much about his overseas duty. Over a period of time I got to know that he had had seven recurrences of malaria from Guadalcanal and had apparently taken some shrapnel in the shoulder. It wasn't a bad wound, but a buddy of his at the hospital told me he kept it secret for two or three days until it became infected by the jungle atmosphere and was considered serious enough to earn him a Purple Heart. Later, on Tarawa, he caught dengue fever, a terribly painful disease in which all the joints in the body—knuckles, knees, toes, backbone—swell up.

Then there was something about his asthma. All told, he was just a plain worn-out warrior in need of a long healing period.

I arranged a party of girlfriends to go to the Oak Knoll Hospital to see his play. To my surprise, it was a terribly funny show, acted with skill and abandon. Loved the plot. A Marine detachment was shot into outer space, where they formed a colony on a distant planet. After several centuries the colony lost contact and they were eventually forgotten. Life was eternal out there. Every day for hundreds of years, the Marines woke up to reveille, did close-order drill, were spit and polish, and held inspections. They were rediscovered and returned to Earth. The last act, in which they discover sex with women, was hilarious. But after looking over the world, they opted to be returned to outer space and do close-order drill forever.

I don't know why I kept dating this guy. He was a bit of a blowhard. Most Marines have a problem with modesty. I think I was also enchanted with being able to go out with enlisted men and finding out they weren't all hairy apes. After I saw Gideon's play, I began to wonder. What is it drawing me to him?

> I'll be seeing you
> In all the old familiar places,
> That this heart of mine embraces,
> All day through . . .

I hope there is still slow dancing when Roxanne and Penelope start dating. Their old mom can teach them the yins and yangs of it. A good part of my slow-dancing career had been in the arms of some ambitious young officer trying to zap the Admiral's daughter. A lot of random clutching, sweating and, oh shit, here comes his erection.

But on the other hand, comrades, slow dancing can run a very close second to you know what. PFC Zadok really knew his way around the back alleys and gutter fighting and on a dance floor. He held you firmly but fairly, his antennae alert to pick up the faintest signal. After I decided I liked the way we fit, and stopped fighting it, I'd just wrap myself around him, feel his cheek, breathe hard, and sway like there was only one of us moving for two.

He knew a restaurant, within his means, over the bay in San Francisco. El Globo on Broadway, in the Italian North Beach section. It was actually a Portuguese bar with rooms over the top for visiting seamen. Behind the bar were a half-dozen booths in a room that served a family-style dinner for ninety-nine cents with wine.

We were getting quieter and quieter every time, just holding hands and looking at each other through the candle's flame.

"How's all this going to go down with the Admiral? Me being an enlisted man. And a Marine?"

"The Admiral and I are not that close. I don't know. He had a ship shot out from under him at Midway. He's seen too many of his own boys die and too many Marines scraped up from the beach. He's lost a lot of his bigotry."

"You want to keep on seeing me?"

I was about to say, "I'm not ready." That's what I'd always said before: "I could really go for you, buddy, but I'm not ready. Paris and all that." I didn't answer him.

"You want to hear a real deal breaker?" Gideon asked.

"Shoot."

"I'm a Jew."

I don't know what he had to go through to say that, but a strange moment arrived between us. Suddenly it wasn't fun and games any longer. I made a smart-assed remark like, "I thought you were some kind of weirdo."

Gideon looked into the bar where a serious arm-wrestling contest was going on. "There's our dinner and gas money. Lend me a couple of bucks, we'll split the winnings."

Oh, that little bastard was deceptive. He pinned three Portuguese sailors, all twice his size, and scooped up fifteen dollars from the bar.

I had access to a girlfriend's car, which was in drydock most of the time because of the gas rationing until Gideon came along. He hustled enough ration stamps to keep the tank full. We got outside and I knew I'd have to give him some kind of answer.

"Let's drive to someplace quiet," he said. "There's something I want to show you."

With all his bravado, Gideon had scarcely touched me. I felt very comfortable about being alone with him. I drove up to Twin Peaks. It was a rare night without fog and we could see the entire Bay area and bridges.

"Taken many poor sailors up here?"

"Oh, quite a few, but you're my very first Marine Jew."

He didn't kiss me. I learned later that was all a part of the bastard's strategy. He opened a large manila envelope and took out a small stack of pages.

"What's that?"

"The first chapter of my novel. I'd like to read it to you."

I found myself shaking. Everything was twinkling out there and an eager young man was sitting opposite me ready to throw down the gauntlet and challenge the world.

"What do you call it?"

"Of Men in Battle."

When he finished reading, I just came apart and wept uncontrollably. It was so beautiful. I looked at Gideon Zadok, hard. Lord, what was this all about!

"Oh buddy," I cried, "you've got me going."

Gideon reached out and touched my cheek and told me not to cry. I never felt anything like his hand before. No one has ever touched me that way since, but him.

> *In that small café,*
> *The park across the way,*
> *The children's carrousel,*
> *The chestnut trees,*
> *The wishing well,*
> *I'll be seeing you,*
> *In every lovely summer's day . . .*

"I love you, Gideon."

"Me too, Val. And you're going to live to see them all standing up and applauding when I enter the room. Even the Admiral."

TEA WITH MOTHER at the stroke of four, Garden Court, Palace Hotel, and "try not to be late, dear." Afternoon tea, gentle music under a high glass roof, amid flowers, potted trees, and fountain. Jane Ballard belonged in the Garden Court. She was pure Renoir in a frilly French collar and one of her smashing straw hats. Mother was a pale beauty, born to wear lavender and long strings of pearls.

"Hi, Mom."

"Hello, darling."

A catch-up on the news. Father had been given the temporary rank of vice admiral and now commanded a task force, hundreds of ships. It was a monstrous-sized command, a fitting climax in the closing days of the war, to end a distinguished career.

Sweet Sister Ellen's drinking problem had oozed out of the closet. Fred had been overseas for two years now and Sweet Sister Ellen was apparently doing a little of this and a little of that on the side. Thank God Ellen had Mom. But she'd always had Mom. It was Ellen's deliberate pissant decision. I was envious, no doubt. It stuck in my craw.

Tom's Peruvian wife was about to have their fourth child. Would we ever get to see them? Maybe, after the war. That wasn't just idle talk. The Admiral had softened up a bit. He was corresponding regularly with Tom. Really! Bulldog Ballard relenting!

The evening before, Gideon and I had pooled our resources and taken Mother out to Shadows Restaurant on Telegraph Hill and he'd unleashed his charms on her.

"What do you think of him, Mom?"

"Oh, he's a charmer, all right. Very clever boy."

"I'm crazy about him."

"That's rather obvious. How far is this thing going to go?"

Silence. The orchestra switched to a medley of sentimental British war tunes . . . "The White Cliffs of Dover" . . . "When the Lights Go On Again." Tea arrived with "A Nightingale Sang in Berkeley Square." Mother lit her long thin cigarette with a gold lighter embossed with a Navy ensign. Twenty-fifth anniversary present from Sweet Sister Ellen and Fred.

"Waiter," Mom said, breaking the growing awkwardness.

"Yes, ma'am."

"Take this damned stuff away. I'd like a bourbon on the rocks, a double."

I had an aversion to drinking. Mother and the Admiral drank enough for me. But we were getting down to brass tacks and nasty words could be in store. I dreaded it. "I'll have a whiskey sour," I said.

Now properly fortified, Mom popped the question. "Are you sleeping together, dear?"

"Sort of."

"I'm afraid I don't understand."

"We're lying together and we want to, and we don't want to. We kind of do and we kind of don't. We're going crazy. Cripes."

Mother's glass lowered a full inch and her eyes became slightly watery as the whiskey hit its mark.

"What next?"

"I want you to like him."

"You intend to marry this boy, don't you?"

I shrugged.

"The Admiral and I have discovered that young people are absolutely certain of their emotions and convictions. They're also bullheaded and deaf. I take it we're not being consulted, only informed."

"I'll listen," I said.

"Gideon is extremely ambitious and he could be talented. I'm not a proper judge of that. I read his pages last night. They're very crude. It takes years and years to become a writer. This boy hasn't graduated from high school. He can't get into college. He hasn't got a chance in hell of becoming a novelist with that background."

"I knew you wouldn't understand."

"No, I don't. He has a better chance of swimming across the Pacific. I suppose in time we'll learn to live with a Jewish son-in-law. But neither the Admiral nor I will accept your unhappiness."

I felt a sudden rage! "Mom, that's a damned laugh. Neither one of you have known I've been alive for the last ten years. All right, so he doesn't become a writer. I love him for dreaming about it. For daring it. Whatever, he'll make a good living. I want him for the way he loves me . . . for the way he touches me."

Mother just stared at me, as though she had been struck.

"I need him for his tenderness," I said.

She twiddled with her glass, spinning the ice cubes around, then held it out quickly as the waiter passed. She had been caught off guard. Darling Val never argued with either of them.

"That's very unkind," she said.

"All right, Mom. When was the last time the Admiral was tender to you?"

"Oh, don't you know, darling, he and I have had our wild nights in the Orient. He knows his way around my body. Why the hell is it that all young people can't believe their parents ever made love to each other?"

"Me," I said, not believing the words were coming from my mouth. "What about loving me?"

"Great men have great weaknesses," she answered. "No, don't interrupt me, Valerie. Your father is an honorable man and a patriot. He's one of the greatest in the world at what he does. And I don't believe he's ever been unfaithful to me in over thirty years. Perhaps I gave him too much and you too little. Families of men like these always have to pay a price. Do you really think your young man, Gideon, is all that much different from your father? I said don't interrupt me, Val. . . . The Admiral never got a word of love from his own father in his entire life. He doesn't know how to say 'I love you.' But he does love, in his own way, and God knows I do. This man—your father—when he stands on the bridge of his flagship, a battle wagon, and puts a pair of binoculars to his eyes, he sees ships from horizon to horizon. Carriers, battleships, cruisers, destroyers, planes overhead, submarines below. He, Bulldog Ballard, is the commander! What can I, as a wife, give him to compare? Just keep him fit and understand his weaknesses and love him for what he is."

"Things are different with me and Gideon. The world is becoming different. This is going to be a two-career family. The minute he earns enough by writing, we're off to Paris for me to finish my schooling."

"Oh, Val, my darling, do you really believe that Gideon doesn't have the same kind of ambition as your father? Do you really believe that you can match him if he starts to fly? To be on the bridge of that ship, he must have peace in his home. Maybe there is a brave new world beginning. I hear talk of it all the time, but I don't understand it. I'm just a plain old Navy wife. My career is my man and that's been more than enough for me."

"Mom. We were married last week."

She turned ashen. We were both underage. They could annul it if they wanted to.

"I'm sorry you didn't think enough of us to come to us. Maybe you'll manage your own family better than I managed mine."

She left quickly to go to her room and cry it out. It was the first time in my life I had ever made a real defiant stand against my parents. Now, I was frightened.

GIDEON AND I had a tiny third-floor walk-up flat over a Chinese grocery on Larkin Street, on the edge of San Francisco's tenderloin. Thirty-five dollars a month, furnished.

My introduction to my new father-in-law was a five-page letter, not unlike the Rocks and Shoals (the articles governing the United States Navy).

. . . I don't know how much my sonny boy told you about his happy childhood in Philadelphia, but we are a very progressive family. I have no objection whatsoever that my son marries a *shiksa* (gentile) but he should not forget he is Jewish.

Enclosed are the recipes to make gefilte fish, *matzo brie, borsht, gadempta fleysh, tsimmes,* etc. when we meet personally, I'll give you a test.

Mainly, you should see to it that Gideon writes to me every week. I hold you responsible. And it wouldn't hurt a thing if you also correspond with me.

I don't know why Gideon is boycotting Philadelphia. What's so great about San Francisco?

From Gideon's mother, a strange, simple message, "How could you do this to your mother?"

Gideon didn't want to go back to Baltimore and Philly, even for a short visit as the war was coming to a close. "I'll go back," he said, "after my first book is published, and I'll drive home in a Cadillac."

Before the war ended, an event took place that should have tipped me off that I had married a wild man. Gideon had wangled a transfer from the hospital to duty at a supply depot in San Francisco. At that time the San Francisco *Examiner* and other Hearst newspapers were pushing for Douglas MacArthur, a soldier, to become supreme commander in the Pacific, placing him over the Navy and the Marines. A terrible front-page editorial was headlined MARINES DIE NEEDLESSLY and cited MacArthur's skill at keeping down Army casualties. Of course it did not mention that the Marines were given by far the most dangerous islands to invade. Gideon and some three hundred enlisted Marines paid a visit to the *Examiner.* When the editor phoned the Shore Patrol for help—what do you know, not a single Navy or Marine officer of authority was left in town.

As the police arrived, I was told later, Gideon, as spokesman, grabbed the editor by his necktie and said, "The first cop that enters, we're taking your presses apart."

Result, the *Examiner* printed a retraction and the rest of the Hearst papers canceled the editorial. I recall this incident because it was the first time I saw Gideon refuse to back down, a situation that often would recur.

A BEAUTIFUL LETTER came from his sister, Molly. Molly wrote that she had waited for this day for so long. She said that many people loved Gideon and he had many good friends and caring relatives, but in a strange way, he was always very much alone. Molly said he desperately needed one person in this world he could call his own, someone to watch over him. And Molly wrote that she loved me because I loved Gideon.

Did I love Molly's baby brother? Did I love him! Oh, I know all newlyweds are moonstruck with the wonderment of discovery, but we devoured each other. My tightly controlled emotions, disciplined by the untouching hands of my parents, had locked in my ability to show affection as effectively as if contained in a steel box. I never realized how tight it was and how tightly controlled my emotions had become. Love, deeply buried, erupted from me now.

We were slightly crazy. We tried everything, read every sex book we could get our hands on. He loved to make me blush when he came across something strange.

As soon as we sat down in a restaurant, our hands were under the tablecloth. We'd duck into alleyways. We'd make love on the ground in Muir Woods, just a few feet off the main walking path. Some of this doesn't sound so wild now, but it was the 1940s, and modesty and whispers ranked over candor. Crazy costumes, mirrors, fantasy. Our fertile minds were seeking all the time. The first Christmas he was out of the service, we had a two-foot tree, pending poverty, and glorious, glorious love.

And then the dawn came up like thunder from the hoary hills of Oakland cross the bay!

We were mainly living on dreams, youthful ignorance, and veteran's and unemployment benefits. I thought he would plunge into his novel. He tried for a short time, but finally threw it into a drawer and seldom took it out. Some call it writer's block. I call it fear. He couldn't admit to that.

Gideon embarked on a series of gigantic ventures, guaranteed to change the world. Only the world wasn't quite ready for him. He formed a bogus Marine veterans' organization with a membership of five, which enabled him to get a charter from the state, giving him nonprofit status and a number of veterans' perks. The little bastard went out and rented the San Francisco Opera House to present his new play. He hustled scenery, costumes, got feature articles in the newspapers, received a waiver from the musicians' and stagehands' unions, passed out handbills, elbowed his way onto radio programs, wrote rave reviews in which he quoted from nonexistent papers in Chicago and New York. Result: seventy-four dollars in the box office and a thousand-dollar debt.

This shook him up so, he hid away in a fight gym in the tenderloin, played pinball machines every day, all day long, for three months.

Next, it was a veterans' newspaper. This afforded him space to write. He wrote the entire paper, including four columns under different names. He telephoned far into the evenings, hustling ads from local businesses. It took six months for this enterprise to sink and add another thousand dollars to our debt.

Next came publication of a magazine offering "job opportunities" all over the world. The bunko squad came looking for him.

After which he wrote skits for a number of cabarets around North Beach. These were quite funny social commentaries. Unfortunately, the customers liked their entertainment a little more in the raw.

I was so damned in love with the guy that I believed each and every one of his cockamamy schemes right up to the day they busted.

And then I confronted him with those two magic words, "I'm pregnant."

A COUPLE OF fight trainers he had befriended at the gym sent him to a Teamsters local and Gideon became circulation district manager for the San Francisco *Call-Bulletin*, an afternoon newspaper. He had between thirty and forty newspaper boys working for him in home delivery. Between my morning sickness and Gideon having a regular job, we were back in the real world and little by little climbed out of the hole.

I had hoped that he would return to writing his novel, but the early disasters had left him gun-shy. He did write constantly, every spare moment, but they were short fiction and nonfiction pieces. He kept between fifteen and twenty of these constantly circulating in the mails from publication to publication. In the next two years, he collected four hundred and twenty-two rejection slips.

MOTHER AND I had kept in touch through the occasional letter and phone call. As I went into the eighth month of my pregnancy, we received a sudden message that she and the Admiral were going to pay us a visit. Panic city!

Our apartment, such as it was, was scarcely large enough to hold my belly. It had a closet-sized kitchenette, a one-person-at-a-time bathroom, and an all-purpose room with a pull-down Murphy bed. We ate at a card table on fold-up canvas director's chairs.

I had dolled the place up with a couple of my own splashy paintings, some wild color, posters, and gypsy wall hangings. In addition to its collection of saloons, muggers, hookers, and other sleazy characters, the tenderloin had a number of flea market-type shops and used book and record stores. Some polished-up bric-a-brac and filled bookshelves gave the place a kind of kinky charm. Outside our window, life in the raw played out daily human dramas—fire trucks shifting gears on our hill rattling our building . . . wife beaters . . . husband beaters . . . drunks passing out in our lobby . . . warring gangs of alley cats . . . and a couple of self-employed ladies of the night down our hall. I knew Mom and the Admiral were going to choke when they saw where and how we were living.

To my surprise, they didn't seem to give a damn. My own insecurity was quickly replaced by concern over the way my father looked. He was dying. That accounted for the sudden peace visit. He had cancer and I was grateful they had come. Mom told me he had refused all pain medication. "With the pain," he had told her, "at least I know I'm alive."

Well, don't you know that two years of dreading this visit was all for naught. It turned out to be the most wonderful evening I had ever had with them. We blew everything on the meal. The El Globo Restaurant put up a stupendous pot of take-out bouillabaisse and sold us the vino wholesale.

The room was bathed in candlelight flickering from Chianti bottles which had grown wax hairdos six inches thick, and there was a background of operatic music. We all proceeded to gorge ourselves and get loaded.

The Admiral and Gideon talked about the invasion of Tarawa like two old war buddies. Gideon had seen it from a Marine's point of view and researched it further to use in his novel. The Admiral was impressed as hell.

"Well, why aren't you working on your book?" Father asked with a bluntness I knew only too well. "It's not going to write itself."

I don't think any of us were ready for Gideon's answer. "I'm scared," he said.

"Scared? To write?" Mother asked, with honest innocence.

"Everything I've ever wanted or dreamed of since I was a little boy depends on that book. What if it fails? Sometimes I think that if I didn't make it, I'd want to die. I just can't go through life being nobody. So, I'm scared."

The room became terribly quiet. The Admiral looked long and hard at Gideon. "I know exactly what you're saying," he said.

The record ended. Gideon switched it off.

The Admiral filled his glass again and spoke, as though to himself. "I've never known a sane man who wasn't afraid. I've never known a great man who didn't have to conquer his greatest fears."

It came time for them to leave, too soon. Gideon said goodbye and tastefully left the three of us alone. Mother would come back when the baby was due. We all lingered at the door. We had never lingered before over farewells. The Admiral patted my shoulder as though I were a junior officer who had done something commendable.

"You are glowing with happiness, Val. I'm glad. That boy is a good boy. I've seen a thousand like him, burning inside. He's picked a rough passage for himself."

"Will he ever do it, Dad?"

"He'll face that book when he has built enough courage to face defeat."

"Oh, Dad!" I cried and flung my arms around him. I wanted to tell him that there was so much we hadn't ever said to each other. And now he was going to leave! Forever. Just when we were starting to say hello.

The Admiral's hands remained at his side as I held him. He was awkward in my embrace, not knowing what to do. I longed for him to put his arms around me. He couldn't. Yet I realized that he understood everything. And I suppose he did love me, in his own way.

I'm glad the Admiral lived long enough to see Roxanne born. He was in a wheelchair then. There wasn't much left of him. When they put her into his arms, he held her quite tenderly for a long time . . . and he looked at me and smiled . . . as though he had been holding me.

GLORY, GLORY, HALLELUJAH! And yet another easy monthly payment book bites the dust. We were now the proud owners of our own sofa, a Monkey Ward fridge, and a secondhand Model A Ford, for which we paid eighty dollars cold hard cash. Now comes the Great Valerie Santini balancing act!

Do we go for dishes, towels, silver, and linens?

OR

Gideon longed for one of those new long-playing record machines.

HOWEVER

Roxy needed a ballet costume.

AND

If we could only get six more months out of the front tires.

If it all went according to schedule, we would have everything we ever wanted and it would be all paid off in three hundred and forty-five years, down considerably from the last accounting of four hundred and six years. We were making headway.

I hid money so that every week we had enough left over for a movie and a Chinese or El Globo dinner. On payday I'd hide another two dollars in nickels and dimes around the apartment for my own clothing fund and mad money.

Gideon's job paid pretty well, seventy-five dollars a week. Otherwise it was rotten. He detested it, but he never brought it home, no matter how terrible his day had been.

Being poor was a new and growing experience for me. What I hadn't realized was that you could be poor but deliriously happy at the same time. Every night when I heard him take the stairs three steps at a time I'd shiver a little bit. We'd meet in the doorway or out in the hall and he would hold me like we hadn't seen each other for weeks. As soon as the apartment door was closed, he'd feel my backside or wherever he could get with his hand under my dress (I didn't make it too difficult for him). In a few minutes Roxy would have him pinned down on the floor, fishing through his pockets for her prize.

I put Roxy to bed early. She was coming down with the sniffles. Besides, tonight was going to be a super special time. Mom and Dad were reading *The Kinsey Report* on human sexuality and were trying out something a little kinky. I mean stuff that twenty or thirty percent of the people were already into.

There was a little something else going on too. I skipped a period every now and again and usually it wasn't cause for alarm.

Candlelight on the card table. *La Bohème* on the record player. *I've wanted it back so many times, Gideon. Where did it go? Jesus, we were so happy.*

I served him wearing a knockout front-button sweater. He stared at me so adoringly, I blushed. For a long time I'd wondered why Gideon married me. I was on the tall side, blond, with a terrific pair of tits. I knew it made him feel good when I was at his side. He was proud of me, my college education, my old man being an Admiral. Through me, Gideon was thumbing his nose at something in his childhood. He wouldn't talk about it, just as he wouldn't talk about the war.

We talked about everything else. We couldn't wait to be alone and talk. He was a very funny guy when he got a little tipsy and he knew something about everything going on in the world. A lot of times we'd talk without words. He'd put his arm about my shoulder and lay my head on his chest and we'd listen to those secondhand records and sip vino.

"You've been looking awfully beautiful lately, Val."

He unbuttoned the sweater front and did all those nice sweet things to my breasts . . .

"We pregnant?" he asked.

"Yes."

"Hey, how about that! I wouldn't mind another little girl."

"How come?"

"Little boys have to be little men the minute they're born. The pressure is on for them to be tough—don't cry—look how strong he is—he'll be a hockey player, that one."

"But I want your son."

"But I don't want my son to go to war," he said. And I knew this came from way back and very deep.

"I've been thinking, honey. I can take a few brush-up art courses. You know, I really don't have that many credits left to get my teacher's certificate," I said.

"There's a ten-dollar pay raise coming and I'm getting an extra fiver a week as the union shop steward. Let's try it this way for the time being."

Roxanne ran a little temp and had a bad dream. I took her to bed with me and Gideon sacked out on our paid-for couch. During the night when she was restless and woke me I could see Gideon, his eyes open staring at us, so filled with love.

"Hi," I said.

"Hi," he answered.

"Squeeze in with us, honey," I told him. I pushed my backside against his tummy and his arm went around the both of us. When Roxy's fever dropped, I wished for an endless night.

GIDEON AND I had this crazy notion about living in Marin County, over the Golden Gate Bridge, even though it meant a long bus ride to the city. We would spend his days off driving around Marin, fantasizing that our dream house would appear.

Mill Valley was a sweet, cuddly little town with redwood stands, woodsy trails, running brooks, zillions of flowers, and an artsy village center.

Henry Perkins was a real estate salesman who worked the poor side of the tracks. He had long deduced from our Model A that we weren't going into the high-rent district.

The house Mr. Perkins found for us was actually an abandoned week-end cottage and, as we say in the trade, needed a bit of work by a handyman. But dammit, it had a spacious yard with a big madrona tree and a front porch meant for a swing and the living room had a fireplace and there were really nice schools within walking distance and . . . the price was right.

"Seven thousand four hundred dollars," Mr. Perkins said, consulting his little book. Gulp!

"How much down?"

"This little beauty has a full G.I. loan. Nothing down and about a hundred bucks closing costs."

"How much are the monthly payments?"

"On a 4 percent loan it comes to . . . let's see. Forty-one dollars and six cents a month, principal, interest, and insurance."

Our hearts were in our throats. We had a hundred and four dollars in the bank.

What mistakes Gideon didn't make as a carpenter, he made as a gardener, a painter, a plumber, and a bricklayer. But we attacked our little witch's cottage until my belly got in the way, and by the time Penelope was born we had a warm, cozy, tiny piece of the world with a garden filled with roses.

GIDEON HATED his job. I mean, he hated it with a passion. Home delivery in newspaper parlance conjures up a nice, clean-cut, all-American image of yapping dogs and picket fences and smiles on the faces of satisfied subscribers. Why, some of our presidents were newspaper carriers, the classic apple-pie road from rags to riches.

It was a shit job.

There was an ugly circulation war among the four San Francisco newspapers. The game was rigged so that the newspaper boys got screwed right, left, and center.

District managers like Gideon came under unbearable pressure from an unsavory circulation department on the one side and the need to protect their paperboys on the other. His department floated on antacids and ulcer medication. Someone had a heart attack every six weeks.

Gideon and some of the other district managers became just as sleazy fighting the paper and seeing to it their boys didn't suffer losses. To make matters worse, the men elected Gideon as the union shop steward so he had every other district manager's misery to contend with as well as his own.

Winters were wet in San Francisco, but neither paperboys nor papers came waterproofed. The department became such a meat grinder that out of forty district managers, Gideon was third in seniority in a few short years. There was an inevitable moment when things reached a point where a wildcat walkout was being planned. This could mean bare-knuckle time, because the paper kept a lot of ex-fighters and toughs around to deal with such unrest.

As a ringleader of the "agitators," Gideon was transferred to a fully certified skid row, a district of poor blacks, poorer Hispanics, winos, prostitutes, several save-your-soul missions, V.D. clinics, and five candy-store robberies a night.

"HI, MOM!"

"Hello, Val. I just set my bags down. Can you make it for cocktails at six in the Garden Court? Gideon can join us for dinner when he gets off work."

Mother and I had grown close, or at least as close as we were able. She adored Penny and Roxy, and Gideon never failed to bring a twinkle to her eye.

Scotch is one of the unsung perks that comes with motherhood. Lovely stuff. Over drinks in the Garden Court, Mom and I made plans for the girls to spend a month with her in Coronado when school was out and I'd join them for the last couple of weeks.

Mother was too elegant to come out with the forbidden subject, so I did.

"He doesn't write anymore. When we first moved to Mill Valley he did some short pieces. The job has just taken all the starch out of him. To say nothing of the rejections. Oh God, I hate rejections. They are death sentences. How many death sentences can a man take?"

"Do you think he's done with it forever?"

"Right now I do. He'd have to find another job. Maybe if he could get something in Marin, he would start writing again. As for me, I've decided to go back to school and pick up my credits as soon as we have Penny in kindergarten. Between the two of us, we can become comfortable in time."

Mom grew uncharacteristically quiet and managed a sad smile.

"What's on your mind, Mom?"

"Somewhere along the line, we all give up the dream, I suppose. The Admiral didn't, but on the other hand he didn't try to take a trip to the moon alone. Somehow I thought Gideon was going to make it."

"We're still very much in love. Sooner or later he'll get his job situation squared away. Maybe he'll try again."

"The longer he waits, the tougher it becomes. And what if he realizes he'll never be a writer?"

"Maybe Gideon got in over his head. Anyone who goes into writing has to find out somewhere along the line, he's either naïve or insane. It's not going to be the end of our life."

ONE MORE San Francisco winter and Gideon changed. A lot of his cockiness and bravado had turned into sulkiness. The fire in him was dying out and he was trying to find the way to cope with his defeat and still keep going.

One night he was packed home between a couple of his buddies, pissy-assed drunk, too crocked to drive the car. Was this a new phase of our marriage, or was the old Marine just bidding fond adieu to writing?

We did not communicate for a week, except through the girls. On his day off, he came into the kitchen sheepishly lugging his typewriter.

"I want a new typewriter," he said. "How much can we swing?"

Pencil went to paper. Jesus, there was a dress I wanted so badly—I'd saved thirty dollars in hidden nickels and dimes. We were still paying off the washing machine.

"Three dollars," I said.

Gideon got six dollars a week allowance. He'd cut it to five. The same day he took the Underwood to an office supply store in San Rafael. It was so old it had a right-hand carriage throw.

"This is the down payment. I can afford five bucks a month. Can I get a new machine?"

"I've got some real nice reconditioned models . . ."

"I need a new typewriter. I've got a long book to write. I'll throw in an autographed copy when it's finished."

"I don't get rich from these kind of deals, buddy."

"Yes or no?"

"You're serious about this writing. I never sold a machine to a writer before."

"You're fucking A I'm serious. Marine's honor."

Gideon had said the magic words. The store owner was an ex-Marine. They stick together like Jews. Gideon came home with a Smith-Corona, unlocked the manuscript drawer, and took out the first pages of *Of Men in Battle*.

WHAT HAPPENED to my man in the next three years, I wouldn't have wished on a dog. Gideon arrived home about eight at night and he wrote in a little attic alcove until two or three in the morning. The alcove held a card table and the typewriter. It was situated next to a small bedroom belonging to the girls. His typing became their lullaby.

He was usually so exhausted he couldn't speak coherently or walk down the steps alone. I had to undress him. On his day off, he'd work at the typewriter for seventeen or eighteen straight hours.

And so it came to pass that one night he wrote THE END and then he dedicated the manuscript to his "long-suffering wife" and the two of us got stiffed and agonized through a monumental hangover.

Next came the prelude to hell. Writer's death. Rejection. Every trip to the post office box, you enter with fear in the throat, in the chest. Days and weeks and months go by and then—POW! . . . that terrible little half sheet mimeographed form arrives saying "This doesn't meet our current publishing needs." Most of the time the signature is so blurred you can't decipher it, other times there is no signature at all, just the form. No word of encouragement, no compliment, no hope. No explanation. Writing a personal letter apparently would mean no time for an editor to enjoy a martini. The publishing term for unsolicited manuscripts like Gideon's was "junk mail," the "sludge pile."

Occasionally someone wrote a smart-assed heartless note: "This is perhaps the worst manuscript ever produced in the English language," or "Try a nice trade, like plumbing."

I got sick of seeing Gideon being beaten like this. He became too numbed for tears, but I didn't. Our lives were being savaged by nameless, faceless bastards. Well . . . enough winters and springs and summers and autumns pass and somewhere along the line, if you are persistent, you pick up a friend or two. The West Coast editor of Summerfield House, Donald Howard, thought enough of the book to send it to New York with the recommendation, "I know it needs a lot of work but I have a hunch about this writer and would like to spend the time helping him clean up this manuscript."

To which the publisher answered, "Forget it. It would take two years to straighten up his grammar and spelling. You've got better things to do." Obviously Howard didn't have clout, but he did have mercy and called Gideon to his office.

Gideon was down. I mean really down. His eyes showed constant pain and sorrow.

"I think I can show you a few things that will help this manuscript," Donald Howard told him. So Gideon squandered our vacation to go over to San Francisco every day for an hour or so and he and Donald went through the manuscript sentence by sentence. It was filled with overwriting, loose ends, failed characterizations, bad construction. The manuscript began to look like a herd of elephants had crapped on it. But Howard insisted the good far outweighed the bad. Gideon had an inborn, God-given talent for dialogue, for power and drive, and a sense of rhythm and timing and mostly—an enormous love of humanity.

"The question is," Howard said, "do you have the balls to write it over, one more time?"

And so he climbed the stairs to the attic, kissed the girls, ate at the typewriter, and was put to bed by me.

And then came the rejections again . . . six more of them . . .

WHEN GIDEON got off the bus and saw my face, he knew instantly.

"There's been an accident. Penelope is in the hospital."

Mom held us together. Our little girl lay in a coma for two weeks, fighting for her life. I cannot write, or even think about it. There is no pain to compare, no fear to equal. We were tough and brave for each other . . . but Mom held us together . . . and my guilt nearly drove me insane.

Days and nights ran together . . . that awful hospital corridor . . . the grim face of the doctor . . . all those tubes and bandages and monitors . . . her beautiful little face one huge bruise . . . no flutter of recognition . . . oh God, Penny, speak to Mommy, just once . . . please . . . nightmares of her running into the street . . . "Penny! The bus!"

Another midnight . . . I staggered to the coffee machine numbed, another setback. Across the hall was the chapel and the door was ajar. I sat down on the rear bench . . .

Gideon was near the altar, unaware of my presence . . . I'd never seen him in a church or a synagogue . . . he didn't think much of religion . . .

"God!" he said with a voice so anguished I could scarcely recognize it. "I don't know if you're there. I don't know if you've ever been there . . . I was told when I was a kid not to ask for favors from God . . . only to ask for strength and wisdom. . . . I've got no strength left . . . look, man, you listen to me, fucker—I never asked to come out alive at Guadalcanal or Tarawa, did I? I wanted to ask you to let Pedro live, but I didn't . . . but . . . but . . . God . . . I can't handle this . . . I know, man, you don't make any deals but there has only been one thing in my life I really wanted, to be a writer . . . if you don't take her, God . . . I'll work at that fucking newspaper the rest of my life and I won't complain, okay? I swear I'll never complain about not becoming a writer . . . man, that's all I can give you. Please don't take my baby . . ."

IT TOOK a long, long time and many nights of tears and dread, but Penelope fought through it. She was her father's daughter. One day, almost to the year, Penny and Roxy and I waited for Gideon at the bus stop. Penny handed him a telegram. FORGIVE DELAY. WE ARE MAKING AN OFFER FOR YOUR BOOK TO BE PUBLISHED AS SOON AS POSSIBLE. LETTER FOLLOWS. SIGNED J. BASCOMB III, EDITOR-IN-CHIEF, REAVES BROTHERS PUBLISHERS.

WE WERE SUDDENLY in a new world with stunning fury. Gideon coped with it all quite easily, like an old friend he'd been waiting for. He quit the newspaper with a lovely touch of understated dignity. The fellows at work were terribly proud to see one of their own leave by the front door and not have to be carried out feet first. They gave him a beautiful suitcase, a dictionary, and (so I heard) a raunchy stag party.

His newspaperboys cried openly. They chipped in and bought him a rather expensive butane cigarette lighter and told him they were sorry they didn't have a nickel left over for the card. When he stopped smoking, he continued to carry the lighter with him, always.

Oh, he had a few blowouts, to be sure, and there were a couple of times I had to send the Marines out looking for him, but by and large I felt he would ease into his new status comfortably and certainly nothing was going to change between the two of us. Maybe I should have objected to his prolonged celebration, but the guy had worked so long and so hard for it, I decided to leave it alone. I talked it over with Mother, who'd had more than a little experience of her own. She'd come to love Gideon and didn't think it was a good time to clip his wings. Anyhow, I knew Gideon would always find his way home.

I wasn't entirely happy with the plans for his second novel. Gideon had become intrigued with the people who inhabited San Francisco's tenderloin and had done a number of short character sketches which he wanted to build into a novel. He enjoyed hanging out in the crummiest bars, with the fight crowd, or getting into a little card game with the small-time hoods, and listening to the hookers' tales of woe. It wasn't exactly my cup of tea, but I decided to keep my peace and let him work it out with his editor.

I didn't cotton to his idea of going over the Bay to the tenderloin to live while he finished his research, and pretty much decided that this would be where I would draw the line. Maybe, by the time he had to make a decision, he would have changed his mind.

As for me, Valerie Zadok wanted peace, a nicer home in the hills of Sausalito overlooking the Bay and San Francisco. Maybe we could afford a sailboat. We always had one when I was growing up in Coronado. And, up in the loft, Gideon would be pecking away at his typewriter. San Francisco venerated writers. We would be a big new part of the scene. What wonderful things lay ahead. Maybe I'd even pick up the paintbrush again and try my hand at a few canvases.

Well, so much for pipe dreams. The first rude awakening came a few months later when he received the galleys of his book from the publisher to make corrections.

Reaves Brothers Publishers was an old-line, medium-sized house which had been dominated for three decades by the powerful and "legendary" Martin Reaves. The old man was declining rapidly, losing his iron grip, and with no heir apparent the company broke up into warring factions.

The editor-in-chief, Jed Bascomb III, was a Boston type who had been brought in by the old man to fill the role as number one gofer. When the old man's health deteriorated, J. Bascomb III got delusions of grandeur. However, he proved more of a manipulator than a man of any literary integrity. Gideon's *Of Men in Battle* was apparently a major cog in Bascomb's scheme to make a name for himself.

Gideon had written the novel in a breezy and whimsical style all his own. He inserted a first-person narrator who jumped in and out of the story at odd moments. It was quite out of the ordinary and also quite daring. J. III obviously didn't want to take a chance and, without consulting Gideon, simply lifted the narrator out of the novel. The first Gideon knew about it was when the galleys arrived.

J. III MUST have felt pretty certain of his ground. He knew the book's history of rejections and doubted if Gideon would give him any problems.

He had picked on the wrong Jew.

We were so starved for success and now we could taste it, feel it, smell it. I prayed Gideon wouldn't upset the cart at this stage.

I don't know who Gideon communicated with, but after two days of pondering without sleep, he came into the kitchen with blood in his eyes.

"It's no use, Val. I can't do it. I'm not going to release the galleys until they agree to change the book back to the way I wrote it."

God! I thought I'd drop dead, right there, on the spot! I personally couldn't see that it made that much difference. Moreover, the people in New York certainly had more experience in these matters than Gideon. Worst of all, what if they refused to publish? All the punch-drunk nights, all the rejections, all the years of struggle and fear, down the drain.

"I think we'd better let them have their way," I said shakily.

"Not you too, Val."

"Don't make me a traitor, Gideon. Honey, they're just trying to improve the book."

"I don't believe you, Val."

"And I don't believe you. You're just looking for a fight."

"If they're too stupid to understand what I'm trying to do—"

"Shut up for once! There are other people involved in this. Maybe that's why this damned thing has been rejected fifteen times. Maybe once, just once, they know better than you."

"I can't believe that you don't understand!"

"I understand, Gideon. I understand. I peeled your clothing off every night. For your sainted information, we have just about spent the thousand-dollar advance and you've quit your job against everyone's advice. I have something to say about this book. My blood is in it too."

"Strange! Strange! You went through all this with me and you haven't got idea one what a writer is supposed to be."

"Take that lily-white banner and shove it up your ass," I screamed. "We can't eat ideals . . . Look . . . look . . . let's cool down. Honey, nobody's going to know if they change it."

"I'll know," he cried, poking his thumb into his chest. "They've put me at the crossroads. They want me to go left, I want to go right."

"But don't you see—when you're stronger, when you're established, you can retrace your steps and go any way you want."

"Val, you're crazy, baby. Once you compromise, you can never get it back. You've got to put your foot down and make your fight when you're hungry. Once you're fat, you'll always do as they say."

"Oh God . . . Oh God . . . all those God-damned nights . . ." I just bawled. "Oh shit . . . shit, shit, shit." I felt his hand on my shoulder. "Please, honey."

"I can't, Val," he said. "I—uh—uh—I'll go down to the union next week and see about getting back on one of the newspapers. Don't . . . don't worry about me . . . I've got to walk it off for a few days . . . I'll be back. I wish I could explain what being a writer means to me."

Gideon didn't have to explain. We'd live it out, bloody battle by bloody battle. He sent Bascomb a telegram refusing to release the galleys, left the house, and disappeared for three days.

"MOMMY! Daddy's back!"

Lord, he looked like he'd been in a flophouse on skid row. I don't know how I felt at that moment. Like throwing my arms about him. Like hitting him over the head with a chair.

"Union's going to put me on the *Chronicle,*" he said. "I'll be driving a truck temporarily. No problem getting back on. Just lose a little seniority."

"You don't have to," I said. "The publisher has agreed to your demands."

MARTIN REAVES died before *Of Men in Battle* was published. The house was ripped to pieces. J. Bascomb III replaced publishing skill with cunning, candor with deceit. Without a program, no one knew who was talking to whom.

Gideon really needed someone now, to guide him through the coming months and give him some direction for his second novel.

Of Men in Battle had built a sizable advance sale to the booksellers and was to become the first novel in history to be sold with a money-back guarantee. Gideon had left the newspaper with an understanding we would get six hundred dollars a month from the publisher in advances, so he could begin the tenderloin novel and we could stay afloat until regular royalty checks caught up with us.

The money failed to come in, even though the book went back for a third printing before publication. So here was Gideon with a book about to go onto the bestseller list and we had to take a second mortgage on the house.

When a Hollywood sale and screenplay were offered by Pacific Studios, we grabbed it in order not to sink.

I don't know the answer. If his publisher had kept his word, Gideon might have passed up the screenplay job and started *The Tenderloin*. I didn't know and neither did he. It had become a matter of survival and the studio salary of seven hundred dollars a week seemed like the end of the rainbow.

For me, my dream of tranquillity was shattered, forever. I was locked in with a warrior.

GIDEON

San Francisco Bay Area, 1953

FROM THE TIME I was a little guy I rehearsed the moments of future glory a thousand and one times. When it did happen, I, Gideon Zadok, would be ready. During the dark years, the fantasy of reaching the top had become an overwhelming driving force that kept me going.

Now, it began to happen. Dream after dream came true. Val enjoyed some of it—the TV shows, the newspaper articles, the good reviews, the recognition and attention. For the first time, I saw a completely different side of her. She was very uncomfortable with the spotlight on her. She wasn't getting the kicks I was getting.

For years, when I was working on the newspaper and writing in the attic in Mill Valley, I would get to a radio every day and listen to the Mary Margaret McBride show. She was a pleasant little fat lady who broadcast from her flat on Central Park South in New York and interviewed an author a day who was having a new book published. When I was summoned to her show, *I was ready*.

I was ready for my suite at the writer's mecca, the Algonquin Hotel. Bloody suite cost over twenty bucks a day, but what the hell. I was ready when I was invited to lunch at their famed Round Table, graced by the literary lights of the day. Halfway through the meal I realized these assholes took their one-upmanship seriously. *The New Yorker* crowd. Would-be Oscar Wildes. I stopped the show with a couple of blunt, crude remarks to watch them gag and turn pale. Val didn't catch the drift of my humor at all. In fact, she was furious with me.

"I suppose you think your vulgar Marine gutter talk was amusing."

"Oh, for Christ sake, Val. Don't you see what a bunch of fakes they are? The whole goddam gang of them haven't written anything for ten years. Who in the hell are they to dictate public taste?"

"You had a chip on your shoulder the minute you entered New York."

"This scene runs on too much bullshit. Look at the bullshit at the '21' Club. Look at the bullshit with the owner himself, in person, ushering us past the peasants into the chummy Cub Room reserved for the hotsy-totsy elite. The publisher picked up a tab of over sixty dollars— over sixty dollars. For what? Bullshit."

"Relax, buddy, enjoy," she said. "You've made it. Stop waving a red flag. Everyone knows G. Zadok isn't a member of the establishment. Take a cold shower."

Maybe Val was right. I'm nice to most people. I just don't like phonies. I was just mixed up. I wanted to be me but I was having difficulty finding out who me was. I couldn't hang out around the newspaper and suck on beers at the corner bar anymore. My old buddies looked at me differently these days. Like I was some kind of tin Jesus, or something.

Are guys like J. III my new life? Fight/, don't fight. I don't know how I'm supposed to act.

"Rough transition, Gideon," Val said. "They'll find out how tough you are soon enough. So, relax."

"Yeah, I guess I'd better."

"How about you and me taking a walk up Fifth Avenue to look for the real Gideon Zadok?" she said.

"The real Zadok's in this room with you, baby, and he wants to put you flat on that bed."

"You crazy guy," she said, taking my kisses.

I stroked her hair later and kissed her a lot and found myself looking out of the window down on Forty-fourth street. It was hysterical down there. "Getting the first book accepted is like getting shot out of a cannon. I guess water has to find its own level."

She sat up in the bed. I never got tired of looking at her. "You'll be okay," she said. "You're really a nice guy."

"There's a pile of good plays on here. I want to see them all."

I settled down and enjoyed all those things I thought I was ready for: the interview with *Variety*, the 50,000-watt clear-channel station, the bow on "The Ed Sullivan Show," the blurb in Winchell's column. Be graceful, be decent. Remember, buddy, none of it means a damn if anything is wrong with Val or Penny or Roxy.

The war had been over for nearly a decade and I hadn't returned to Baltimore. Now I was ready. Kid's stuff, I know, but I rented the biggest, blackest Caddy convertible and drove down for the long-delayed family reunion. When I parked it in front of my sister Molly's house, it took up half the street. All the kids gathered around it and gawked and the neighbors tried to steal a glimpse of me. I went up to them and gave them hugs and they blushed and stammered. Yeah, it was nice and everyone enjoyed it. The champ was home! The American dream lives!

In *Look* magazine there was a photo of Radio City's Rockettes in their dressing room reading *Of Men in Battle* all in a pretty row.

And an A.P. wirephoto of the heiress Barbara Hutton getting off the plane in Vegas to get another divorce, with a copy under her arm, and one of Floyd Patterson reading it on the night before he creamed Hurricane Jackson.

There was my first autographing party at Stationers Book Store in San Diego. San Diego. Of the early moments of the early days of the victory tour, this was the answer to my wildest dream.

I'd done my boot camp in Dago. Back then I was a kid, seventeen, and war had just broken out. I had enlisted in the Corps. It was in Dago that the writer's dream took on first reality and life. I now had something to say to the world. I'd walk Broadway past the Y and the sleaze joints and get pissed on a fake I.D. card. And in Dago I had my first lay by a whore.

I'd get on the ferry to Coronado and find a place off by myself and ride until liberty was about up and I'd dream of the story I'd tell someday.

The El Cortez Hotel crowned a small hill near Broadway. I'd look up to it, a symbol of rank and affluence, and I'd say to myself, "someday." Dago was a war-hardened town that had sent off hundreds of thousands of boys to do battle in the Pacific. Now, over a decade later, it stopped for a moment and bowed to Gideon Zadok, Private, USMC.

The day before the autographing party, I entered the Marine Corps base and was whisked to the commanding general's office and I stood next to him while the graduating recruit battalion passed in review.

"We're proud of you, Marine," he said to me.

Sounds like the old boys' club stuff, I know. Schlocky. Corny as hell. But I'd written a new and different kind of war book. Most of the war novels had expressed deep hatred for America and the services. God knows I hated the war, but I didn't hate the men I fought it with. I loved them and I respected my officers and I knew why I was fighting. I was glad the Corps was proud of me.

Val and I had left the girls in Coronado with their grandmother and we took a suite at the El Cortez. We had dinner in the Skyroom restaurant with all of Dago and all of her ships and planes and lights spread below . . . and for the moment, I was king of the hill.

"You look so pensive, honey," Val said.

"Lot of things running through my head," I answered.

Later that night, we made some of the randiest love of our marriage. It started in the cocktail lounge. Val came in first and took a table by herself. In a service town like Dago, drinks start appearing like magic when a single lady enters a bar. She rejected them with thanks.

Enter great new American novelist looking for a pickup. I befriended the bartender and surveyed the room.

"Any action?" I asked.

"Little slow tonight," he said.

I nodded toward Val.

"She alone?"

"She's not accepting."

"What's she drinking?"

"Whiskey sour."

"Fix me up one."

"I think you're wasting your money."

As I sidled over to her, she crossed her legs enticingly.

"Hi. Your drink," I said.

She looked me up and down. "Thanks, but no thanks. You're a little short for my taste."

"I'm tall in the saddle," I said, taking a seat opposite her. (Tonight Val was the wife of a Navy flier out in the Pacific, somewhere.)

"Writer, huh?"

"Author. One of the best."

"If truth be known, I've already turned a trick here tonight. He didn't do me much good."

And so forth and so forth and so forth. When I whisked her out to my suite two drinks later, the railbirds at the bar gawked and the bartender gave me a V for victory sign. Nothing, fellows, really nothing.

It was two in the morning. I couldn't sleep. Val flicked on the bed lamp.

"Honey, you're dressed."

"I've got to get some air," I said.

"Everything okay?"

"I'm just a little on edge about tomorrow. I won't be out long."

I walked down the hill toward Broadway and stopped in front of Stationers Book Store. The window held several dozen copies of *Of Men in Battle*, along with a blowup photograph of me—my first author's photo, pipe, patches on the elbow of a corduroy jacket, the whole thing. *Meet the Author, Autographing Party, Friday at 2 P.M.*

Was I really standing there! So much flooded through me. The old memory of Broadway came alive and the street was filled with hundreds of swabbies and gyrene recruits and I could hear the voices of my buddies pretending they were tough and having fun. Seventeen years old, a long way from home, and all the world out there ahead of me. *Meet the Author.* What beautiful words . . . meet the author . . . you don't know me, do you? I was one of those bewildered kids sick to the stomach from too many Singapore slings.

It was empty. Not a soul around. My books in the window. I started to cry.

"Looking for company, mister?"

It was Val. She'd thrown on a dress and coat and followed me from the hotel.

A squad car pulled up and one of the cops jumped out.

"What's going on?"

Before I could answer, he saw my photo in the window.

"Hey! That's you!"

"Jesus! Hey, Sean. It's the author! Gideon Zadok. We heard you over the radio this evening. This broad bothering you?"

"She's the mother of my children."

The cop had been a Marine. He wouldn't hear of us walking back up the hill. We had a couple of drinks with them in the old Mexican section and they drove us back to the El Cortez. I took their names and addresses and said I'd send them books.

Although the evening ended up with laughs, there was a disturbing undertone. The instant Val had broken my reverie before the store window, I felt put upon. I wanted to be alone, dammit, alone with my buddies. I wanted Pedro to be proud of me now.

Why was I so ticked? Val and I had shared everything. Or had we? I'd never told her about Pedro.

April 10, 1953
My Son! My Son!
The first copy of your novel was received by me with its beauti-

ful inscription. Confidentially, I don't like, too much, the colors on the cover. And for why were they trying to hide your name?

Nevertheless, your leap into American letters comes as no surprise to me. From the time you were a little boy I helped you grow, encouraged you and now the fruits of our labors have been realized. My son the writer! And I, a humble paperhanger, a celebrity in my own right. I did not have any chance in my life to achieve in the arts, so you will realize for me, all my dreams.

Every night now we have over to our humble apartment, friends, filled with good wishes. "How will Gideon react when he is famous and wealthy?" Some would like to believe that Gideon will become like all other celebrities, go live in luxury, forget the little man and soon his writing will decline in quality and he will adapt his writings to the taste of the less literary minded. But *we the majority* categorically defeated that school of thought. *We* the majority are convinced that fame and riches will never degenerate Gideon, because Gideon Zadok the writer is bigger in heart and mind than money and the gilded objects, that Gideon Zadok the writer and human being will never forget the people he came from.

My wife, Lena, your stepmother, who loves you as her own son, says she is afraid she will have to buy a ticket and stand in line to see you and that her borsht and knishes will not be good enough for you to eat. So son, you should reassure her by return letter and tell her you plan to come with the family immediately to Philadelphia and put her, and everyone else's fears to rest. You still like borsht and knishes? No? And also, son, you should always mention her in your letters as she is sensitive. Say something personal and nice. Lena says we should have made a child together so we could have a genius of our own.

And what do you have against Philadelphia? Why are you avoiding?

You will forgive in advance a few observations and advice from me. Although the circumstances of life kept me from being a writer, I am still considered an educated and literate man. So, thank you and think over carefully, namely:

Stay away from red baiting.

Try to make your next book more profound, with deeper thinking and more meaningful characters. Your plans to write a book about fighters and prostitutes frankly doesn't sit too well with me.

You should be thinking more in terms of Jewish themes and themes of the struggles of the working class.

Don't make so much dirty dialogue. It is untasteful.

I have many, many, many more criticisms of which I will advise you in my forthcoming letters, for only through criticism will you grow.

You will have thousands of fans in Philadelphia. I wish you wouldn't snub so much this town. Perhaps you will even consider moving to Philadelphia as it is more of a literary and cultural center than so-called San Francisco and God forbid you stay in Los Angeles, a notorious center of anti-Semitism.

I have given your address to a number of relatives now desirous of making your personal acquaintance, although many of them snubbed me for years. I hold no grudges. You are now my personal representative.

And now, to a serious subject. There is a feeling among intellectuals that once a writer makes his debut in Hollywood, his literary abilities, his ambition to write important subjects becomes negligible, that he is degraded, that he gives up his talent, his name, for what? Money? Glamour? And soon his name is forgotten once the glitter of gold and diamonds is before his eyes. Of course, Hollywood has the genius to produce good artistic and educational pictures, but the ignorant masses instead prefer sexy *shmattes*.

And lastly, being in Hollywood doesn't mean you must not write to me every week. And now that Valerie is a woman of leisure, she should also write more regularly. It is the fourth commandment that she should write. She believes in the ten commandments, doesn't she?

Your loving father,

Nathan

P.S. My love also to the girls. I hope they don't become corrupted by the glitter of Hollywood. Otherwise I and Lena are fine, with the usual aches and pains of old age.

Before I left to do the screenplay in Pacific Studios, I wanted the comfort of knowing I would return to writing my second novel. I sent an outline and the first two chapters of *The Tenderloin* to J. Bascomb III and asked for a contract. I found out that J. III didn't trust his own judgment. He edited by round table and his reply consisted of the reports of five editors . . .

"A one-shot novelist."

"We'd be better off letting our option lapse."

"A sad commentary from someone starting so promising a career."

"Zadok is obviously turning into a junk writer."

"He'll never be heard from again."

J. III wrote that despite these reports, he would publish *The Tenderloin* anyhow, when it was finished, because anything of mine would do fairly well after my first novel.

This was a pretty crude way for an editor-in-chief to behave, but he wanted to put me down for "going Hollywood" and he also wanted to be certain I only got a minimum contract.

I phoned for a week. He was either out to lunch or in conference or otherwise engaged, so I wrote him that I wanted out of Reaves Brothers, in my best Marine language.

Val was outraged. "They'll know about your letter all up and down Madison Avenue. Haven't we had enough trouble finding a publisher?"

"You're asking me to stay with those sons of bitches after what they think of my new work!"

God damn, there were some things that Val just didn't understand about me. Compromise, back down, keep quiet. God damn, Val! Don't you ever get mad at anyone but me?

I put out a call for a literary agent, not really knowing one from another. I can't say why I settled on F. Todd Wallace. He had a veddy/veddy uptown manner and represented some good authors. He reminded me of those jerks at the Algonquin Round Table, but he obviously was one of them and knew his way around the literary scene. And that name, F. Todd Wallace—INTEGRITY, like the Rock of Gibraltar.

"Can't go wrong with old Todd."

As time unfolded I might as well have been represented by the Mother Superior at a Carmelite nunnery. Anyhow, I'd never have to deal with J. III or that bloody house again.

I left ahead of Val and the girls, to get set up at the studio and find a place for us to live. It was on a sour note. Things I always believed that Val would understand automatically—she didn't understand at all.

Hollywood, 1954–1956

THE ACTUAL FILM DEAL on *Of Men in Battle* had been made by my Hollywood literary agent, Sal Sensibar.

From our first meeting, I realized Sal was a back stabber who might well have been in the white slave traffic if he hadn't been a literary agent. Sal had terminal cases of diarrhea of the mouth and megalomania. Nevertheless, I liked him. We came from the same side of the tracks, way back when. As long as I remained a marketable writer, Sal Sensibar would always find work for me. He liked *things*, lots of *things*, *things* with big engines, *things* that sparkled, furry *things* to drape on his tawdry wife and tawdry girlfriends, huge *things* to swim in.

When Sal dined me at Chasen's and Scandia, back to back, I knew I was the bright new boy in town. The restaurant prices automatically signaled the value of the writer. Advice was doled out in huge globs. Some of it was even worth listening to.

Sal gave it to me straight. The studios usually pacified the author with four to six weeks' work as a little icing on the cake in order to get his general ideas, nothing more. Few producers were ever serious about letting a novelist complete his own screenplay.

"Remember, Gideon, what you have written is preserved forever between the covers of a book."

"Sal, I'm going to do this screenplay."

"I'm not saying you're not," he said, "but you got to bear in mind a studio might buy a book for any number of reasons—as a star vehicle, because a director likes it, for its title value, or just as a rough outline for a film. They own it. You sold the rights to them. They're not obliged to make a faithful rendition."

"Why are you telling me this?"

"I like you, Gideon. Get through this alive and we'll both make a lot of money together. But don't go in there with any *farcockta* ideas of grandeur."

THE FIRST DAY at Pacific was awesome! I had passed through the gates of a place of glamour and power second only to the White House. I was assigned to an old-time staff producer, Kurt von Dortann, who had come over during the Lubitsch era when monocled Germans were all the rage.

Von Dortann had some great early successes. In a weak moment, after a big hit, the studio chief, Stanley Gold, gave him an ironclad ten-year contract worth millions, in order to keep him at Pacific.

When von Dortann started to bomb with one picture after another, Gold tried every which way to get rid of him. Von Dortann hung in there through public insults, humiliations, and degradations. Gold did everything but kick his shins and slap his face. Von Dortann would merely smile and bow crisply and pick up his paycheck.

What I met was a rag of a man, completely broken, in a haze of memories. Von Dortann still ripped around in a Porsche, but his old Spanish-style estate in Tarzana was like a haunted house, where he would get into his cups every night and bemoan the wife and daughter who had abandoned him. On weekends the place looked like a hookers' convention.

At our first meeting von Dortann confirmed Sal's warning that I was there for a long walk off a short pier.

"No hurry. Don't rush," he assured me. "Just write a treatment of what you think should go from the book into the film. An outline. Forget about the screenplay."

Bullshit, little Eva. *I was ready.* Not that I was planning a Hollywood career, but after a lifetime in cheap sneakers the money, the office, the secretary, the new car, the power, the beautiful little home I was able to lease were like a stroll on the glory road.

You know what the hell it's like taking your wife into a dress shop on Rodeo Drive and peeling off eighty dollars, cold cash, and not feel like you've been hit in the stomach? And not have to say for the first time in your life, "How much is this going to cost?"

I knew all about this place being a writers' graveyard when I came. But dammit, as a poor boy, I wouldn't have been human if I didn't think I'd died and gone to heaven.

So, from day one, excuse me for repeating, *I was ready.*

"Can I get a film run for me?" I asked von Dortann.

"Surely."

"I'd like to see *High Noon* and I want the final script as well."

High Noon, for me, was the ultimate motion picture. It had a perfect, miraculous blend of script, acting, direction, music, art, sound, every element of film. As I watched the picture, I read the script simultaneously. Every few minutes I'd signal for the projectionist to stop and I'd dictate to my secretary the type of shot, what the camera was doing, how the film was scored and cut, sound effects, stunts. I broke it down almost frame by frame.

That was my entire schooling on film writing.

I knocked off a two-page treatment in twenty minutes and then went immediately into a first-draft screenplay. Von Dortann didn't ask to see pages for the four weeks of my employment contract. When he did, I handed him a two-hundred-and-fifty-page screenplay. He gaped in disbelief.

Most of the other writers dragged ass to prolong their weekly salaries. They hated my guts. Tough shit, gentlemen; you sink, I swim. In the history of Pacific Studios they had never seen a novel of this size and scope turned into a screenplay so fast.

The golden moment arrived! I was summoned to the office of the head of the studio and its founder, the almighty Colonel Stanley Gold. My secretary cleaned some spots off my shirt and borrowed a necktie and jacket for me.

The opulence of Gold's office was staggering. The array of "yes" men seemed like something out of a really bad movie. Gold had earned his rank during the war when patriotic fever swept the town.

"Find out what rank they gave Zanuck and Jack Warner."

Thus, Colonel Gold.

"Hell of a piece of work, Zadok. We'd like you to carry on with a second-draft screenplay."

Bingo! I was counting the money. Val! We're rich!

"Cut this thing down to two pounds," Gold continued, pointing to the screenplay. On cue laughter broke out, led by von Dortann.

Stanley Gold was in a folksy mood, retelling a story to me about how his family ran a butcher shop in Chicago and how they cheated their "colored" customers by putting their thumb on the scale when they weighed the meat. More laughter.

He cleared his throat and the entourage leaped to its collective feet. The audience with his eminence was over.

"It's been a real pleasure meeting you, Colonel," I said, "but the next time you buy one of my books, keep your fucking thumb off the scale."

Everyone turned a pale shade of green in unison, while the Colonel mulled that one over. He finally decided it was funny and burst into laughter, at which time the ten others present also burst into laughter.

I HAD A strange, wild, and unique situation working for me at Pacific. For a number of years after the war, many military films had been uncomplimentary to the services. *From Here to Eternity*, *The Caine Mutiny*, and a number of others stuck in the craw of the Defense Department. It all came to a boil when Metro did a picture called *Take the High Ground*. The Defense Department found it too anti-Army and stopped all further cooperation with the studios.

Unless the Army, Navy, Marines, and Air Force provided masses of men, guns, tanks, ships, planes, and equipment, the cost of the big war film was too much for the studios to bear.

Thus far Pacific Studios had been clean and everyone was keeping an eye on *Of Men in Battle.* I was sent back to Washington to go over the script with the Marine Corps and take out the objectionable parts.

The Corps didn't find a hell of a lot wrong. At the end of an easy week, I was ushered into the commandant's office. It was down to PFC Zadok and a four-star general.

"My first duty is to the Corps, sir," I told him. "If the studio gets out of line, I'll let you know immediately."

The Marines had benefited greatly from the novel. I was one of theirs and they trusted me. I returned to Pacific with a golden club to hold over the Colonel's head.

At one point the studio tried to deviate from my screenplay by secretly putting on another writer. I walked out of the studio, leaving a two-word letter on my desk; namely, "I quit." The next day I was implored to return. The Corps had expressed its displeasure.

"We feel that it is in everyone's best interest to keep Zadok on through the filming."

What the hell. The Corps was allowing Pacific to have eight cameras film their maneuvers and landing on Vieques Island in the Caribbean.

Colonel Gold got the message. I don't know whether von Dortann had hired another writer on his own volition or on orders from the studio. I do know he was removed from the film and I suddenly functioned as a part-time producer, in on everything from casting to the final cut. That's the way it goes in this town. When you fly, you fly.

While the picture was being filmed, the studio pulled out several shelved screenplays for me to putter around with. Two dead projects were revived and one of them made it to the cameras and gained me a reputation as a script doctor.

Then came my ultimate coup. I was working late in one of the cutting rooms with the Colonel and we both got blasted and I conned him into a world premiere in my hometown, Baltimore.

"You're the God-damnedest hustler I've ever seen, Zadok."

"I take that as a compliment, Colonel. Baltimore is going to love you."

"I've got nothing against a hustler, as long as he's doing it on my behalf," he said.

I was kept on as a script doctor until the film was released. *Of Men in Battle* went on to become one of a half-dozen great films of World War II and made a bundle for the studio.

As my time was running out I began thinking hard about my next novel. How do I break loose from Val to do my research? Or, was I really using Val as a crutch for my own indecision?

Then came a famous "summons" to Colonel Gold's office. This could cause mere writers to shake, rattle, and roll. What was more, Sal Sensibar had been "summoned" as well. Gold had set the stage for something big.

"I like you, Zadok!" he said after wearing us out with a couple of his cornball jokes. "I like you big!" Sensibar began levitating right there in the office.

The Colonel then offered me a three-year writer/producer contract starting at two thousand dollars a week and ending at four thousand. Jaysus! Jaysus! Valhalla! He had made damned sure Sal was present, in case I had any ideas of rejecting his offer.

Sal retreated, groveling out backward, which was no easy trick.

"You've got me, Zadok," Gold said as a parting shot. "See, I took my thumb off the scale."

Does all this shit sound like dream stuff? Well, I left all the rotten parts on the cutting-room floor. I was a fool to think I was going to be the first golden boy who drifted into town, made a killing, and drifted out without getting my hands bloody. My thirtieth birthday was coming up and I had a lot to think over.

AS WE LEFT the Colonel's office, Sal Sensibar was breathing orgasmically. By the time we reached the parking lot he was having hot flashes, groaning, and his eyes were wild like he'd just seen the glory of the coming of the Lord.

"Romanoff's tonight," Sal said, "eight-thirty." Sal was a toucher, a knee slapper. He gazed into my eyes with all the pathos of a pleading German shepherd and pinched my cheek. *"Bubele,"* he said. That's all he could say, *"Bubele, bubele."* Sal had a stable of over twenty writers, most of them working. I had just replaced the reigning king.

As Sal reached his car, he was hit with a sudden gas attack and doused the fire with an antacid. "Romanoff's, eight-thirty, and don't be late, *bubele,* we've some heavy celebrating to do. Tonight with the wives. Tomorrow, who knows?"

"Aren't you celebrating a little early, Sal?"

"No jokes, no fucking jokes, Gideon."

"I didn't tell Gold I was taking his offer."

Sal's face expressed pain, deep, terrible pain. "Don't make with the jokes."

"Why don't we skip Romanoff's. Let's have lunch tomorrow and we'll talk about it. Calm down, Sal, you look like you've just been liberated from Auschwitz."

Sweat broke out simultaneously on Sal's shirt front, his face, and his armpits. He fished around his jacket pocket for his date book.

"Lunch. How about breakfast? Why not let's talk it over at your house tonight? Why wait for tonight, how about now?"

"See you tomorrow for lunch," I said. "Frascati's, Beverly Hills, okay? One o'clock."

Sal was having a difficult time getting the key into his Jaguar door. I turned and without further word headed back to my office.

"Don't you even want to . . ."

"See you tomorrow."

The writers' building at Pacific was set up so that it could be observed from all directions by the studio police. The only thing missing was guard towers. The Colonel had a number of petty obsessions. One of them was to keep his writers penned in. A few writers around town were beginning to work at home. I planned to make a stand on it, if and when I did another screenplay.

My secretary Belle Prentice was on pins and needles waiting for me to return from my meeting with Gold. A summons from Gold's office was a chilling thing. I stopped at her desk in the outer office.

"Any calls, anything?"

I shuffled through the notes. One from a young lady who wanted me to have dinner with her. She would be the dinner. Another from a tennis partner, Johnny Brookes. Another from a visiting relative who wanted a tour through a studio.

"Call them back. Tell them I've gone for the day."

Belle trailed me into my office. I flopped on the couch. "Will you tell me what happened?" she demanded.

"The Colonel wants me to remain at the studio. A three-year writer/producer deal."

"Congratulations!"

"I told him I'd think it over."

Belle's face saddened. "You've already made your mind up, haven't you?"

"Six months ago. I'll get my crap out of here tomorrow. Do you want me to put in a word for you with anyone in particular?"

"No, I'll just go back to the secretarial pool and take my chances."

"I'm sorry, Belle. You've been real thunder and lightning."

She shed a few tears. We'd had a heavy year together. She'd covered for me a dozen times and even marched into von Dortann's office and chewed him out on my behalf.

She closed the door behind her and returned to her office. I gave a sentimental look around the room. The office had once been occupied by William Faulkner on one of the thousand and one studio projects that never got off the ground. Belle had been his secretary. She used to siphon him out of the gutter, blind drunk. He apparently needed the money.

This wasn't a difficult decision for me. All I had to do was spend an evening with Kurt von Dortann to see what I'd become in three years. What I didn't want to face was the coming shoot-out at home, tonight.

Val and I were having a lot of heavy arguments. A half-dozen times, when I was waging trench warfare at the studio, Val had disappointed me. She blew up at me for refusing to sign the loyalty oath. She could not bring herself to understand that it was an affront to me after having served in the Marine Corps. Later, the oath was judged unconstitutional. It didn't matter—I was still wrong in her eyes.

Val had turned on me when I walked out of the studio after von Dortann put on a writer behind my back. Hell, I was back at work two days later. I was the bad guy for not cooperating with the studio. It was my fault for standing up to Gold.

Val didn't want me to fight about anything that would endanger my jobs with the studios. It hurts to say it, but she was an out-and-out appeaser. Val was happy down there, sterilized by the good life. "Don't Rock the Boat" might as well have been done in petit point and hung over the fireplace.

I didn't want to commit to writing a full-time screenplay until I completed my second novel, so I took short doctoring jobs. There comes a moment in the life of every screenplay when the writer has to take a stand or give away a piece of his soul. When you're dealing with the swollen egos of actors, actresses, and directors, you've got to try to remember that they are the boss—even though they can't read a script, even though their arguments are moronic. They're the boss. When the inevitable showdown came, Val raised purple hell with me for playing it tough.

She really was livid when I turned down a project, a flat-fee screenplay for Columbia for fifty thousand dollars. The project was a piece of trash. Not one bloody word of understanding from her.

I don't know what it was with Val. I'd never seen this in her before. Maybe it was because she had been raised in the Navy where you obey orders and don't make problems.

"What's the difference, Gideon," she argued. "Nobody remembers the name of the screenwriter. You recall what Sal told you the first day. What you've written is between covers of a book and can't be changed. I know screenwriting runs against your grain, but you get paid a hell of a lot for your discomfort."

A lot of nights I drove out to the Holiday House past Malibu when I'd had a fight at the studio. I'd walk over to Paradise Cove, rent fishing gear, and fish from the pier. I was just too damned beat to go home and have her blast at me. Well, you know what follows. I started taking women out to the Holiday House. Lots of them.

What troubled me about the other women was that I felt less and less guilty about it after each brawl with Val.

After Sal drove off, I returned to my office. I dialed home a half-dozen times. The line was busy. Obviously Sal had headed for the first pay phone. That son of a bitch had gotten to Val first. He was chewing her ear off.

Belle came in with tea. I remained on the couch and she took my chair behind the desk and kept dialing my home.

"Still busy."

"You liked Faulkner an awful lot, didn't you?"

Belle smiled. "Secretly, I suppose I loved him. He was a great man, very genteel and soft-spoken. Yes ma'am, Miss Belle, no ma'am, Miss Belle. He always called me Miss Belle."

"How was he able to take Stanley Gold?"

"I sat in to take notes on quite a few story conferences. It became apparent early on that Mr. Faulkner's project would never get off the ground. But Gold kept him on, much like a pet dog. I think the Colonel got off on the very notion that he had control over the mind of a great writer like Mr. Faulkner. He loved to berate Mr. Faulkner, the same as he does von Dortann. The same as he does with anyone who's afraid of him. Mr. Faulkner would go to pieces. He was always at one of three or four bars along Ventura Boulevard. George and I would find him, take him to his apartment, and sometimes we'd have to put him to bed."

"The resolution of fear is one of the writer's greatest reasons for being," I said.

Belle smiled again. "That's from his Nobel acceptance speech."

She answered the phone and covered the mouthpiece. "It's Stanley Gold."

"Hello, Colonel," I said.

"Zadok. I was thinking that it might be time to pop some bubbly. I'd

love to give a little dinner party for you over at my place. How about
Friday?"
"Sorry, I can't. One of my daughters is in a play at school. You know
how that one goes."
There was a long, expected silence. Gold was stashing this rebuff in
his memory book. "Another time," he said, "you'll be around."
I tried home again. The line was still busy.

I PULLED OUT of the studio gate and flicked on the radio, girding
myself for the traffic.

EXTERIOR VENTURA BOULEVARD   DAY

After ESTABLISHING SHOT of the bumper to bumper traffic,
CAMERA zooms in to

CLOSE SHOT of WRITER at the wheel of his TR-3 convertible,
top down. His jacket is on seat beside him. He fishes for, finds, and
lights cigarette and snaps on radio as he inches along in traffic.

FIRST RADIO VOICE (OVER SCENE)
And now for Ernie, Maxine, Dave and all the gang at Mario's the
king . . . Elvis sings "Love Me Tender" . . .

WRITER turns dial

SECOND RADIO VOICE O.S.
The situation at Central High School in Little Rock has worsened.
According to White House sources, President Eisenhower is con-
sidering sending troops . . .

WRITER flips dial again, grunts impatiently at the traffic.

THIRD RADIO VOICE O.S.
Davy! Davy Crockett
King of the wild frontier . . .

ANGLE WIDENS as a chorus of horns sounds in frustration.
WRITER drives off and we

DISSOLVE TO:

EXTERIOR   LOVELY RANCH HOUSE   EVENING

Grounds show some affluence. WRITER pulls into driveway, parks, gets out of car. He is besieged by two young GIRLS wearing Davy Crockett coonskin caps and shooting toy guns. Family dog joins in. WRITER "falls dead" and is pounced upon by daughters. He gets up, throws ball for dog. The three walk to

INTERIOR   LOVELY LIVING ROOM   NIGHT

WIFE is glum. She approaches WRITER obliquely.

WIFE
Sal called. He told me all about your meeting with the Colonel.
(no response)
Well, what are you going to tell him?

WRITER
I told him I'd think it over.

WIFE
Two thousand dollars a week going up to four thousand. A producership by the time you're thirty. What's to think over?

WRITER
(dreads this moment)
I can't be a producer, Val. I'm not cut out for these studio gang bangs. Too much politics. Too much back stabbing. Too many people to deal with. Look, baby, one of the reasons I became a novelist was so that I could work alone. Writing to me is freedom. Freedom!

WIFE
You're a very selfish man, Gideon.

WRITER
I know that.

FADE OUT

Dinner was perky with the girls. Lots of happy things were going on for them. I helped with their homework and after their bath we had a short punch-up and pillow fight.

"Just one half hour of TV and that's it," I said.

They accepted reluctantly.

"I wish we didn't have one of those idiot boxes in the house."

"They've been looking forward to this program all week. So, why make a fuss, every single week?"

The volcano was rumbling within. I went into the living room and took a crack at reading a magazine. Val came in. She was glum. She paced and looked at me, sort of out of the corner of her eye.

"Sal called," she said. "He told me all about your meeting with the Colonel."

I didn't answer her.

"Well, what are you going to tell him?"

"I told him I'd think it over."

"Two thousand dollars a week going up to four thousand. A producership by the time you're thirty. What's to think over?"

I dreaded this moment. "I can't be a producer, Val. I'm not cut out for these studio gang bangs. Too much politics. Too much back stabbing. Too many people to deal with. Look, baby, one of the reasons I became a novelist was so that I could work alone. Writing, to me, is freedom. Freedom!"

"You're a very selfish man, Gideon."

"I know that. Being selfish is one of my job requirements. But I'm not going to be a producer for Stanley Gold, period, paragraph, end of report. There's a few more things we'd better get cleaned up, right now."

"Look at you. You're begging for a fight. Nobody can talk to you when you're in this kind of mood."

"Every time we have something to talk over, you start out by saying nobody can talk to me. Well, a lot of things have piled up. We'd better sort them out."

Val became more and more defensive when there was something to thrash out. Delay it, stuff it in the closet, do anything but face up and get it over with. Half of our life was the unspoken words. I'd get angry and stomp out and when I returned Val would pretend that absolutely nothing had happened.

"I'm going to my office," I said. "If you feel like talking, come on over. Incidentally, I'm going to cut out for a few days for San Francisco. I need to hang out, see some of the guys."

"I can't stop you."

THE OPENING SALVOS had been fired. The silent period now ruled the scene. The ice age was setting in. My office was a little guest cottage on the other side of the pool. I rehearsed my arguments just as I was certain Val was rehearsing hers. The only problem was that neither of us followed the script. She didn't give the answers I expected. Our mouths were set on automatic. Usually within two minutes we'd both blown off course, and sometimes we even forgot what we were fighting about.

I poked about the office. I couldn't concentrate on reading. No use phoning around. Didn't want to answer my mail. Letter from my old man. Better not read it now. Nothing on the tube. I stretched on the couch and continued to present my bulletproof case to the "jury."

One of the unwritten rules was that Val had to give in first and come to me. A couple of times I caved in and went to her first. No way, this time.

At around two in the morning, I could hear the shuffle of her steps. I drew the blanket over me and feigned sleep. A knock, the door opened, and a small light was turned on.

"Honey," she peeped softly.

I grunted as though coming out of a deep slumber. I sat up, stretched, yawned, looked over my surroundings, and "remembered" where I was. Val slipped into the easy chair as I dunked my face and wiped it.

"We'd better start from square one," I said. "When J. III and Reaves accepted *Of Men in Battle,* the only plans we made regarding the future were a few vague mentions of trying to find a nicer place in Sausalito. Soon as the screenplay was done, we'd go back up there and I'd keep writing books."

"Things have changed, Gideon. You've opened up a second career in the studios. We have other options in life now."

"Val, I've got to decide what I want to be when I grow up. I can't be a producer. I'd murder half of the actors and directors I know. Point two. This town is stacked against the writers. What we've gotten into is an endless war to try to retain normalcy in an abnormal town. You haven't mentioned my next novel for months. San Francisco isn't even in your vocabulary anymore. Inch by inch I'm being sucked in, down here."

"For the first eighteen years of my life, I was a Navy brat. We lived on twelve different bases. And for the first eight years of our marriage, we lived a nightmare. We're happy here. I want a home," she said.

"So do I. But it's got to be outside of this magnetic field. I don't know if I can produce books in this atmosphere. This problem is going to come up again and again."

"Suppose you want to write a novel on India the next time, or Alaska?"

"What are you telling me, Val? No more novels? What else is buzzing around in your head?"

She was frightened and didn't want to say what was on the edge of her tongue.

"What else, Val?" I demanded.

"Suppose your next book flops. I don't relish returning to poverty. You have to stay near the studios."

That was blunt enough. I owed my family a living and a home and I had no business dragging them around the world.

"School vacation starts next month. You and the girls come up to San Francisco with me for three months. I'll finish my research and come back here and write the book. We'll decide what to do afterward."

"I'm not going up there with you to be a writer's nurse and whore. I've enrolled in art school."

She unloaded the heavy artillery on me. Subtle but rich with innuendo. What she was saying, silently, was that I had ruined her promising career as an artist. She had made all the big sacrifices for me and now it was my turn.

Val understood one thing. She knew I had a dreadful fear of loneliness. I'd go to pieces if I had to eat a meal alone in a restaurant. If I was in a hotel out of town, I never took my finger out of the telephone dial. I couldn't hack it alone in San Francisco.

"Christ sake, there are art schools in San Francisco!"

"Neither Penny, Roxy, nor I want to be around with your hookers and pimps."

"But that's the book I'm writing! Val, I'm not buying this. For ten years you've complained about the magnificent career you lost on account of me. You're using this fantasy career to lie to yourself. You want to hear it? You don't have the talent or the balls to make it. If you needed it like I need to write, you would have done it ten years ago. Dammit, all it is is a lie to keep a weapon over my head."

WELL, I DIDN'T GO to San Francisco to finish my research. Val knew I wouldn't. Of course, she never set foot in art school either.

So, I wrote *The Tenderloin* in my pleasant little cottage in four frantic months. I really needed double that time, but Sal kept pressure on me and Val had established a fat lifestyle.

When the book was finished, Val found a lovely home on three acres in Woodland Hills that had every yummy thing that any girl would want, forever and ever. Stable, pool, tennis court, big oaks, the works. I'd need a screenplay right away.

Several months later, *The Tenderloin* was published. Do you want the long version or the short version? It bombed. Of all the hurts inflicted on me, none was more devastating than what one reviewer wrote: "Zadok must have written the novel in an orange grove. He certainly didn't go anywhere near the tenderloin."

The Tenderloin was a flat, glossy, imitation Runyon, a superficial exercise for me to zip through and then get back to what was really important in life, making money.

If. If . . . if . . . IF! IF I had taken the three months and gone up to San Francisco, I would have captured the unique lilt and toughness of the place. IF the rabbit hadn't stopped to take a crap he would have caught the turtle. Val and I didn't talk much about *The Tenderloin*. We didn't have to.

A man can lie to his boss, his wife, his children, but he can't lie to the typewriter. Sooner or later truths will emerge. The truth was that I was writing about people who were suffering, but I never felt their pain and the readers saw right through me. It's hard to feel your stomach growl with hunger on two thousand dollars a week. Want to play the novel game? You've got to bare it all.

I was going to dwell in shit city forever. I envisioned the yellow brick road stretched out before me. Producership, maybe with Stanley Gold. Television series, bundles of money involved. Take any ridiculous idea and embellish it with canned laughter. Crap is selling these days like never before.

When I had wept before God begging Him to spare Penny's life, didn't I also swear I'd be a writer He would be proud of? Golden handcuffs. Mink-lined cells. God almighty, Val bought me shirts with my initials on the pockets. My asthma was returning. I hadn't had an attack in fifteen years. Maybe I've got to see a shrink. Fire a shot on Bedford Drive and you'll hit fifty of them.

It had become apparent that with all my bluster, I didn't really have what it takes. I couldn't stomach the sacrifice anymore and I blamed it on Val or Sal or Mal or Gold. Everyone but myself. All right! I haven't got it! Leave me in peace! I HAVEN'T GOT IT!

"HELLO, Zadok speaking."

"Gideon, you old mother. How you been?"

"Junkyard?"

"That's what they call me."

"Oh, buddy, you're a voice for the weary. Where are you?"

"I've got a cottage at the Beverly Hills. I'm on the way to Hong Kong on a business trip. I was hoping you'd be in town."

My spirits lifted. Sergeant Kelly Murphy had been an old Marine buddy. We called him Junkyard because he'd collect the oddest pieces of worthless trash and somehow always get rid of it for a profit. A regular rug merchant.

Along with running his oriental bazaar, Murphy was a hell of a gambler, one of the best crap shooters I'd ever seen. He left the Corps with a sizable bankroll.

Junkyard had done a hitch in the Corps before the war, which included service in the Caribbean. He swore he was going to return there after the war, and he did, in spades. Starting with one small boat, he scoured the Caribbean for war surplus and ended up with a small fleet of tramp steamers and a couple of airplanes. We always stayed in touch, even before my first book was published.

Penny and Roxy adored him, partly because of his extravagant presents. Valerie tolerated him because she'd grown up with so many colorful characters in the Navy. On the other hand, she detested him because when he blew into town I was always bound to go out on a real twister for a few days.

We started out at Tail o' the Cock, and ended up at his cottage at the Beverly Hills, with numerous intermediate stops.

"You haven't drawn a happy breath since you've been down here but I've never seen you like this," Junkyard said.

"I saw six hundred that's six zero zero—screenwriters bow like sheep in the face of a loyalty oath. When I refused to sign, Colonel Gold recited to me, for the first time, those immortal words, 'You'll never work in this town again.' Son of a bitch hired me two weeks later to get a bungled script into order."

Junkyard unpeeled the top of a new vodka bottle. I was on the stuff, straight, now.

"And furthermore," I emoted, "I saw a casting call go out for dumb, big-titted redheads answered by five hundred big-titted redheads who went down on forty-two producers and a partridge in a pear tree."

I banged down some hors d'oeuvres and a shot.

"Speaking of big-titted redheads, the girls should be showing up pretty soon."

"Why don't you give them a call and tell them we'll catch up with them tomorrow night. I think you need to talk to your buddy," Junkyard said.

"I'm running off at the mouth. Better shut up."

"It's hidden down there pretty deep. It's got to find its way out of you, Gideon."

I dialed. "Hello, Brenda, Gideon. Sorry to break your heart, lover, but we're not going to be able to get together tonight. We'll take care of the tab. Hold tomorrow night open. You're a real doll."

I couldn't look Junkyard in the eyes. "Actors," I said. "Ever see a peacock spread its fan and shriek? Horrible sound. You whore writers aren't making me beautiful enough. And the broads come after your nuts with switchblade knives. I owe this Oscar to all the little people, the grips, the cameramen, the wardrobe mistress, but most of all to MY writers."

"You was always a big pain in the ass, Gideon. Always hustling. If it had been up to you, you would have turned the whole regiment into dancing boys and staged the biggest fucking review the world had ever seen."

"Let me tell you something. It's not normal, or human, or decent, to ask a man to write a novel. Three to five years in that God-damned darkness!"

"Then stop crying in your beer and be thankful for what you've got."

"Shit! Go to Hong Kong! I don't have to listen to your shit! You were always full of shit!"

"What's scaring you, son?"

Junkyard was a big strong man and when he grabbed you, you knew it. He took my shoulders and shook me.

"What's scaring you!"

I tore out of his arms and could feel my chest tightening up. I was going to have a goddam asthma attack! He came up behind me.

"We're coming into the beach! The Japs have opened fire! The ramp drops! What's scaring you? Is it the Jew business? Are you haunted by dreams about Pedro? You're the biggest man to come out of our regiment! We're proud when we can just touch you! Now what's scaring you?"

"Loneliness!" I screamed.

It grew very quiet. His eyes were filled with the kind of sorrow he had after the battle. I realized then, I meant something special to a lot of Marines. "God," he whispered.

"It's a terrible fear, so awful. I don't know how to whip it."

"Be a Marine," he said.

"Fuck all, I can't make it."

"You've got to get your ass out of this town and prove you can bear

your loneliness. Look at you, son. You're so unhappy you're going to
put a gun to your head."

"I don't know if I can, man."

"I've got a nice setup on St. Barthélemy. I want you to go down
there and get your shit together."

"I don't know, man, I don't know."

UNLIKE F. TODD WALLACE, Sal Sensibar could smell a deal in the
making from two continents away. He'd go through trash cans, listen
from stalls in the men's room, supply girls for a key lawyer at the studio.
Sal knew what was going on and he didn't learn it from reading *Variety*.

There was a particular producer in town I truly admired, Judd
Schlosberg. Who wouldn't? He had been a wonderchild, running a studio when he was twenty-seven. Later, he became one of the first inde-
pendent producers in Hollywood.

When you meet with a producer and he says, "I have the greatest
respect for the writer," you know the son of a bitch is lying. Judd
Schlosberg probably never uttered those words but he had worked successfully with Maxwell Anderson, Tennessee Williams, and John
Steinbeck. That was really what attracted me.

He usually left his writers alone and a goodly number of his scripts
were lush and translated to the screen with great care and taste. Schlosberg had four Oscars on a shelf behind his desk for best picture, plus the
Thalberg Award for lifetime achievement and the Hersholt Humanitar-
ian Award.

When Sal found out Schlosberg had purchased an obscure little story
about the great Texas gunfighter, John Hardin, from *Atlantic*, I told
him I wanted him to get me the job.

Judd Schlosberg was a short man, barely over five feet, with a kind of
angelic face. His office was a subtle showcase of his achievements, a holy
room topped off with a dozen Remington paintings and statues.

Judd Schlosberg had heard enough bullshit from the lips of glib writers to create landfill for a medium-sized city. I wasn't about to give him
his first snow job.

"You don't have any track record as a Western writer," he said.

"This story could be set on a ship, with a gang of tunnel workers,
with a football team. The whole world is one big cowboy story. There's
no mystery to a Western. I asked for a crack at this because I know
what you saw in the story and what you want out of it."

"What did I see in it?"

"You've got everyone in Hollywood riding in those sixteen saddles. Maybe the whole world."

He knew my perception and approach were exactly like his and gave me four weeks to do a treatment. I took no shortcuts. It was the best I could write. I needed this one so badly I found places my typewriter had never roamed.

Sal turned it in and the agonizing wait began. After two weeks, Sal called. "We've heard from Schlosberg's office. He wants to see us tomorrow at ten."

Heart in the throat time. "How do you read it, Sal?"

"I'm positive he wants to go into screenplay."

FROM THE TIME Junkyard had left for Hong Kong, I never spoke with Val about the gist of our evening. Nonetheless his words preyed on my mind, constantly. If I were to make one last shot at being a novelist I had to find the courage to overcome my dread of loneliness. I knew that there were a raft of other phobias I would have to conquer in order to become a complete novelist. It doesn't fall like manna from heaven.

I had made the decision that if Judd Schlosberg gave me the screenplay I would do it alone in St. Barthélemy. One of the cheapest commodities in the world is unfulfilled genius. All of us want to be known as a unique individual, the one who broke out of the pack. So, you offer yourself up as a sacrifice and what you're afraid of is losing and being thrown back into the pack. One question taunts you. Do you want to have, or do you want to be?

I realized now that I'd have to prove something all my life. I could never go a hundred yards without a barrier blocking my way.

I had run out of time in keeping my plans from Val. Tomorrow Schlosberg might give me the screenplay and I'd have to tell her.

We were at poolside. Val was fixing drinks. She had on high heels and a bikini. Still a dynamite-looking woman.

"Cheers," she said with a kiss. "So, tomorrow's the big day. Why don't we go to New York or Vegas for a long weekend and shoot out the lights?"

My expression must have been grim. She reacted with apprehensive curiosity. "You certainly don't look like the man who has just snared the brass ring."

"Val, I've decided to write the screenplay away from the house."

"If you want to work at the studio, that's okay with me. I'm going to miss having you around."

"I mean I want to go off and write it."

"Holy mackerel, Amos, this is a little sudden."

"For you, not for me. I've been stewing over it for weeks."

"Good Lord, Gideon, you can't do a thing for yourself. You're helpless."

"I know. A lot of things have piled up. The closet needs a cleaning out."

She was getting my drift that I wasn't going to change my mind. She shrugged and loosened my leash a bit, but still held firmly. "So, write in Malibu. I can spend most nights with you and we can have the girls on the weekend. Say, it might be fun, after all."

"Val, I'm going to the Caribbean. Alone."

I don't think she ever expected to hear me say anything like that. Val always had the trump card, my fear of loneliness. When backed into a corner, she never hesitated to use it. It had never failed to work.

"I realize we all need space but being a writer doesn't give you license to abandon your family and home. God, you make me feel I've driven you out. It's that damned book, *The Tenderloin.*"

"It's not you, not the girls, not the studios, not Los Angeles. It's me. Gideon Zadok is treading water. I thought we had given up so much to do the first book, the rest of the way would be covered with rose petals."

"That bastard Murphy put you up to this."

"Nobody put me up to anything. I cried for mercy. I'm lost, Val. Murphy understood. Becoming a true novelist means that I've got to be prepared to give up much more than I've given up till now. I have to do what is necessary to become a writer again who can look at his face in the mirror without cringing. As for now, Val, I'm going wherever my work takes me. If you and the girls can come, wonderful. If I have to go it alone, that's what I'm going to do."

She must have been numbed. I could hardly believe these words were coming from my mouth.

"I may fall flat on my face. I may not have the stuff. But I'm not going out without protest. I'm going to write another book, baby, and I'm going to give it everything I've got."

We were consumed by deadly, black silence.

"You're cruel! You're rotten! You selfish son of a bitch."

She hadn't heard a bloody word! She felt nothing I was pleading for! Val flung her glass. It skidded over the patio. Glad it was plastic. She stood over me heaving her chest and locking her teeth.

"Why don't you enroll in art school?" I said with all the meanness I could muster.

"What about me!" she cried.

"What about me?" I asked.

ALPACA SWEATERS with muttonchop sleeves were the costume of the moment. Schlosberg wore a tan alpaca, Sal a blaring red, and I had on a white one to indicate chastity, modesty, and virtue.

Schlosberg lit a cigar that seemed half his size and he hung on my every word. We seemed to be of a single mind as to where we were taking the story but something was annoying him. I smelled that he had not totally made up his mind. "Up front?" he asked when I had finished.

Oh God, here it comes, the goodbye kiss.

"Of course," I said.

"I like some of your work, Zadok. I like most of what you said here today. Now, I've always treated my writers as adults, until they prove otherwise. I was the first producer in Hollywood to permit writers to work at home. If home be Santa Barbara or New York. I've even let a couple of the Englishmen work in London. As long as we can stay in communication. But Sal tells me you want to write this in . . . uh . ."

"St. Barthélemy."

"Why?"

"Up front? The house of Zadok is tottering. But mainly, I believe it's going to make the script better."

"Are you fucking me over, Zadok? Why is it going to make the script better?"

"I want to create an atmosphere where I can achieve total, absolute concentration. This is going to be a great script."

"Nine out of ten scripts bomb. Who do you think you are?"

We had worked out a flat deal. I would write a screenplay for fifty thousand dollars and I would be paid—good, bad, or mediocre. Okay, *bubele*, this is your big moment, I thought to myself.

"Give me a month to see if I'm doing the story right, or if I'm whacking off on the beach. If you don't get my pages on time or if you don't like them, the deal is off. You don't owe me a dime."

I thought Sal would swallow his cigar.

"You're serious, aren't you, Zadok? Why are you putting yourself through this?"

"Hard for me to put it into words."

"I haven't noticed any overpowering shyness from you."

I shook my head. "You've heard too much shit in this office from too many shit merchants."

"Why, Zadok?"

"When I die, I want one word on my tombstone beside my name: author. I'm not as gifted as a lot of novelists. But I'm not picking soft spots for myself. I'm in a fight to find out if I have the balls and the discipline."

"Well, I hope you win because if you don't, it's going to kill you."

"At least I'll die with a shit-eating grin on my face."

"Good luck, Gideon, I mean that."

I stopped in the outer office to phone Val.

"Hello."

"Hi, baby, we're in screenplay," I said.

She hung up on me.

I MONKEYED AROUND town most of the day, dreading another brawl at home. It was evening when I turned into the driveway. I sensed something was very wrong. Usually our golden retriever hung out by the main gate waiting for me. No Grover Vandover. I opened the front door and called in. No Val, no maid, no girls. I was startled! What's going on here? Thoughts of a robbery or that maybe one of the girls had been hurt ran through my mind.

"Val! Penny! Roxy!"

I heard Grover whimper and made for Roxanne's room. Her dresser drawers were open and half cleaned out as though she had been evacuated in a hurry. Penny's room was the same. Jesus! What's going on! No note on the kitchen board. Knock off this shit, Val!

I saw Val's car in the carport. Did an ambulance come? What the hell? Wait a minute. Val might still be here. I flung open our bedroom door. There it was!

Pinned onto the pillow with a rose lying across it. My special little address book. It must have had fifty to a hundred names of girlfriends, hookers, escorts. There were even phone numbers for some of Val's best girlfriends, the divorced ones. I drew the line at other men's wives. I must have gotten sloppy careless and left it out.

I went outside and looked around. My office, maybe. I opened the door. It was an awful sight. Val had gone through it with a club or knives. Everything was smashed. My bookcases were overturned and the books all ripped up . . . my typewriter bashed to smithereens, the telephone jerked from the wall, my record collection scratched to uselessness, all the windows broken. The stuffing from my couch and armchair had been cut out with a knife . . . all my photographs knocked down and trampled, the curtains slashed.

That's it. The safe was opened. Val had found the combination and gotten the address book out of it. Manuscript papers were shredded and hurled all over the room. The pistol was gone! Wait! My chair filled with bullet holes, the empty gun on the floor.

Valerie stood in the doorway to the kitchenette. She tossed a big-bladed kitchen knife and a baseball bat to the ground and stood, frightfully calm.

My first reaction was one of relief that she hadn't hurt herself.

"Where are the girls?"

She didn't answer.

"Are they with your mother?"

"Yes," she said softly. "Get out. You can have one of your buddies come over and get your stuff."

"Okay."

Oh Lord, that woman was hurt. "Okay," I repeated.

"I had a long talk with some of your lady friends," she said with a twisted smile on her lips. "They said they'd put me down as an extra girl. If there's a big party I can go out and do a few tricks with them. Fifty bucks a pop, three hundred for an all-night party. You don't have any objections, do you?"

"I've been very unhappy, Val. But no matter what happened, you didn't deserve this."

"Does Phil Delaney know you're balling Joany? Did you fuck her in our bed? And sweet little Mary Allen. Prettiest little math teacher I ever did see. Fucking wholesale meat operation!"

"Val."

"Get out!"

"Okay, but there's one thing I want to know. You've known about this for a long, long time, Val. Why didn't you stop me?"

She put her hands in her face and sank to the floor. "Whores," she wept, "whores, whores, whores."

St. Barths, 1956

OKAY, BUSTER, you fought for it, you won it. You now have the
absolute right to go bust your ass on another novel. So, go get it. St.
Barthélemy? I didn't know the place existed or where it existed. The
ultimate romance of the novelist, self-imposed exile. Real Somerset
Maugham stuff.

My knowledge of the Caribbean was formed by Hollywood studios
when I was a kid. So many of our conceptions of life and places were
made on sound stages. Yo, ho, ho and a bottle of rum. Steamy jungles,
miserable black slaves sweating in the sugarcane fields, voodoo rites.
Devil's Island where no man escapes, except in a wooden box. Maureen
O'Hara, so magnificent, so voluptuous. Bruce Cabot—now there was a
villain for you. I'd duel my way, Errol Flynn style, through ten Basil
Rathbones to free my beloved from those driveling, one-eyed, hook-
handed scums.

A blissful haze enveloped me after I boarded the plane in L.A. I
usually became maudlin after a few drinks at eighteen thousand feet.
Val, I've hurt you so badly. I can't even comprehend the visions that
must have run through your mind on the hundred and one nights when
I was away from home.

Maybe I was predestined to go to St. Barthélemy to salvage something, to pay penance. Christ in the wilderness. Val . . . Val . . . I bit
my lip hard to hold back tears for the want of another chance to stroke
Penny's hair and read to her, or the kicks I got watching Roxanne
taking jumps on her pony.

"This is for you, Daddy. I made it in art class."

Remorse was punctuated by the white-knuckle aspects of flying in
the Caribbean in 1955. The trip wasn't for sissies. After Miami, I
changed from one baling-wire airline to another, from Cuba down to
Jamaica and then up to Haiti and over to Puerto Rico to my first
destination, St. Thomas.

I was met by Tex Richie, one of Junkyard Murphy's pilots. Generally
speaking, old, fat-bellied pilots gave me a feeling of security. They had
survived. Tex Richie was old, fat, and spoke with a whiskey-flavored
Southwestern drawl. He didn't exactly fill me with confidence. The
plane gave me even less. It was an odd, dumpy configuration made in

Holland with a push-pull engine in the rear. Tex called it a STOL, acronym for Short Take Off and Landing.

When he put on a thick pair of glasses to read the map, I almost called the whole thing off.

"There's the little mother," he said, holding a magnifying glass.

"Where?"

"There."

SHIT!

"Where's the runway?"

"Oh, it's there all right. All thirteen hundred feet of it."

"Thirteen hundred feet!"

"Hell, ain't no worse than landing on the deck of a carrier. They keep the grass low by using it as a grazing plot for the island's sheep. When it gets down low enough, they sweep the sheep shit off it and use it as a soccer field. Junkyard told me to take real good care of you. They're mowing the field for our arrival."

Reinforced by that bit of intelligence, we took off. The flight was short and choppy. We came to a confluence of islands. Tex pointed out a speck.

"St. Barths."

Good Lord, was he kidding? He flew over it once to see if any emergency panels had been laid out and to check the wind sock.

"God dammit," he grumbled.

"What's wrong?"

"We got a twenty-five-knot tail wind. It's gonna be a good one."

He went out to sea, circled back, and lowered the plane until we were but a few hundred feet over the water, then he banked her almost ninety degrees. At this terrifying angle we were being kicked from behind by the wind. He slowed her till I thought she had to stall and drop us into the sea. Tex held this attitude and the stall warning beeped.

"Motherfucker," he garbled under his breath.

The runway went from the water's edge and then took off uphill into a dead end of boulder-filled hillocks. If we touched down too far up the runway it seemed there was little chance of getting her up in the air again quickly enough.

"Used to have an awful lot of pileups," he said to comfort me.

At the last instant, with the stall button blaring, Tex leveled her out and let her glide. She hit the runway twenty feet in from the water's edge and started an uphill run coming to a halt with—oh hell, a good ten or twelve feet to spare. Piece of cake.

And then I lightened up. At the side of the runway by the shack a pleasant-looking couple stood beside a battered jeep and waved us in. Denise and Pierre Dumont, Junkyard's caretakers. They fussed over me as though I were visiting royalty. Who knows? I might have been the first Jew ever to have set foot on the place.

I really didn't know what I was expecting—a thatched hut, a cave dwelling, a spear-carrying native chief. Junkyard had digs on a half-dozen islands. This one turned out to be a petite but nicely built villa. It obviously belonged to a skilled trader, for it was supplied to the gunwales with everything from bug spray to bourbon. All I would need was one pair of shoes, one pair of shorts, and my typewriter.

The location was primo. Villa Murphy was on a small hillside above a magnificent curve of beach, a bay called St. Jean. It was a three-minute walk from the front door to the strand.

In the next few days I made friends with the Dumonts and their five children, who had their own home a short distance away. They spoke French with a sprinkling of English and we worked out a palatable language. Pierre was Junkyard's man on St. Barths, so to speak.

We jeeped every road on the island in the next few days. It was a speck of a place, a volcanic rock of about eight square miles. Leaping and bounding hills, cliffs, and rockfalls were ribboned by a few dozen kilometers of road, some of cement, some of volcanic rock, and some of washboard dirt. Tire busters, one and all. It was a roller coaster with a few flat stretches here and there with potholes—I hesitate to call them potholes, as they were large enough to make the jeep almost vanish.

A dozen Lilliputian bays were serene on the leeward side and inclined to violence on the windward. Warm water rolled or bashed up onto the most magnificent beaches of wheatfield-colored off-white sands. St. Barths was not what you would call a garden spot, but the ash was rich and there were many wild runs of bougainvillea wrapping around scrub trees and smatterings of wild-flower cover. No turn in any direction was without understated beauty.

There was little fertile land and it was easy to see that the islanders had to struggle to maintain a marginal existence.

Gustavia, a pearl of a little harbor, housed a waterfront quay and a half-dozen dirt streets. Most of the island's fifteen hundred population lived around there. The Select Bar on the quay was the central watering hole.

St. Barths proved to be an anachronism for this part of the world. Because she was so tiny, one by six miles, no sugar plantation ever rooted there and thus the island never had slaves. The inhabitants were mostly of French ancestry from Normandy and Brittany. It seemed more of a misplaced parcel of France. Some of the older women still wore Amish-like bonnets and long black skirts and the men dressed in seafaring blue.

St. Barths had some beef cattle, a smattering of vegetable and fruit plots and, of course, the bountiful sea. There was intense trade with a radius of neighboring islands. One got the idea quickly that black market, white market, and free market were the key to existence. Junkyard had a small warehouse in Gustavia. It lacked very little.

Some wealthy French had found St. Barths. Yachtsmen had wandered on it. There were a few dozen small villas in spellbinding cliffside locations, including a half dozen belonging to Americans. One is always leery of being an outsider and crashing their solitude. I needn't have worried. "Junkyard" was the magic name. He had shipped in most of the building materials for the homes erected since the war. Because it was a place where every outsider came looking for the same thing, friendships formed easily, and the islanders were just about the nicest people I had ever met.

Life was unencumbered with the problems, values, and intricacies of modern civilization. There was some electricity, always unreliable, of the home generator variety. One school, one doctor. Otherwise there were no telephones, waterworks, or sewers.

Directly below Villa Murphy, St. Jean's beach was split in half by an enormous boulder of lava that ran out to the sea. On this outcropping, built on several levels, was the single hotel, the Eden Rock, consisting of five rooms. I befriended the owner, a flier named Remy de Haenen who had pioneered the airstrip. His wife, like Denise Dumont and most of the women, was a superb chef, making little miracles of meals with the lean pickings from the fields.

Otherwise there was a lot of beach to meditate on, a lot of sunsets to watch, a lot of conversation at the Select Bar. I don't know if anyone ever called me by my name. I was simply "the writer."

How utterly strange the way things turned out. I came girded for battle, to scale or bash down walls of fear I had erected all my life. When I opened my eyes on St. Barths, the walls simply vanished. Instead, St. Barths opened its arms wide and caressed me and told me, "Take off your pack and stand at ease, Marine, and be afraid no more."

I learned to shut out of my mind anything that distracted me from my work. I could go for days without remembering Penny and Roxy. This was my fear, remembering. It was a revelation that I had the capacity to forget.

This was what I came to find. The conquest of loneliness was the missing link that was, one day, going to make a decent novelist out of me. If you are out here and cannot close off the loves and hates of all that back there in the real world, the memories will overtake you and swamp you and wilt your tenacity. Tenacity, stamina . . . close off to everything and everyone but your writing. That's the bloody price. I don't know, maybe it's some kind of ultimate selfishness. Maybe it's part of the killer instinct. Unless you can stash away and bury thoughts of your greatest love, you cannot sustain the kind of concentration that breaks most men trying to write a book over a three- or four-year period.

I learned this barefoot on a screened-in veranda on Villa Murphy. Nothing on this planet existed but the words I was putting on paper. I didn't even exist. I had no needs but food and sleep. I had no reason to live, except to create by writing.

I ran the beach at sunup, thinking, talking to myself as I ran.

"Hey, writer, how's it go?"

I'd wave and keep running.

I would talk out my next day's work to myself watching the sunset. And when the sun went down I drank hard. Once in a while the words wouldn't come. I'd take a day off and Pierre and I went fishing and he taught me to sail.

Sometimes loneliness would strike like the suddenness of the lightning storms. I would not permit the pain to overtake me.

Things were starting to happen now that I had longed might happen when I was a little boy. When the electricity failed, I wrote by candlelight. When a hurricane wrecked part of the villa, I wrote from a room at the Eden Rock. I had reached a level of obsession, consummation—not of this planet. I wrote when I had fever. I wrote with hangovers. I wrote when some damned fine-looking women came prowling around.

I had envisioned St. Barths as a hell island where I had to serve a sentence. Instead of imprisoning me, it liberated me in so many ways. I had learned that when you have accomplished, without fear, an ability to go far, far, far inside yourself, relive the emotional starvation and lovelessness from parents during childhood, you have come to know a certain awesome splendor. Without it, you cannot reach for eternity as a writer. Paying your dues to attain it becomes so frightening, so gut-wrenching, it guarantees you years of sleeplessness and nightmares. I had to find it or never hope again.

Every so often Tex dropped in in his stupid little Dutch STOL. For a time I expected divorce papers, but they never came. I filled my letters to the girls with happiness. One day I gave Tex the first draft screenplay to send to Schlosberg, and then I dared to start thinking about a novel. Christmas was coming and so were Penny and Roxy. Tex flew me over to St. Thomas to fetch them. With my screenplay on Judd Schlosberg's desk, I allowed myself to become excited, to reenter the world. St. Barths wasn't forever, but I wanted my girls to know the place.

We worked out St. Thomas as a rendezvous because Val's family had a number of retired Navy friends there who could keep the girls till I arrived. We radioed ahead to get them packed and down to the airport.

I was totally unprepared to see Val when we landed. I thought she would fly part of the way but expected she would vacation in Jamaica, which she loved as a girl.

After an uproarious hello from the girls, Tex showed them around the plane and I went aside with Val. We shook hands and then I kissed her cheek. She didn't resist, or show any hostility. I hadn't thought of her much. I hadn't let myself. I had known my guilt was stuffed down and would erupt, but not till after I'd won my tussle with the screenplay.

Maybe she was expecting me to look like a bearded, rum-soaked beachcomber. I was really tan and fit.

"You look great," she said.

"Not much to do except stay healthy or go to seed. I . . . look—I didn't expect to see you, Val. Let me catch my breath."

"Sure. How's the work coming?"

"I turned in the first draft screenplay a few weeks ago. I should be hearing soon. Sometimes it's tough to get a message to me. Where are you heading, anyhow?"

"I'm staying on St. Thomas. Mom is going to join me in a few days."

"Roxy wrote that she had a stroke. How is she doing?"

"Not too badly. This will be her first trip. She's having a little trouble with—never mind."

"Well, you give her my love, will you?"

"Sure."

"Any special instructions about the girls?"

"No. They're dying to be with you. They've missed their dad."

"I've got a good time planned. I have a record player that works most of the time. I plan to run them through an opera and a symphony a day and I've got a half-dozen books I want to read to them. Really hit it lucky. I'm not working right now so we'll do a lot of beaching and bust open lobsters. Don't laugh but I even sail a little."

"You? Sail? I'll bet you're good."

"I'm terrible. So, there's a lot of kids their age. Everyone seems to get along with the language problem. They'll have a good time."

I became a little uneasy and looked over to Tex. He gave me a high sign, "Anytime you're ready, boss."

"We'll be back on Friday, the second. I'll try to radio ahead and let you know."

"Oh, I meant to tell you. No scuba diving for Penny. She can snorkel but the doctor said he didn't want any pressure on her head."

"Yeah . . . well, pleasant surprise seeing you. Have yourself a happy holiday and . . . look . . . would you be interested in taking a hop over and seeing how the other half lives? Tex will run you back when your mom arrives."

"I'd love to come over," she whispered.

"Better get in touch with the people you're staying with . . ."

"I mentioned to them and to Mom that there was a chance in a thousand I might wind up in St. Barths. It's fine with her."

"Well, then let's go get you a bag packed. You don't need much."

"It's already packed. It's in the terminal. Gideon, we're going to be able to . . ."

I put my arms about her and held her.

FROM THE FIRST MOMENT at St. Barths, my love affair with the island had started. I had pushed myself, beyond myself, out to a supernova called writer's isolation. But for me, a horny little Jew, no place can be paradise without a woman. Now, it was paradise. The island conquered my girls as it had conquered me.

"Where on earth did you find this record, Gideon?"

"In a back closet, all covered with dust."

"Seventy-eight RPM's . . . holy cow."

"It's the latest thing on St. Barths."

We danced on the veranda, so tightly.

I saw you last night,
And got that old feeling,
When you came in sight,
I got that old feeling,
The moment you passed by,
I felt a thrill,
And when you caught my eye,
My heart stood still,

Once again I seemed to feel
That old yearning,
And I knew the spark of love,
Was still burning . . .

"Hey, Marine, you're moving in a little fast."

"That's me, baby. Stick with me. I'll take you over the rough spots."

"What did you say your name was?"

"Zadok, Gideon Zadok, and I'm going to be a great writer someday."

With all the beauty and magic around us, there was still terrible unhealed pain between Val and me. We didn't talk about it much, but it was there. When people have inflicted such hurt on each other for so long a time, there must be scar tissue and bad dreams that will never go away. Were we strong enough, did we have the capability of love so powerful that we could endure black memories of the past, tuck them into a remote corner and never let them haunt us again? Could Val and I make it to the end? The moment I saw her, I knew I wanted to try.

Tex returned in a week with the message that Judd Schlosberg had lined up radio time to speak to me on Guadeloupe. The big island, which administrated St. Barths, was a hundred miles or so to the south and was more in touch with the outside world.

We could easily round-trip it in a day and it would be fun for the girls. Basse Terre had a bazaar to drive them crazy. I went to the shortwave radio center at the central post office.

Oh, my, my, my! Those exquisite words. "We love the script. We want to do the picture."

Schlosberg wanted a few weeks of changes, nothing major. Could I get back after New Year's?

"I'll be there."

End of transmission.

I was halfway home! Now, I dared dream openly of the novel.

ON THE WESTERN end of St. Barths, Mount Vitet rose a thousand feet above the sea. Sometimes the jeep won the battle up the road, sometimes the road won. We had to climb the last half hour. We were both weary from welcoming in the New Year with a party for two.

The expanse of water below us held a scattering of islands, little volcanic wonderments blasting up from the seabed millions of years ago.

Val perched on a rock and crossed her legs and threw her head back

to catch the breeze. The sweat shone off her face and neck and bosom. I
unbuttoned her blouse.

"God, they taste good sweaty."

She held my head to her. "You crazy. I'm so happy we're all going
back together."

"Me too," I said.

"You'll miss this place, Gideon."

"I was lucky to find it. God forbid I never come back. I was lucky.
I'd like to freeze time now, here. Val, you're beautiful."

"Shucks, man, you're going to make me cry."

You can make love to a hundred women, but no one feels like the
woman who gave you your children.

We sat for a long time hanging onto the last images. "Val, I once took
a girl up to a hilltop a long time ago. A place called Twin Peaks in San
Francisco. We were kids. I told her I was going to be a great writer
someday and I read her the first chapter of a book I was going to write,
someday."

"What happened to her?"

"We got married but we didn't live happily ever after. Along the way
I got messed up. Then, I found an island called St. Barths and it taught
me to go back and do what I was supposed to do in this world. I'd
rather come back here and live like a fisherman and write what I want
to write. You know what I mean?"

"I'm starting to understand what you're about, Gideon. I'd like to
believe I can keep you but I don't know. I haven't got a hell of a lot of
confidence anymore. You're a tough number to handle, buddy. You've
got a trillion volts running through you. I swear I don't know if there's
a woman in the world who can ever really bring you peace."

"Val, I'm sorry for what I did to you."

"I know that, Gideon. You don't have to say it."

"I do have to say it. I've got to hear myself saying it."

"I made you do a lot of things that drove you away. I'm not all that
clean," she said. "We've both done numbers on each other. Can we
make it? I wish I were more certain."

"I brought you up here because we started once on a hilltop. I know
where I'm heading. I'll find out why, when I'm there. I thought this
would be the right place to tell you."

"Well, here we are," she said shakily, afraid of what wild, crazy
scheme I was going to come up with.

"I've never talked much about my childhood," I began.

"I know. Sometimes I wondered if you ever had a childhood. It's been like a wall around you."

"You know how it is. You spend the second half of your life getting over the first half," I said. "There are doors I'm opening a crack, one by one. I opened a door marked, 'Danger, Tarawa and Guadalcanal, enter at your own risk.'"

"I think I understand," she said.

"There's a big, fucking iron vault door inside me. It's marked 'Jew.' I have to open it and go inside. I don't know what the hell I'm going to find in there. You remember me talking about my Uncle Matti?"

"Just a little. He's the one who went to Palestine. Hero. Killed in the Arab riots of 1939. That's about all I know," she said.

"That's about all I know, too. But I sense something dynamic happening. I sensed it the moment I opened the vault a crack. I—I want to go to Israel and find out. I'm not totally sure why but it's magnetic, pulling me. It's like the Old Man upstairs," I said pointing to the sky. "He's telling me to go. It's an instinct I have to follow. I denied I was a Jew several times in my life. It's been around my neck like an albatross all my life. I've got to free myself and I believe there may be a great book just waiting for a writer."

She shook her head and laughed a little. "You take the cake, old buddy."

"We can make it if we lease the house and you move down with your mom. The way I figure it, it's going to take about six months to research. If I think it's going to go longer, or if I decide to write the book there, I'd want you and the girls to come to Israel. It's going to be tight, but if we count our pennies we can hack it."

Val stared at me for ever so long. She was on the brink of tears. She had no illusions but that we were in for a long, terrible struggle. "You won't settle for less, will you? You've got to win."

"I'm afraid so."

"You son of a bitch," she whispered.

"Val, if you can't or don't want to handle it, let's say goodbye now, like buddies."

"And after Israel? Timbuktu?"

"Maybe."

"Gideon, I'll keep up with you as long as I can. You go with my love. I'll wait for you to send for us."

IT BEGAN as a low rumble. Flashes on the horizon looked like heat lightning. Valerie blinked her eyes open. She recalled that when she was a little girl and the family was stationed on Guam, earthquakes and lightning storms were a common occurrence. It was the same kind of sounds and flashes as she heard now. She instinctively braced herself for the ground to start shaking but it didn't. Only the rumbles and flashes continued. Then she could hear faint popping sounds.

Val flung off the sheet and fumbled for the lamp. It was nine o'clock at night. Wait, let me think. It all came back. Gideon had left early in the morning to go out on a raid with the Israelis. The day had dragged by torturously. Dr. Hartmann had come by to check on her again and given her a shot to settle her down. She had fallen into a deep sleep.

"Mommy, come up to the roof," Roxanne cried, running into the room.

By the time they got up, Grover had joined a choir of dogs howling from one end of the Sharon Plain to the other. From their elevation they could make out a horizon being lit by cannon fire some seven or eight miles away. From here the sounds and sights seemed like a playland.

The bombardment went on incessantly. Nearly an hour passed before any of them moved or spoke.

"Is Daddy there?" Penny asked.

"Yes."

"Why?"

"He's looking for something," Val answered.

Roxanne began to cry. Her mother held her tightly. "Daddy always makes it home," Val said.

WHAT GIDEON HAD not anticipated was the speed with which the raid was executed. There was no dusting off a stack of old contingency plans, nor was there a surplus of battle-ready troops standing by. A dangerous target had been selected, one that would make all the necessary military and political points to the Jordanians. The Jordanian police fort was just across the border, only twelve miles from downtown Tel Aviv, on the outskirts of Kalkilia, a city of twenty-five thousand inhabitants.

During the day, elements of the Israeli Paratroop Brigade assembled from all parts of the country. Some had interrupted hard training and arrived at the staging area extremely tired. Yet they were the best available troops.

The raid went well in the opening stages. There were no natural barriers to cross at the border and the forward units moved over easily.

The Kalkilia police fort was illuminated by Israeli searchlights from two miles' distance and support artillery fire opened up from a tank detachment.

In the normal flow of battle something always went awry. The plan sprang leaks and all hell broke loose. The sky stayed lit with cannon bursts until 0300 but small arms fire could be heard until daybreak.

Val and the girls had slept in fits and snatches. It was six in the morning when Val spotted Mr. Zimmerman, an assistant manager from the hotel, wheel his bicycle up the path toward the cottage. She was too terrified to move.

Mr. Zimmerman was a friendly old codger. He delighted in running messages to the Zadok cottage in exchange for a few words of gossip. Val had seen a concentration camp number tattooed on his arm—one of the first times she had seen such a thing. She cried softly for several nights and understood so much about Israel in that single incident.

"I just got a telephone call from Mr. Zadok," he said. "He said to tell you he is all right and he would be home in a few hours."

Val screamed and collapsed against him.

"Mr. Zadok was on the raid last night?" he asked.

"Yes."

"*Oy, mein got.* Sit down, Mrs. Zadok, please sit. I make you a glass tea. Oh, it was a very bad one. We had almost a hundred boys casualties. *Nu*, what can we do? Thanks *got* Mr. Zadok wasn't hurt."

The terrible wait was done. Val brought herself under control with the help of a wallop of that awful brandy. As color returned to her cheeks she managed a smile.

"Bad news, I'm afraid," Mr. Zimmerman said. "We're closing the hotel down. If Mr. Zadok will come to my house this evening, I give him a key to the side entrance and show him the fuse box for his room. We want he should keep his office."

When Mr. Zimmerman left Val rushed around the kitchen trying to find something to bake, something to clean, something to defrost. Strangely, as if they knew, the neighbors began to gather.

THE GIRLS ran toward the jeep and flung their arms about him.

"Better not touch me," Gideon said, "I'm all stinky."

He was, in fact, putrid. His eyes seemed far away, still reflecting a recent horror. He plopped down at the kitchen table. Val served him some cake and juice and shooed the neighbors out. He was too exhausted to chew. Gideon pulled himself up and swayed down the hall to the bedroom, made it to the edge of the bed, doubled over and held his face in his hands.

"Dad's okay. He needs some rest," Val said and closed the door. She wanted to go to him, but somehow couldn't or didn't. He was a naughty boy who had run out into the street and was pulled to the sidewalk by a mother who first kissed him, then slapped him. He didn't have to put them through this.

Val was unable to temper her anger. "Well, I suppose you finally got to feel it," she said. She really hadn't wanted to say that. It just came out. "Well, I felt it too," she went on acidly.

"Okay, I deserve to be kicked in the ass," he mumbled.

"They've closed down the hotel," she continued, wanting to hit him with bad news.

"Can't it wait!" he snapped.

"Sure, it can wait."

"I better take a shower and try to get some sleep." He fumbled for the buttons of his combat jacket but his fingers would not function.

There was a period of quiet, long enough for the venom to pass from her. She came to him and sat on the floor before him and rested her head on his lap.

"Simon was killed. So was Ben Dror. Zev lost both of his legs."

"Oh Christ," Val sobbed.

"It was a real fuck-up."

"Oh, honey, honey," she cried. "Poor Shalimit. She's going to have a baby . . . oh, honey. I'd better go see her."

"I saw her along with the battalion commander, this morning."

"God dammit," Val cried. . . . "Oh, honey . . . oh, damn." She got to her feet and stood over him and tousled his hair. It was sticky. "You're a real mess, buddy," she wept.

"I'll clean up."

Alpha Company of the Lion's Battalion was sent out to bypass the fort. They set up an ambush on a hillock overlooking the road into Kalkilia in the event the Jordanians tried to reinforce the fort.

It took longer to capture and blow up the fort than expected. With the timetable fucked, the battle plan went out the window. It was just like at Tarawa when the first wave of Marines failed to reach their objective. Officers and men in little groups had to improvise.

The Jordanians sent a unit of the Arab Legion toward Kalkilia but did not play sucker or fall for the ambush. They went off the road, encircled Alpha Company, and had them trapped.

Only after the balance of the Lion's Battalion retreated for the border did they realize that Alpha Company was surrounded by the Legion and being chopped to pieces. The rest of the night turned into a frantic effort to break the encirclement.

It turned into a bloody mess. Infantry, artillery, tanks and, later, planes had to try to open a hole. The Arab Legion hung tough when they realized they could annihilate an entire Israeli company. If they succeeded, they could claim victory. Translated into Arabic, this would make Jordan and King Hussein a more dangerous and adventurous foe.

About dawn some Israeli tanks and half-tracks broke through to Alpha Company. The dead and wounded were loaded on. Some of the dead were tied to the tanks. Alpha Company did make it back but twenty-eight boys had been killed and thirty-five wounded.

The Israeli raid succeeded but it was a terrible toll for a small country where everyone knew everyone.

Val pushed Gideon's chest gently and made him lie down on the bed, then unlaced his boots and tugged them off and unbuttoned his clothing.

"Golly, I haven't undressed you like this for years. Remember when you were writing your first book? The girls wouldn't fall asleep until they heard your typewriter. You'd come home from work and go up to the attic and write till two or three in the morning. I'd come up after you, but you'd be so tired you couldn't make it down the stairs by yourself, and I'd have to undress you."

She tugged him out of his clothing.

"Help me to the shower, baby."

"Just lie back," Val said, "just lie back."

Valerie pulled her blouse over her head slowly and unsnapped her bra and wiggled out of her jeans and stood over him.

"What a time to be looking at tits," he said. "I'm a goddam animal."

Valerie lay on top of him, covering him.

"It's so crazy. They're dead. But I want you."

She wrapped herself around him as best she could, blotting up his sweat with her body, kissing and licking the grit and dirt from his eyes and cheeks, rubbing her hair into the circles of sweat staining his neck, gripping him with her legs.

"Fly away, buddy," she said, "fly away."

IT HAD BEEN a sticky wicket from the beginning. When Gideon first arrived in Israel, he promised the Israelis that he would not seek out intelligence from the Americans or carry it back to them. In exchange the Israelis agreed to give him the help he needed to research his book.

Rich Cromwell, the American CIA station chief, badgered Gideon for information from time to time, without success. Gideon knew that without earning the deep trust of the Israelis, he would never get the information he needed to write the novel he wanted.

The call for a luncheon date at Cromwell's Ramat Aviv villa carried an unmistakable sound of urgency. Gideon never failed to marvel at the lack of discomfort American Embassy personnel "survived" in. Now, take the huge silver bowl in Cromwell's foyer. It brimmed over with petite calling cards, in the language of the caller and in French.

Israel was a tiny country insofar as the number of embassies, legations, and consulates was concerned. Yet, when one figured that each country had an ambassador, first secretary, second secretaries, chargé d'affaires, military attachés, cultural attachés, economic attachés, special missions such as the Point Four program, trade missions, purchasing missions, an endless stream of visiting scholars in endless conferences to produce endless wisdom, and Jewish philanthropists, investors, orchestras, dance troupes, and everyone received a welcoming and departing cocktail party, that was a lot of caviar and crackers. Then there was the

Fourth of July, Bastille Day, and the Queen's birthday, and every country had a national holiday, particularly the newly liberated African
nations (the Africans really threw bashes), and because every legation
bought everything duty-free, livers collapsed like sand castles at high
tide. Everyone had a big silver or cut glass bowl or native basketweave
in their foyer, and everyone coming for a visit left a petite calling card,
in two languages. One could reasonably count on a minimum of twelve
hundred and sixty-one cocktail parties a year.

Rich Cromwell looked like a semi-rumpled, silver-haired old Yalie,
which he was, who would be far more at home in a blue blazer on Cape
Cod. Two-letter man, old Rich, hockey and lacrosse. A middling State
Department foreign service employee, who clipped a few coupons from
his inheritance, he rose no higher than a consul general post in Peru. He
drifted to the CIA for a more fulfilling way of life.

Cromwell knew of Gideon's lust for prime rib and plumped him up at
lunch to a fare-thee-well. When the amenities were done, Rich generally
switched on his "sincere" mode. This afternoon he passed right over
sincere and went directly to grim. Gideon sipped on his after-lunch
Scotch slowly, lest he have a violent reaction to his sudden reexposure
to it.

"What happened on the Kalkilia raid?" Rich began.

"Now, how in the hell should I know?"

"Come on, Gideon. This would make you the only one in the country
who didn't know where you were on the night of the tenth. Your buddy
Simon Galil got hit by a stray bullet. He was standing right next to
you."

"What are you on my case for, Rich? You've been briefed, rebriefed,
and debriefed. Christ, a minute-by-minute report has been in all the
papers. It was a military operation. Some things went right. Some
things went wrong."

"We all know about your arrangement with the Israelis and we've
respected it."

"However," Gideon said.

"However, it's getting down to the short strokes."

"And?"

"You're a Marine, Gideon."

Oh balls, he's going to Semper-Fi me, Gideon thought. Old Cromwell
had been a Marine major, not too high a rank, not too low. Just right
for a mediocre Yalie.

"Rich," Gideon said, "I know we shared the big war together, the war to end all wars, you as a major and me as a PFC. So here it is, as one old buck-assed gyrene to another. I don't know doodly shit."

Gideon sensed that hardball time was coming up. Rich needed some intelligence, badly.

"Don't be so modest, Gideon. You've got better lines into the Prime Minister's office than President Eisenhower does. Your pals read like Who's Who. You chum around with Teddy Kollek, Moshe Pearlman, Beham, Jackie Herzog . . ."

"This may be difficult for you to comprehend, but they don't rush out of cabinet meetings to brief me."

Cromwell didn't believe him. He digested his frustration and decided to take a bold step. "I'm going to level with you," he said. "This place is about to blow up. You may have it within your power to help prevent a catastrophe."

"I'm listening," Gideon answered quietly.

"I'm going to give you a scenario, a secret scenario. Maybe you can fill in some of the blank spots."

Careful, Gideon said to himself, careful.

"Dayan, Golda, Peres, and Moshe Carmel flew to Paris a few weeks back."

"What's so earthshaking about that? France is Israel's major supporter and supplier," Gideon answered.

"It was a secret mission. They flew via Bizerte in a reconverted French bomber to avoid all civilian airports. Now, I'm talking about Israel's Foreign Minister, Transportation Minister, Chief of Staff, and Peres, the architect of the French connection. They met at the home, not the office, of Louis Mangin in Montparnasse," Cromwell went on. "On the French side were Foreign Minister Pineau, Defense Minister Bourges-Maunoury, Director General of the Defense Ministry Abel Thomas, and Chief of Staff Eli with four of his closest aides."

Gideon managed to listen without expression.

"France and Britain want the Suez Canal back, right?" Cromwell said.

"I suppose so."

"Israel's interest is getting Nasser's troops out of the Sinai, opening the Red Sea to their shipping, and stopping the terrorist attacks from the Gaza Strip. Now, let's make an educated guess what these people were discussing."

"I don't know that this meeting even took place, Rich. I know you're implying some kind of joint military action."

"Against Egypt," Rich said.

"Hell, it could be. From the looks of it, Jordan seems to be the target."

"A decoy," Rich said. "We think Jordan is a decoy and we take umbrage that two of America's closest allies are planning a military action without consulting us."

"It's all over my head, Rich."

"Here it is, Gideon, straight and unvarnished. You're an American. You can get us the answers to a couple of very frustrating questions. We think the British and French aren't consulting us because they're afraid we'd stop them."

Gideon popped out of his chair, tipped the Scotch bottle into his glass, and considered Cromwell's theory. "Why is it in America's interest to stop two of her allies from taking back an international waterway vital to the West and why is it in our interest to keep the Suez Canal and Red Sea closed to Israeli shipping? Like, Rich, I don't follow you."

Cromwell had succeeded in the first step, getting Zadok to discuss the matter. "The instant England and France make a hostile move against Egypt, the Soviet Union is going to plunge headlong into the Middle East to play hero to the Arabs. We don't want Russia in here any deeper. It's Egypt's canal. Nasser owns it. We don't give a big rat's ass if England and France don't get it back. Are you starting to get the drift of America's interest?"

Gideon gave a noncommittal gesture.

"What happens when the Kremlin advises the British and French that five hundred Russian missiles are trained on Paris and London and are going to be fired if they set foot in Egypt? Who's going to get to clean this mess up? I'm talking about the probability of a Soviet-American confrontation. Eisenhower does not want to go to war over the Suez Canal, nor do we want the Russians arming every two-bit Arab dictator in the Middle East. Now, let me ask you one more time. Are Israel, France, and England planning an attack on Egypt? Yes, or no?"

"I don't know," Gideon rasped.

"I think you're a liar."

"I don't know. How could I know?"

"I don't want to be crude but you've got a lady friend in the Prime Minister's office who translates all the top-secret documents into Hebrew. Everybody in Israel knows that Natasha Solomon is your mistress. In fact, you didn't make much of an effort to cover it until your family arrived."

Gideon sat again and fidgeted uncomfortably.

"You could find out if you wanted to," Cromwell pressed.

"Natasha wouldn't tell me. No way she would tell me."

"All right, Gideon, sit on this one. Israel is going to mobilize. She's calling up the reserves the day after tomorrow."

The thunder of Cromwell's announcement fell on him, hard. The book. Val. The girls. Ruined! Everything's ruined!

"I personally like you," Cromwell said. "You might need me to help you get your family out of here. Things could get very tight."

"Mind if I have another drink?"

"Help yourself." Cromwell jotted a number on a slip of paper and handed it to Gideon. "Private line. It's scrambled so you can talk freely. However, you make your calls from a pay phone. Keep in touch every day and let me know if you have anything to tell me."

Gideon scarcely heard him. He slipped the note into his pocket, his head reeling, trying to find a way, any way, to salvage the wreckage.

EVACUATION
October 27, 1956

AN UNSEEN HAND swept over the land of Israel gathering up men from the fields and shops, from the offices and factories. A Hebrew code word spoken at news time over the radio sent men of a particular reserve unit scurrying to their homes where they took weapons from a locked closet, packed a bit of food, took their own winter coats and blankets, kissed the family goodbye, and headed quickly and quietly to the bus stop or hitched a ride. Units assembled in predestined secret places, a clump of woods, a kibbutz or moshav, or someplace away from the probing eyes across the border. It all took place in a silent, ethereal way without histrionics. Most of the reserve units were then moved into defensive positions along the border, freeing the standing army to go into the attack.

Transport was gleaned from city streets and highways. Vehicles were stopped at roadblocks, checked off a list, and the driver given a receipt for his confiscated car or truck. He continued on by hitching a ride. A good part of the bus system left the streets and highways to staging areas for the motor pools.

This was an army of poorly equipped militia which had to travel on the shaky wheels of aged buses, laundry vans, flatbed and stake trucks, ancient civilian automobiles, taxis.

Essential committees assembled all over the land and reviewed the
emergency plans to keep vital services going with volunteer skeleton
crews. This was the role of the older citizens. While the reservists were
away the water had to keep running, the electricity humming, the
schools and hospitals functioning, food supplies moving from farm to
city.

The entire country moved in this ominous, silent, deadly rhythm.

AFTER LUNCH Gideon drove the jeep into Tel Aviv where Moshe
Pearlman, a reserve colonel in the Prime Minister's office had commandeered space over an auto agency and was in the process of converting
it into the military press, censorship, and spokesman's office. It was
alive with activity, laying in as many new telex lines as possible.

Gideon's literary agent in New York had again failed to come up with
assignments, so he sent a dozen telex messages on his own to the newspaper syndicates asking for work.

From there, Gideon drove to the defense complex and turned in his
jeep for the duration, then hitched a ride back to Herzlia. Valerie and
the girls were making a game of putting blackout paper over the window.

In their neighborhood, mostly consisting of South African Jews, the
men had simply disappeared. "You and Mr. Zimmerman seem to be the
only men left," Val said. "What do you think, hon? Is it going to blow
over?"

Apparently the CIA didn't think so. Gideon shrugged. "I'm not worried," he lied.

Gideon kept a typewriter at home and took a whirl at writing. After a
dozen crumpled pages hit the trash can he gave up.

"Switchboard at the hotel is shut down," he said. "I'm going to run
over to the village and make a few phone calls."

As he jogged toward the village center, Gideon's mind went strangely
to something other than the call-up of the reserves and the deteriorat-
ing situation. He was thinking of his meeting with Rich Cromwell and
particularly the stinging words about him and Natasha Solomon.

Back home in L.A., Gideon had always managed his extracurricular
affairs with discretion, or so he thought. He controlled them from start
to finish, never crossing a certain line of involvement, always pulling out
before it became too serious.

"You're a rotten bastard, Gideon," a young actress had told him.
"You deliberately make a girl fall in love with you then you let her

down, always the gentleman. And you run home and pull the draw-
bridges up."

Gideon had arrived in Israel determined to stay clean. Israel, he discovered, was quite sophisticated about bed hopping, General Dayan
being the most prolific lecher in the country. Even Ben-Gurion was
rumored to have a mistress, now and again.

Well, he hadn't planned to fall in love with Natasha, but he did. For
the first time in his life, he went out of control for a woman. There was
excitement, madness, daring exceeding anything he had dreamed of.
Here was a woman who could match him, make him do what he had
made other women do. These were arms he couldn't walk away from on
his whim. He knew jealous anger and went into rages for the first time.
He behaved, at times, in a manner he had disdained in other men.

Rich Cromwell said everyone in the country knew. Did Valerie know
as well? She never let on that she did. Had some bitch made a sly
inference at a cocktail party? Had Natasha herself let Val know
obliquely by being overly sweet and patronizing? After all, it wasn't a
state secret, only delicious gossip.

Val had come to Israel, done her best, loved him hard. She didn't
deserve another humiliation. He wanted to leave Natasha. He tried,
really tried. Each time he tried they ended up in a wilder reunion. This
was a sweet moment in his life he would never know again. He didn't
have the strength or the real desire to walk away.

GIDEON PULLED up panting at a tiny corner café where Mrs. Mandel
greeted him. He opened the soft-drink cooler. No ice.

"The ice truck was mobilized," she said, "so was my Harry. I'm
closing down until this thing is over with."

Gideon unsnapped and slowly drank a soft-drink concoction. Satisfied no one else was around, he went to the wall phone and dialed Rich
Cromwell's private number.

"Hello."

"Hi. This is your old gyrene buddy."

"Anything we should get together on?" Rich asked.

"No, no new information. Just checking in."

"I'm glad you did. We're calling for the evacuation of all Americans."

Sweat streaked from Gideon's forehead into his eyes. He wiped it but
he stung from the salt. Keep your head, he said to himself. He sipped
the soft drink to moisten his dry mouth so he could speak.

"When's this going to happen?" he asked shakily.

"Starting tonight. We're flying over some transport from the Rhine-Main base in Germany. They're already en route. Embassy, consulate, missions, and Point Four personnel are being jerked out of the country. Otherwise, a destroyer is on the way to Haifa to take out civilians working here and tourists. That might take a couple of days."

"Holy shit."

"Planes are due in around ten or eleven tonight. Get your family to the airport. I'll see that they get on tonight. Otherwise, it might be a Chinese fire drill."

"I don't know . . ." Gideon mumbled.

"This isn't coming through as a request, Gideon. It's orders. Eisenhower is pissed. P-I-S-S-E-D. If you stay, you're on your own and you could run into some real problems."

"How about my dog?" Gideon said for no reason.

"I don't think so. Look, got to run. Get to Lydda by nine o'clock and look me up."

The line went dead.

GIDEON STRIPPED OFF his shorts and shirt and stood under the cold outdoor shower for a short eternity hoping the water would suddenly give him strange powers. He wrapped a towel about his waist and walked toward the cottage as though it were his last mile.

"Hi, baby, where are the kids?"

"Playing with the Ben Josephs."

Val turned from the sink and saw him. He was ashen. "You shouldn't run in this heat," she said.

He averted her stare, went to the fridge, and devoured another bottle of soda pop. "I just talked to Cromwell," he whispered.

"Sorry, honey, I can't hear you." Val turned off the faucets and wiped her hands. "What did you say?"

"I said, I talked to Cromwell. Val, we've been ordered to evacuate."

It didn't register. "Evacuate? Where, how, when? Is this part of some kind of maneuvers?"

"It's not maneuvers. We've been ordered to evacuate the country."

Val was horror-stricken. She uttered a little peep and gripped the sink to steady herself. Gideon sank to the table, his head lowered, his eyes on the aggregate floor studying the designs abstractedly. He looked up slowly. She was over him.

"Where? When?"

"Tonight. Probably someplace in Europe. Planes are on the way from Germany."

She appealed to him with her eyes. "Please tell me it's a bad joke," she was trying to say. He shrugged. "We don't have to go," Gideon said.

"What kind of crazy business is this!"

"There seems to be a lot of spite involved. Eisenhower is furious with Israel. Jerking the embassy people out like this seems to be more of a warning than anything."

"What do you think?"

"I don't think we're in any danger, but it's something I don't want to be wrong about. What really disturbs me is how this must all sound over the news at home. I guess I'm thinking about your mother and my old man. If there's one chance in a million of the girls getting hurt, we can't take it."

"You're right, it would kill Mom on top of her stroke," Val said slowly, allowing reality to take over her fright.

"Settled, then. Better start packing up for you and the girls."

"What about you?"

Gideon shook his head. "There's no way I can leave."

"Why?" she asked. It was a devastating, all-encompassing, "WHY."

"I can't, you know I can't. I'm . . ."

"You're what!"

"I'm a Jew . . . I represented myself here as a fighter . . . a Marine . . . *Of Men in Battle* is their second bible. . . . I can't tuck my tail between my legs and jump ship with the women and children. It wouldn't sit right."

"To whom wouldn't it sit right?"

"To myself among others. Who in the hell would ever believe a word I wrote in my book?"

"Fuck your book!" Val yelled.

"Whatever you say, whatever you think, is right. I've messed up, in spades. Even if I could make myself believe it was morally right to leave, we still have problems. We've got to salvage something out of this. You're only going to be able to take a couple of suitcases."

"Don't give me that shit, Gideon! Your pals can pack and ship the rest of the stuff."

"Baby, we are broke. I mean dead-ass busted. I've got to try to get some of the lease money back. Maybe, if I can sell the car to a foreigner on a passport-to-passport deal, I can raise a few thousand dollars. We've got three thousand in Israeli currency in the bank. It's going to take some real manipulation to get it converted."

"Dammit, let's just leave," she cried.

He didn't hear her. She didn't hear him. "I've got a dozen cables to get on the wire. I've got to pick up some writing assignments," he mumbled.

"Let's just go!"

"We've barely got hotel money for you in Europe."

And then they stopped their soliloquies and stared at each other. "What about the rest of it, Gideon? Are you going to find the hottest combat unit in Israel and wing it out with them?"

No more needed to be said. The confrontation was spoken with eyes. What about Natasha Solomon?

Val accepted the reality as though the life had been squeezed from her body. "What about Grover?" she asked, barely speaking. "He's sick."

"I was told I couldn't get him on the plane. I'll take him in to Dr. Klement and do everything I can to bring him out with me, later. If not, I'll find him a good home."

Val looked around desperately as though she were waiting for the hypnotist to clap his hands and wake her from her nightmare. The girls were standing in the doorway, gaping in disbelief.

"How much did you hear?"

"We have to leave," Penny said.

"Go to your room and lay out only the most essential things on the bed," Valerie said with sudden firmness. "Dad will send everything to us later."

"Grover!"

"I'll do everything I can to get him to you as soon as he's well."

Roxy broke and wept.

"Roxanne," Valerie said sternly, "we've got to tough it, so pull yourself together, girl. There's a long night ahead."

"Yes, Momma . . ."

EACH ITEM of clothing was rolled up tightly and jammed down into a pair of Gideon's Marine Corps seabags. It was amazing how much they were able to pack in.

Gideon told them that during the war, just before they went into combat they would wind a roll of toilet paper around a pencil and keep stretching it tighter so that five or six rolls could be compressed into a few inches in diameter.

The six o'clock news came on, with a chilling announcement that a blackout was now in effect. It was Grover Vandover who picked up on the growing tension as neighbors arrived, but the dog was feeling too low to protest with much more than a whimper.

Some of the neighbors brought dollars from their hidden stashes and exchanged them for Israeli currency to help the Zadoks. Everyone gave Val a letter to be mailed to South Africa or elsewhere when she was out of the country. Farewell embraces as Gideon finished painting the headlights of the car to comply with the blackout. He muscled the seabags into the trunk just as the sun set.

The four of them were suddenly standing by the Ford, looking at the cottage. They had barely settled in and it was over with. As they closed the doors, the situation hit them with a sickening thud. Gideon hesitated as though a last-minute reprieve might save them, then he switched on the engine.

The car probed into a suddenly blackened countryside, bypassing a Tel Aviv that no longer seemed to be there. He had taken the route a hundred times on the way to Jerusalem but never in darkness.

Gideon gripped the wheel tightly and strained to pick up any little familiar landmarks. The car suddenly banged into something and bucked hard. He had driven up and over a curb. A few minutes later they went off the shoulder of the road and barely missed sinking into a ditch. Val drove them out while Gideon pushed.

Good. A familiar straight road for a while. Val took the Uzi gun off her lap, set it on the floor, and wrote a list of things he had to do. The girls forced their way through *The Little Brown Song Book.*

There was once a man
With a double chin
Who performed with skill
On the violin,
And he play'd in time,
And he played in tune,
But he never play'd anything
But Old Zip Coon.
Old Zip Coon
He played all day,
Until he drove his friends away;
He played all night
By the light of the moon,
And he wouldn't play anything
But Old Zip Coon.

Gideon slammed the brakes on. Jesus! He had almost dead-centered a donkey and cart. Fierce words were exchanged in Hebrew and English. No one understood the other.

"Come on back in the car, honey. We haven't got time to get into a fight now," she said.

"Shmuck!"

Just a song at twilight,
When the lights are low,
And the flick'ring shadows
Softly come and go.

He inched to a stop, apparently lost. Dammit! Seemed to be an intersection ahead. He walked up and found the road signs. Blessed relief. Lydda Airport—4km.

They were passed through the security gate and reached the parking lot just before nine o'clock, coming upon an eerie scene. The main lounge of the aged terminal was clogged with fleeing diplomats and their families. The place was lit by candle and lantern light casting a yellowish glow over piles of hastily packed suitcases and confused, disorganized humanity. Talk was in whispers, as though an enemy were listening. No one seemed to know anything.

Gideon carved out a place for Val and the girls and set out to find Rich Cromwell. He located him up in the tower. He flashed a false credential, one of a half dozen he carried, and shoved his way into the control room. The confusion there seemed as rampant as it was in the terminal. There had been word of American evacuation plans and a lot of unidentified blips were spooking the radar screens. The situation was worsened by the standoff between the Americans and Israelis. The Americans wanted no cooperation, not even data from Israeli patrol planes.

"Hi, Rich, how's it going?"

"You tell me," he said.

"It's not exactly America's proudest moment. Hard to tell whether the rats are deserting the sinking ship or the ship is deserting the sinking rats," Gideon said sourly.

"Did you register?" Cromwell asked, ignoring the comment.

"No."

"There's a desk in the cafeteria. Tell them your name is on the CIA list. I'll hunt you down in a while; I want to talk to you." Gideon had been leery of the special treatment. He was certain that Cromwell was going to have one more crack at him for intelligence data. He didn't like it.

Val had used her wits, packing a deck of cards, some jacks and a ball, and mini-chess and cribbage boards. She also had thrown together some sandwiches and fruit. The latter proved inspirational as the cafeteria had been stripped down to the last crust of bread.

The air grew thick from too many people and too much cigarette smoke. As the moments oozed by, a surrealistic pall dulled the place further. With each new rumor sudden flurries of loud talk broke out above the whispers.

Eleven o'clock . . . eleven-thirty . . . the rest rooms were becoming unusable.

Numbness set in. It became unearthly quiet.

Gideon put Roxanne on his lap and hugged her and rocked her.

"Where are we going, Daddy?"

"I'm not sure, darling. Probably across the sea. Italy, or maybe to Germany."

"I'm scared."

"Well, that's natural. But you've got a lot of people watching out for you."

"How?"

"There are a lot of planes out there making sure the skies are safe. It's going to be a while before we know the rights and wrongs of this thing. But you've got to be proud you're an American. Why, your country thinks so much about one little girl, they're coming from thousands of miles away to take you to safety."

"Why can't you come?"

"I . . . I've got work to do, darling. Mom and I decided you ought to go because of Grandma Jane and your *zayde.*"

Midnight.

Valerie dosed the girls up with Dramamine and a mild sleeping prescription and soon they fell into a deep slumber curled up on the seabags.

Val and Gideon were wordless, their thoughts jumbled and disconnected. Val's hair had become disheveled and her eyes listless.

She was unaware of Gideon's patting her. Her mind was on the list. Did I put a note for him to cancel my hair appointment? Not to bother, the hairdresser is in a reserve unit . . . did I pack Penelope's medication . . . sure I did, I must have . . . the minute we land I'll find the nearest U.S. Naval facility and they'll get a message through to Mom . . .

She studied him in the low light. The weight of the world seemed on his shoulders. He needed a word. He needed to be comforted, absolved. Oh Lord, what was he facing up ahead? Dammit! Gideon and his God-damned ambition. Comfort him, hell—comfort me. I should talk to him. Honey, don't do anything foolish. You can't write the book if you're dead. Come back to us, honey. I love you. Why can't I say I love you?

Gideon tried to work himself up to a pep talk. Someday, he thought, you'll be so proud of this. It's all going to be worthwhile. I'll write the greatest—oh shit, forget it, Zadok. That's all she needs now, a rah-rah Zadok speech from me. Val, I'll make it up to you. I swear it . . .

Wordless, numb.

One o'clock.

Rich Cromwell tapped Gideon on the arm and signaled for him to follow. They went into a side office. Gideon looked at the assemblage. The three military attachés from the embassy glared at him as Cromwell closed the door behind them.

"Shit," Gideon said, "the KGB interrogation team."

"Two hundred French six-by-six trucks arrived at the Haifa port about four hours ago. Somebody is getting ready to transport a lot of troops somewhere," the naval attaché said.

"I didn't clear the shipment," Gideon snapped.

"On the other side of the field here," Rich said, "a dozen French Ouragan fighter planes have landed and they're painting the Star of David over the tricolors."

"Are they going to attack Egypt or not?" the army attaché demanded.

"Is this why you told me to bring my family here? To hold them hostage?"

"We've got a message the Egyptian fighter planes are off the coast," Rich said.

"If I knew," Gideon snarled, "do you think I'd let my wife and daughters fly into them?"

Cromwell's nerve snapped. "You God-damned Jews had better get this question settled of whether you're Americans or not!" His pinkish cheeks turned crimson as their little red veins bulged. He shook his finger at Gideon menacingly. "Now listen, Jew boy, you'd better give it to us and give it to us right."

"Go fuck yourself, you rumheaded cunt. We Jews have paid our passage to be Americans, to make America great. We are the most loyal community America has. You mother-fucking Nantucket-Pasadena lily-white plaid-pants pious Jesus bigot. Up yours, Cromwell!"

Gideon turned to leave.

"Don't go away mad," the naval attaché said. "We were just trying to make sure."

"Are there Egyptian planes out there or not?" Gideon asked.

"We've got some unidentified blips. The Israelis are up patrolling. We'll know soon. We're not supposed to be cooperating with them, but we're bending the rules."

"Sorry about what I said," Rich said.

"I'd like it better if you didn't believe what you told me," Gideon answered, and left.

ONE-FORTY A.M. The Israelis reported that no hostile craft were in their air space or off the coast.

A distant drone was heard, causing an instantaneous stir as everyone staggered to their feet and strained to hear. They're coming! They're landing!

Six awkward-looking C-119 Flying Boxcars were followed in by three Globemaster C-124s, opening their jaws to swallow up the refugees.

Gideon carried Penelope while Valerie guided a staggering Roxanne to the outside where they were counted off. He went back and returned with the seabags. An airman assisted them up the ramp. Val, Penny, and Roxanne were buckled in on folding canvas seats, twenty to a side. The airman tapped Gideon on the shoulder, indicating it was time to leave.

"Happy landing, baby," Gideon said.

Val just nodded. Gideon started down the ramp.

"Gideon!" she called. He turned. "I love you," she said.

For some reason people had become uncomfortable with all the Israeli coins in their pockets which they couldn't spend anyhow. A bucket was passed around and soon it was half filled. An airman handed it to Gideon on the tarmac. In a moment the ramp was pulled up into the craft and the jaws of the plane clamped shut.

Runway lights shot on long enough for the planes to push skyward and disappear.

THE AMERICAN BOXCARS and Globemasters cleared the Israeli coast and turned toward Athens into heavy squalls that sent them into violent plunges. People began vomiting. Completely fatigued, Val held on to the girls, white-lipped, fighting her own nausea. Rain found its way into the cabin, adding to the misery. Unsecured luggage skidded and banged about.

"Mommy!"

"It's all right, honey. Hang in there!"

GIDEON CLOSED the living-room blinds tightly by unrolling the canvas sash, lit a candle, and picked up a packet of letters overlooked during the packing.

Grover Vandover came from the girls' room, where schoolbooks were open, beds turned down, bathroom in slight disarray as if someone had just taken a shower. Everything in place but the people gone. Like a mining town abandoned after a sudden disaster.

Gideon tried to coax some food into Grover Vandover. No dice. He took the dog's temperature: 104°. His most urgent business was to get the animal into Tel Aviv to the vet.

"Come on, buddy, let's get some sleep," he said to Grover. His bedroom was in disorder from the speed with which they had packed. The bed rumpled from her afternoon nap. He stared at it. It had been a good old bed.

"I can't stay here," he mumbled.

He put Grover in the car and took the short drive to the Accadia Hotel. It loomed on its cliffside setting like the grim white elephant it had become. No abandoned Scottish castle was eerier, and it was made more so by the low muffle of the sea.

Gideon opened a side door, put his fingers over the flashlight to cut its beam, and edged down to the basement to the fuse boxes. If I throw the wrong switch I could light up the whole damned place, he thought. He decided against it.

Gideon and his dog took a long, dark, scary walk up four stories in pitch blackness to his office. He bolted the door behind them and lit some candles.

A flash of dreaded loneliness returned. He reached for the phone to call Natasha but remembered the switchboard was closed. Gideon snuggled beside his dog on the couch but his eyes were wide open. He stared at a print on the wall as though he had never seen it before, then rolled to his feet, yawned his way to the desk, and poked through the mail. A letter from his father.

Gideon stared at his father's envelope. He opened it.

My Dearest Son,
   My wits have come to an end. Ten days without so much as a
line, a comma. Ignoring and torturing me in such a way, I assure
you, is not good for my health. If it is necessary that I should
come begging, consider that I have begged. Ten days. It is impossible for you to be so busy. I reject the idea.
   I have heard from my landsmen (people who came from my
home town) of Wolkowysk. Some of them are among the great
pioneers of Israel, such as your late Uncle Matthias (Matti), while
others have escaped from brutal Nazi horrors. All of them are
wonderful people. I love them. From the Wolkowysk community
came a great many intellectuals, rabbis, poets, writers, etc., a
small but very vital community. They have asked repeatedly to
honor you with an evening but are feeling like so many *shmattes*
(rags) and *shnorrers* (beggars) by your evasions that you are too
busy. It would especially be good for Valerie and the girls to learn
of their great cultural accomplishments and particularly so they
shouldn't go around thinking that you are an elitist snob . . .

Gideon crumpled the letter angrily in his fist and felt his breath
growing short and his chest tightening. He took a Tedral pill to stem the
attack.
   "Dad," he cried from his foggy weariness, "for God's sake, I'm in
trouble. Tell me I'm good. Tell me you're proud of me! Where is my
wife? Where are my girls? Dad, I really need somebody to hold my
head."
   The rumpled letter trembled in his fist. He took aim for the trash can,
then laid the letter on his desk and straightened it out and put it in its
file.
   Dawn.
   Gideon rolled up the wooden blinds and watched the sea outside as
daylight came. He stood over the candles and worked up enough breath
to blow them out, then wobbled to the couch. His heavy eyelids could
no longer remain open.
   "Daddy," he said as sleep conquered him. "Daddy, I'm so cold. I'm
so cold. Daddy, warm me up . . . Daddy . . ."

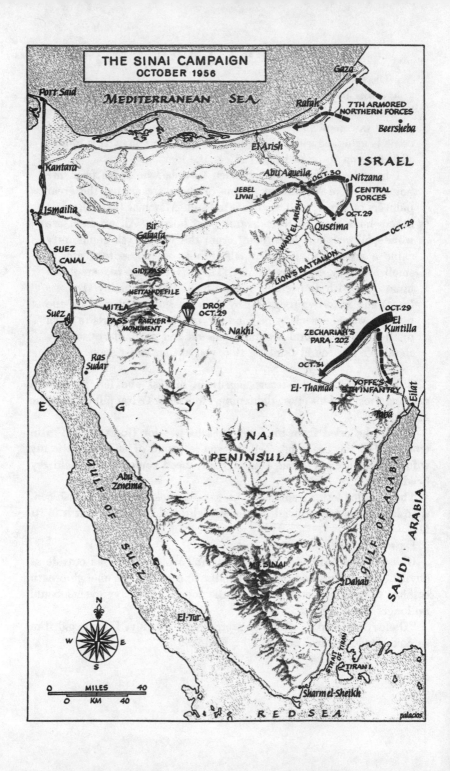

THE SINAI CAMPAIGN
OCTOBER 1956

GIDEON

THE FORMATION of Dakotas plodded deeper into the Sinai, crisscrossing the paths of Moses. The sun made its final gesture, blinking behind the mountains.

The cabin of our plane plunged into darkness. Heat of the day rose off the desert floor and clashed with night air spilling down the mountains. As the formation reached a risky altitude of five hundred feet, fits of turbulence awakened even the deepest sleeper.

Major Ben Asher, the Lions' commander, waved his hand for Shlomo and me to come up front, where they were crammed in over the navigator's desk.

I did a double take, staring at the pilot. I hadn't noticed before, but the pilot was a woman. Ben Asher read the latest message and beamed.

"Hello, writer, squeeze in. Everything looks good now. Our aircraft report no Egyptian air or troop movement along the entire Canal. They haven't got a camel's ass of suspicion."

As Shlomo and I worked our way back to our seats, one by one the paras awoke, yawned, belched, smacked dry lips, fiddled with adjustments on their gear, patted their weapons as though they were girls' backsides, and chatted about the promising news.

The cabin grew so dark I had only vague outlines of their faces. A few of them were bearded, like lions. Many wore kipis on their heads and had opened prayer books and bobbed and weaved, even though they could not read the words for the darkness.

I was suddenly struck by unadulterated, all-consuming terror. I felt
my entire body locking up and feared that normal movement was gone.
The perspiration salted my eyes and my lips turned into dry eroded
cakes. I became afraid to breathe too deeply for I knew that when I
exhaled I would whimper out loud.

My heart pounded audibly as the plane climbed abruptly from under
the Egyptian radar range to the jumping altitude. Shlomo's hand
gripped my arm.

"You'll be all right," he whispered.

"What's the Hebrew word for Geronimo?" I asked.

"Geronimo?"

"That's the American paras' battle cry. Aren't we supposed to give a
bloodcurdling yell as we jump?"

"Believe me, you'll find something to scream," Shlomo said.

The resolution of fear is one of the writer's greatest reasons for being.
What does a man fear most? Being tortured? Being locked in a ward
filled with lunatics or a prison filled with rapists and murderers?

Add to these fears the fear of a surgeon's knife.

Some years back on a routine physical examination my doctor found
a tumor in my chest, maybe the size of a baseball. It was lodged between my lung and aorta. A few days later I was in Denver unpacking a
small suitcase at Rose Hospital, with surgery to commence after several
days of tests.

Val and I were separated at the time. We had to split every so often; a
week, two. We always got back together. I was in Denver with Georgia,
a screwball divorcee who had been married to a musician, among others.
Musicians, as we know, did much pioneering in the use of uncontrolled
substances. Georgia was a very classy lady, one of the first female oil
executives at that period. She loved a wild time and had a real thing for
writers. We were very comfortable with each other, never talked of
marriage or heavy-duty commitments.

When the tumor was found, I talked the doctor into letting me out of
the hospital every night so I could cuddle in with Georgia. What the
hell, the surgeon must have thought, the poor bastard is probably
loaded with cancer, so why not?

The only drug of note going in those days was marijuana. New Wave
stuff. Georgia had a lot of musician buddies and a source of pot. At first
I thought it grew hair in your teeth or made you jump from tall buildings. There was a movie about it in the old days called *Reefer Madness*
and it scared the hell out of me as a kid.

Cancer? So, why not a little marijuana? I reverted to a lot of macho, Marine Corps bullshit. If I was going to die, I was going out with bravado.

Every night I jumped the hospital and Georgia and I would get high and hit every sleazy joint in Denver. Don't laugh when I say Denver. It was still part cowboy town and knew how to take care of a fellow who had had a long dry spell on the dusty cow trails. Raunchy as it gets.

The day before surgery I conned my way out of the hospital on the promise I'd be back by early evening. So, who watches time? Georgia and I always loved playing fantasy and we had pretty fertile minds. We made up a wish list and damned if she didn't go up on the runway at Jake Foxe's, the local strip joint, on amateur night. And Georgia put on quite a show. I got off watching the guys at the front table and she got off watching me get off and damned if we didn't pick up another stripper—but that's another story.

What has this morbid tale of lust and vulgarity to do with the resolution of fear? I recall the exact fraction of a second it happened. The three of us were crossing Colfax Avenue. We were making for a little private club-type hideaway of black musicians to find more substance.

As we were waiting for the signal lights to change, the thought of tomorrow's surgery flashed through my mind. I said to myself, If I could magically change my condition and trade places with anyone in the world at this moment, who would it be?

Churchill? Babe Ruth? Clark Gable? Who would I be? The answer was Gideon Zadok. Facing an operation with less than a fifty-fifty chance of survival, I just wanted to be me . . . with a girl on each arm getting blasted and heading for a whorehouse motel. I was satisfied with what I had done with my life . . . won a big battle . . . written some very fine stuff . . . never compromised as a writer. I had remorse for my sins and tried to pay them off by being a good man. I faced the rotten side of me head-on. In sum, I was damned pleased with myself and I guess I was ready to die.

In this very strange, wonderful moment waiting on Colfax Avenue for the lights to change my fear vanished. No regrets. What a wonderful way to go into an operating theater.

Sometime after midnight and before dawn I returned to my hospital room. The anesthetist was in a rage. I confessed to the various ingredients I had ingested.

"You've got some milkshake in you, Zadok. One more night like this and you won't need surgery."

The operation was postponed until I was detoxed—with an armed guard on my door.

But the main thing was—I wasn't afraid! I wasn't afraid when they wheeled me through those moonshot sliding stainless steel doors. I wasn't afraid as the anesthesia swept over me . . . "So long, world, it's been a real slice."

The wind at the Dakota jump door jolted me. I stood at the edge. I was not afraid! I hurtled out into space, then slowed. All about me chutes billowed open like a fleet of sailboats setting spinnakers.

I wanted to freeze the moment forever. Maybe even reverse my direction and float off into galaxies unknown.

As the formation of Dakotas banked and raced back to Israel, their engines hushed and faded altogether. We were alone, far behind enemy lines. I became aware of the flapping of the chutes and little whumping noises that abruptly ended the short but magnificent odyssey.

Real world below! Laborious grunts, curses, sharply delivered commands. I had kept my legs in good shape over the years, if not my liver, but my knees had been trashed out from years of skiing and motorcycling. Most writers try to imitate the tough-guy image. Having neither the desire nor stomach to murder unarmed animals, I drifted away from my imitation Hemingway routine and let myself become Gideon Zadok, whatever he might be. But it had all come too late to save the knees.

My feet barely brushed the ground when my body swung over like a pendulum and I whammed down hard on my right hip and was dragged along a stretch of ground. It had been much easier than I contemplated —or so I thought until I tried to move about.

Although my hip was numbed from the blow, I was still able to wrestle with my chute and Shlomo was all over me getting me unharnessed.

JESUS! GOD! I'D DONE IT! I FELT GREAT! GIDEON ZADOK! YOU'RE GREAT! GREAT! GREAT!

When Shlomo and I hugged each other like reunited refugee brothers, I realized my celebration was premature. I collapsed in his arms, then fell to the ground. While Shlomo helped me test my leg, the battalion was engaged rapidly in the organized chaos that follows a night drop. Officers and NCOs snapped orders in Hebrew that were responded to with amazing speed and efficiency, considering the blackness. They gathered into units at a rendezvous point around Major Ben Asher.

Shlomo assisted me as I hobbled to a medical tent where the injured

were being collected. There were a dozen of us, mostly sprains but a few
serious injuries.

Dr. Schwartz and a medic ran a flashlight over my body. My hip was
ballooning and darkening, but after a few excruciating tests the doctor
felt there was no break or fracture.

"What is it?"

"Nice, plump hematoma. You broke an artery that will collect a
quart or so of blood."

"Prognosis?"

"It's going to be painful for the first night but in three days or so you
should be able to start moving around."

The doc lifted my shirt in search of further injuries and shook his
head as he saw Natasha's handiwork on my back.

"What the hell did you land on? A cactus?"

"Wound from a previous engagement," I said.

"Remain here with the injured," he ordered and went to the next
man.

The officers gathered around Ben Asher as the Lions secured the
landing. There was some argument and confusion among them. Apparently we had been dropped three miles off target.

So far, shithouse luck. No response from the Egyptians, who we believed were holed up inside Mitla Pass. They certainly must have seen
and heard us come down. Ben Asher ordered his crack outfit, the Recon
platoon, to move up close to the Pass and prevent any Egyptians from
breaking out, then looked over the injured. The final tally was remark-
ably low. We had assorted sprains and bruises and only two paratroopers with broken legs. There was no way the injured could keep up with
the rest of the battalion which had to force-march and dig in behind the
Recon platoon. Two squads were left to guard us as the battalion moved
out.

There were to be continuous air drops of supplies during the night,
including jeeps. If and when they arrived, the jeeps could move the
injured up to battalion.

A night of feverish activity lay ahead for the battalion to reach the
proper site and set up defenses. The precise place was the Parker Monument, a stone near the eastern end of the Pass.

So here I was, at long last, the wandering writer in Apache country,
with a basketball-sized hip and the exhilaration of the parachute jump
knocked out of me. Out here in Moses' bailiwick with the Lions. How
romantic. The numbness was wearing off and pain was ascending.

Where were Valerie and my daughters? And Natasha? She was probably at the Prime Minister's office, drawn and strained, waiting for word that the para drop had succeeded. Some triangle I had created. Oh shit, man, the pain was really coming on. I'd been enough of a hero for one day.

"Shlomo?"

"Yes?"

"It's starting to hurt like hell, buddy. Soon as Doc Schwartz is free, maybe he can give me something."

"Something" turned out to be a shot of morphine. Merciful stuff. It took over in minutes. Time began to pass in irregular flights . . . I dozed and woke up fuzzy to the sounds of low-flying aircraft. Supplies were being parachuted in.

"How's it going?" someone asked.

It was impossible for me to focus. "That you, Shlomo?"

"Yes."

"I'm on queer street. Actually, it feels pretty wild. What's happening?"

"Battalion has reached the Parker Monument. The Egyptians sent out a patrol for a look. We drove them back into the Pass. Well, everyone in Cairo knows we've arrived."

He helped me to a sitting position and I luxuriated on a few sips of water.

"You might as well go back to sleep," Shlomo said, "they aren't scheduled to drop the jeeps for at least a couple of hours." His voice sounded hollow and far away. . . . I leaned back on a pile of rolled-up parachutes . . . soft, lovely . . . all things had become hazy . . . really weird . . . hey, Penny, how about Daddy reading you *The Little Engine That Could* . . . I could feel her sweet soft little cheek against mine . . .

. . . why, Roxanne old bean . . . you're getting to be a woman . . . Girl Scouts having a slumber party, giggling and shouting from the guest cottage . . . there were three little bras in the freezer, some joke . . .

Roxanne wants a formal gown? She's barely twelve! Well, Dad's going to the dress shop with you. I don't want anything risqué . . .

. . . you see, I never got my tuxedo but by God, my girls are going to have the most beautiful gowns money can buy! Gideon's daughters are knockouts! I never did get to the prom—wonder what happened to the girl who invited me? What was her name? Phoebe. Yeah, Phoebe. I loved to dance with her; she'd make all the guys have hard-ons in two minutes—they'd limp off the dance floor . . .

. . . sorry, Phoebe, I won't be able to take you to the prom, but thanks for inviting me, huh . . .

. . . I read that letter so many times, I knew it by heart. Why did I keep it in a top drawer and read it again and again?

Philadelphia, March 10, 1940
My Dear Son Gideon,

Finally I received from you a letter after a week of an empty mailbox. Do you know what that can do to a father, especially a sensitive, loving father like myself?

You have demanded of me that I supply you with a T-U-X.

Before I knew what T-U-X means, I had to find out. I had a hard time because all my friends are working people who likewise have no knowledge of a T-U-X.

When it was finally explained I was horrified, shocked at your ideas of grandeur. I don't know whether you mean to get a job as a hotel porter or a servant for a millionaire family or become a music hall entertainer or work in a nite club. For what purpose do you strive for a T-U-X? To become a Charlie McCarthy dummy?

Anyhow, it is not something you should become involved with and I am sorry that I have to refuse you. It sounds to me like you are intending to go every night to a party.

Gideon, my sonny boy! You may think that I am old-fashioned, but I am not. I am an advanced modern thinker. I know the desires and moods of a young man but there is a limit to everything.

I never refused you a school ring, and I should have . . . but, the reason for the delay is that I am again financially tied up and second, I inquired the price of such a ring and it should not— definitely—cost $9.00. You will be cheated to pay $9.00.

If you need so bad a suit clothing or other *necessary* things, I always do my best to see to it you should have it, even though there are delays due to finances but don't be misled or ill-advised that a T-U-X is the only thing you must have. Don't forget that the tux alone is not the end of it but the beginning. With a tux you will be asking for more money to go with girls to those places where a tux is required.

I beg of you, sonny! Do not be misguided. Think straight and listen sometimes to my advice. You are young and you can make the best foundation for your future life if you will listen to me and not go wrong. Take my advice and you will be thankful to me some day. After all, I have no other children to give advice and love to.

Your job now is school so you should not be all your life, a manual worker like me. Incidentally, didn't you tell me you were cleaning the locker room at the school? Isn't that enough for you to pay for your T-U-X?

I know I was supposed to see you in Baltimore next week but I can't come. I have a cold and I don't think it will be better in time. Besides I am financially strapped for a train ticket and the doctor said I shouldn't travel. I am thinking of you, mainly, so I shouldn't give to you my cold.

So tell your girlfriend that I am not old-fashioned.

I will not forgive you for not writing, so you had better write twice every week.

So long. Remember, I love you.

Your loving father,

Nathan

P.S. In addition to the regular $3.50 a week I am now paying support to your mother, I enclose an extra fifty cents for you. Sorry I can't see you. Write!

"HEY, Gideon, wake up!"

"What . . . wha . . . wha . . ."

"Get yourself together, Gideon. You're crying like a baby in your sleep."

I leaned against Shlomo and wept. . . . "Sorry . . ."

"Hey, forget it. It's the morphine."

"We're in the middle of the Sinai, right?"

"Yes."

"Sorry, I'm really wacko."

"How's your leg?"

"Don't feel any pain."

A piercing chill cut through me, sending me into sudden and rather violent shakes. It was bitter cold. Shlomo wrapped me in a pair of blankets and beat on me until I warmed.

"Desert really gets cold this time of the year," Shlomo said.

"I'm freezing . . . I'm freezing," I said, praying for that blissful stuff to take me over. The painkiller surged through me and the floating sensations began again, only the coldness wouldn't go away. Damned I'm cold . . . "Daddy . . . Daddy . . . I'm freezing, Daddy . . ."

Philadelphia, 1926

Little Gideon's mittens were soaked through. The numbness of his fingers matched the numbness of his nose and his toes.

"We'd better go home and get you warm," Molly said.

"No," he answered, "I want to finish the snowman."

"Come on," she said, picking her brother up. His weight forced her to tilt for balance as she puffed through the snow, out of Fairmount Park to the sidewalk. She looked right and left for streetcars and automobiles and seeing an opening, ran across Parkside Avenue.

She set Gideon down, took his hand and half dragged him up the four flights of stairs to their flat. Pain was setting in in the little boy's extremities, and by the time they reached the door he was crying.

The odor of frying liver and onions reached their nostrils as Molly opened the door. That meant two things. A payment had been made to the gas company and the stove and hot-water heater had been turned on. It also meant that Momma had given the butcher enough on account for her to make a purchase. When they fell too far in arrears, Momma would send Molly and Gideon to the grocer or butcher to play on their sympathies. Sometimes the butcher was feeding his own family on scraps but couldn't stand the stares of children who were obviously hungry.

"That child is not a well child," Momma said. "You shouldn't have had him out in the park for so long. You should get a spanking."

"He's fine, Momma, just a little cold," Molly said, unbuttoning Gideon's dripping jacket and laying it on the radiator. Momma went to the hot-water heater and lit a match. The fire flared on with a whomp and a hiss. Oh boy, hot baths, Molly thought. She stripped her brother and bundled him in his big wool robe with the Indian teepee designs on it, closed off the alcove curtain and changed herself, as well.

As they waited for the water to heat up, Momma opened the icebox and gave each of them a slice of apple. Momma bought old fruit that was about to spoil from the pushcart vendor and could often pick up a half-dozen pieces for a nickel or a dime.

Gideon ate shivering. They heard the slow, familiar steps of Nathan agonizing his way up the stairs. Nathan was Gideon's daddy, but not Molly's. She did not remember her own father.

Nathan entered and, without greeting, set his dilapidated briefcase on the table. He was a small man, barely five feet tall. His long, thin face was permanently etched in a pinch of dismay.

Gideon slipped off his chair and stood in front of his father and stared up at him until Nathan had to become aware of his son's presence.

"Daddy, I'm cold," the boy said.

For that moment, Nathan set aside his own misery, picked up his son, and held him on his lap. He rubbed warmth into the boy's fingers and toes and wrapped his arms about him and rocked him back and forth tenderly.

Nathan sang the words of a lullaby in Yiddish. The child was a little bird and should not be frightened, for his mother and father were guarding the nest.

Gideon smiled and laid his head on his daddy's chest and lingered. It was to be the lone memory of physical contact and affection from his father.

PART TWO

SHTETL BOY

WHITE RUSSIA

Wolkowysk, 1906

SOPHIE ZADOK stopped kneading dough for a moment, wiped her hands on her apron, and rocked the cradle to soothe her screaming infant.

"You're a beautiful thing, little Reuben," she said, pinching his cheek. She sang in a sweet voice a lullaby about the parent birds guarding the nest. A change of diapers and a tit and Reuben was content.

It had been a good cradle, holding all seven of her children, four boys and three girls. Miracle of miracles, all of them survived. The cradle was permanently at stoveside during the day for warmth and because it was where Sophie spent most of her waking hours.

Nathan, the eldest, who had just turned ten, stood by the door for a moment and listened. He had heard his momma sing that song to six of his brothers and sisters. He didn't remember her ever singing to him. Maybe he was too young to remember. More likely, he thought, she never sang to him.

Nathan was a small, frail child, often sick and endowed with a nature that was perpetually surly. He never seemed to engage in laughter. Not that there was that much for Jews to laugh about.

Yet, there was relief from the misery, ecstatic outbreaks of pure joy. Not a week passed without a wedding or *bris* or *bar mitzvah*. There were the holidays and the Sabbath as well, for happiness. But happiness eluded Nathan.

Although his father, Yehuda, was considered part of the clergy, the family was not nearly as fanatic in their observances as the ultra-Orthodox and sects of Hasidim. Sophie had adamantly refused to shave her head and wear the traditional married woman's wig when she wed her husband. Her defiance was considered a serious matter for a time, one that tested the wisdom of the rabbi and the elders.

Wolkowysk was a small city, partly modernized and industrialized and not so isolated and therefore a bit more advanced in its thinking. Other girls, too, were rebelling against the iron dictates of rabbinical tyranny.

Nathan was happy his mother had won because she had beautiful hair which she twisted into a large bun in the back of her head. When times became desperate, she would cut off some of her hair and braid it into a switch and sell it to the wig shop. It always grew back, but each time it was a little grayer.

In Wolkowysk the younger boys and girls were now allowed to dance with one another at celebrations. This was a very modern innovation. Nathan tried it a few times but he felt awkward and ashamed because the girls were always taller. He was afraid to touch them because he knew it could lead to trouble and he wondered why the boys in his class talked about girls so much. Didn't they all realize that the matchmakers were on the prowl, watching the children from an early age for a likely *shiddach* a few years down the line? If an arrangement were made for Nathan he could end up just like his mother and father, doomed to a life of poverty and fear. He would do better. He'd escape the Pale one day and become wealthy. Then all of the family would have to come to him and bow before him. He would be kind and generous to them, despite the way they had mistreated him. This would be his delicious revenge. He would be nice to Momma but quite stern with his father. As for his brothers, he'd make them crawl. This was Nathan's great dream. His sisters would come humbly before him and beg him to put up a large dowry so they would be able to capture an important husband. Oh, the power he would exert!

Nathan stood over the cradle and poked his finger in the baby's stomach, ostensibly to draw a smile, but he was too rough and Reuben screamed his displeasure. Sophie slapped Nathan's hand and admonished him to do his chores. He backed away from the crib wondering how many more babies they were going to have.

Nathan carried two buckets of water in from the pump, wobbling under the weight of the yoke, then gathered wood from the shed and stoked up the stove, which was both hearthstone and slave master of the house.

Today was window-washing day. Where were his brothers Mordechai and Matthias? Probably playing stickball or, worse, that *goyim* game of soccer. Nathan didn't like to play the games. He was afraid of getting roughed up. That damned Mordechai knew how to avoid his chores, and when things weren't done Poppa always blamed Nathan, often with a clout to the ear.

Mordechai, who was a year younger, was the bright scholar, the apple of Yehuda Zadok's eye. Even now, with Nathan earning a ruble a week as a runner for the savings and loan office after school, Mordechai didn't have to fill in with chores at home. Nathan often fantasized punching Mordechai half to death, but his brother was larger than he and very mean.

There were big celebrations when sons were born, but Nathan liked it better when he had a new sister. The girls didn't get so much attention and at least they grew up knowing how to work.

Rifka, Sarah, and even little Ida always had busy hands. Sophie prepared them to be homemakers almost as soon as they could walk. Before the daughters came, Momma did everything: baking and cooking and making the candles; sweeping and scrubbing and washing and ironing; mending and dressmaking; bearing children and nursing and mothering; keeping the vegetable plot and running a kosher home. Sophie was a splendid *balabosta*. How she managed to make ends meet was through incredible manipulation. And she taught her girls, early and well. Nathan frankly preferred his sisters for another reason. As a male, he was allowed to boss them around.

YEHUDA ZADOK was the *shohet* of Wolkowysk, the ritual slaughterer of chickens, an ancient profession first dictated in the Book of Deuteronomy. Each chicken was accorded a brief benediction, then dispatched quickly and with the least amount of pain and in a manner to assure they were kosher.

The tool of his trade was a ten-inch knife with a blunted end. He had a half dozen of these, made of the finest German steel and honed to exquisite sharpness. Yehuda kept them in hand-tooled leather cases which he carried in a little black bag along with other paraphernalia of the trade.

When Nathan was very young he enjoyed going with his father to the slaughterhouse behind the poultry market and watching him at work. His father's hands were sure and swift like lightning. He did the bird in with one clean stroke across the neck, plunged it into a vat of hot water, said a prayer, and plucked it clean in a matter of seconds. It was a matter of great pride that Yehuda never left pinfeathers in his birds. The rabbis periodically examined Yehuda's chickens to assure his proficiency and never found an improperly killed bird.

Nathan's early fascination turned sour when he realized his father was grooming him to follow in his footsteps. He didn't want to spend the rest of his life slitting chickens' throats, especially when he felt that Mordechai would end up as a rabbi.

Moreover, his father's bloody hands and bespattered apron always had a chicken smell. Even the weekly ritual bath at the *mikva* failed to completely deodorize him.

Yehuda was paid a few kopeks for each bird. In a good day he could pocket a few rubles, scarcely enough to sustain his family. He found a variety of odd jobs, mainly sharpening knives and scissors, to augment the family income.

There were benefits. He could take out some of his pay in chickens, so there was usually enough to eat. Sophie knew how to utilize every part of the bird, except the parts that were not kosher. Extra chickens were traded for carp at the fish market or vegetables and milk from the gentile farmers. Even during the years of drought, when half the chickens died of heat prostration, there was some food on the table.

The main benefit of being the *shohet* was that it was an honorable, if undesirable, profession. Life in a *shtetl* town centered around the synagogue. Yehuda Zadok was a learned man in Talmud and his job accorded him a certain communal respect.

The synagogue had a rigid social structure. The building was always constructed so that the most sacred place, the Ark, was on the Eastern Wall which faced Jerusalem. Seated along the Eastern Wall, according to rank, prominence, and respect, were the rabbi, cantor, and other town dignitaries. The last seats were reserved for the *shohet* and the *shammes* or sexton.

The townspeople sat in the main body of the building facing the Eastern Wall. The closer to the Ark, the higher the communal rank. Wealth, of course, could acquire such a seat. Behind the first rows were the ordinary people and the poor. Farthest removed, along the Western Wall, were the beggars, town misfits, and visiting strangers. A small balcony, veiled off by latticework, was reserved for the women.

Yehuda Zadok was gentler than most of the heads of households. Generally the father's outlet against eternal frustration was to impose an authoritarian reign. Corporal punishment of children was common and wife beating was not uncommon. Yehuda seldom whipped his children, except when the futility of daily existence periodically crashed down on him. But his hands were always swift in delivering a single clout to the head or yank on the ear, usually Nathan's.

A crisis was brewing in the Zadok household, as Nathan and Mordechai were reaching an age where plans were to be made concerning their future education. Until now, his sons had attended *cheder*, a small one-room school connected to the synagogue. The subjects were Yiddish and Hebrew and, later, the Talmud.

The *cheder* was little less than a glorified cell; the teacher often a cruel ignorant authoritarian. His reward was to hold power over ragged, half-starved little boys. The hours were exhausting and the rabbi or teacher ruled with a leather strap. Textbooks were a few tattered volumes and modern methods and subjects were unknown. Nathan had been an adequate student, a survivor. Mordechai was singled out as exceptional and received tender treatment. By the age of nine he was a veritable fountain of Talmudic and religious knowledge.

The next stage would normally be to go up to yeshiva, a larger school, which also taught state-approved secular courses in Russian and mathematics.

Yeshiva posed a serious problem for Yehuda Zadok: there was a tuition of a ruble and fifty kopeks a week as well as other expenses for books and materials. A rich man's game. It was boiling down to making a choice between Nathan and Mordechai. As the oldest, Nathan was entitled to attend yeshiva first, but two sons in an advanced school was a luxury that a *shohet* could scarcely afford. Yehuda had been thinking all along of sending Nathan to a trade school so he could help with the family finances until he became a *shohet*.

Nathan had a secret listening post into his parents' discussions. His cot was against the wall next to their bedroom. If he stayed up late enough when they spoke, he could hold a glass against the wall and make out their conversation.

"It would be unfair to deprive Nathan of yeshiva," his mother argued.

"And it would be criminal to deprive Mordechai," Yehuda retorted.

"So Nathan is not by any means a genius, he is still our oldest."

"What am I? The Baron Rothschild? Sophie, we'd not only be sending the wrong head to learn, but we'd be losing a ruble a week that Nathan earns. We are elastic, but elastic also breaks. Since the Lord singled me out for personal abuse, it is reality that we cannot put two boys through yeshiva at the same time. It takes no rabbinical court to tell which son is which."

"And Matthias, and one day, Reuben?"

"So, by the time they are ready for yeshiva, Nathan will be a *shohet* with a full salary."

Sophie rushed in to argue the injustice of it but her case was as thin as the wall.

"Besides," Yehuda said as an afterthought, "it is sometimes beyond difficult to be nice to that boy. Nathan is bitter. If only he didn't wear a face like rhubarb."

Nathan heard it all. He clenched the sheet in his little fists and wept on the pillow. I'll show them! I'll run away from home! I can make two rubles a week peddling to the army camp.

Yehuda became more interested in his wife. Their lovemaking had fascinated Nathan at first, the way he was fascinated by watching his father kill chickens. Over a period of time their grunting and slobbering had grown grotesque. He had overheard Momma speaking among the women. She really didn't like doing it. Her insides were bad from having so many children and it caused her great pain. Yet she could not deny her husband. Nathan covered his ears. His father was sounding like an animal.

LIKE MOST CHILDREN, Nathan was of the belief that his mother and father were either ignorant or naïve about what was happening in the world around them. Yehuda Zadok had long mastered the art of contemplation while he prepared chickens for kosher. He was aware that certain past and present realities dictated future realities.

Yehuda was a boy of six when the pogroms of the early 1880s flared up throughout the Jewish Pale of Settlement. His hometown, Kiev, had a particularly odious history of persecution. Forever seared into his young mind was a horrendous night when the Cossacks stampeded the Jewish quarters and bashed in skulls, burned down synagogues, and looted and raped in an unrestrained frenzy of Jew hating—behavior encouraged and supported by the church and the czarist government.

Yehuda tried to get to the synagogue to rescue his father, who had entered the burning building to save the sacred Torah scrolls. The boy was caught by a pair of drunken Cossacks, severely beaten, and left for dead.

His body eventually healed but his brain had sealed in, and was condemned to perpetually replay, the sight of his father's smoking corpse.

WHEN ISLAM came to power in the Arab lands in the seventh century, the main Jewish population of Europe was centered in the Rhineland where they lived a precarious existence and were continually victimized by Papal-inspired scourges.

During the Crusades of the ninth, tenth, and eleventh centuries, legions of rabble were recruited in the Rhineland for the fight to regain the Holy Land. Maniacal monks, supported by a perverse church, whipped up an ignorant peasantry into blood orgies against the Jews, then marched off under the banners of Jesus Christ on their sacred mission to save Jerusalem from those other heathens, the Moslems.

In a desperation to escape, hundreds of thousands of Jews fled eastward into the feudal serfdoms of Poland and Russia. Most came at the invitation of the nobility, who needed Jewish skills to establish a middle class of merchants, craftsmen, bankers, physicians, and men of commerce, all areas where Jews excelled.

Jewish history in Eastern Europe was to be enveloped in an eternal pall of gray. When the Russians of the north halted the advance of the Moslem armies from the south, reign over all of Russia fell to the Czars of Moscow in league with the Greek Orthodox Church. Jews were offered the dubious opportunity of converting to Christianity. During the Middle Ages, thousands of Jews were burned at the stake for rejecting the honor. Conversion attempts were so unsuccessful over the ages that Catherine I unleashed a series of pogroms in the early 1700s which climaxed with the expulsion of a million Jews from Russia to Poland.

An era of wars and conquest was launched by a successor, Catherine the Great, with the result that Poland was repartitioned a number of times and Russia reinherited the Jews who had been previously evicted.

Thus started a never-ending series of laws banning Jews from trades and ownership of land, and excluding them from Moscow and St. Petersburg where they were considered to be in competition with Christian professionals.

It all evolved into the establishment of a huge reservation in which the Jews had to live and beyond which the Jews were forbidden to go. The Pale of Settlement consisted of a million square miles from the Baltic to the Black Sea, one monstrous ghetto where they were trapped, divorced from the mainstream of Russian life, and reduced to basic survival.

This was the birth of the *shtetl*, a string of towns and small cities open to Jews. Although the law of the Czar was all-powerful, the *shtetl* towns themselves gained a certain autonomy. The Jews ran their own social and health programs and religious courts, spoke the unique Yiddish language, operated their own schools and printing presses, and mainly kept each other alive through a magnificent system of charity.

With Jews restricted to a few basic crafts and trades, boycotted from higher education, facing a constant barrage of suppressive laws, and subjected to the outrages of pogroms, *shtetl* life was a birth-to-death privation.

A few Jews were able to slip through the net and were given dispensation to live in the great cities, but they were the rare cases. Such permission was granted to a handful of the wealthy or talented or cunning whose value to the Czar made them the exceptions.

Despite the shabbiness of dress and humbleness of home, life in the *shtetl* had a magnificent and vital heartbeat. Much of the *shtetl* was in the grip of the tyrannical rabbis and cults, but otherwise there was harbored a smoldering genius of unmeasurable magnitude. Toward the end of the nineteenth century, a new rhythm overtook the *shtetl* and it was relentlessly probing to liberate itself.

The pogroms of the 1880s became the flashpoint. Feeling neither love for "mother" Russia, nor loyalty to the Czars, the Jews bolted out of the country in massive numbers after the latest series of state-approved blood baths.

AFTER HIS FEARSOME beating during the Kiev pogrom, Yehuda Zadok seriously considered emigrating. His older brother, Samuel, had fled Russia for the questionable alternative of becoming a pushcart peddler in Chicago.

Samuel Zadok pushed his cart well—right out of the seething cauldron of Chicago into a small, mobile mercantile business that followed the silver strikes in Colorado. This resulted in a small general store in the frontier town of Denver. His oldest son had been accepted into a university to study medicine and two other sons were going to follow to college. America! America! What a wondrous place. Even Samuel's daughter was earmarked for higher education. Can you imagine?

For a time Samuel urged Yehuda and his other close kin to emigrate, but Yehuda was a child mired in the *shtetl* without the necessary ambition or courage to wrest himself loose from the grasp of his narrow, tortured life. After all, what could a *shohet* with a growing family do in America? That *shtetl* was a pitiful and marginal way to go through life, but at least it was familiar. America was a wild and frightening place. Here in Wolkowysk, Yehuda knew he could always scrape through and he did have that seat on the Eastern Wall.

His brother Samuel left an abundance of needy relatives in Russia and he was as generous to them as he was able. Often the international postal money order had kept Yehuda from going under. Yehuda accepted, but never asked. He had made his own bed.

A new idea was making headway among the Jews and that was the resettlement and redemption of Palestine. Many of the younger people chose the Holy Land and left with a spirit of pioneers. The movement to Zion was small by comparison to the flood going to America, but it carried extraordinary zeal.

The return to Zion was codified by a Viennese Jew, Theodor Herzl, at a convention in Basel, Switzerland, and soon had organizations in every *shtetl.*

In 1905, the year of Reuben's birth, another series of pogroms erupted. General discontent was spreading all over Russia and somehow the venom was turned against the Jews, as it had always been. In the neighboring city of Bialystok the suffering was particularly horrible for the Jews at the hands of the army.

Breezes of change became winds of change. Yehuda Zadok was wise enough to know that his sons would probably want to emigrate. He had silently prepared himself to let them go. All of them, except Mordechai.

Mordechai was the flesh of his flesh, the soul of his soul. A young man immersed in Talmud, immersed in Yiddish, prepared for *shtetl* life. Although the *shtetl* was splintering, some, like him, could never leave it. He was determined to salvage his own life and perpetuate it through Mordechai.

When Nathan's turn at rebellion came, Yehuda was ready. Irreversible forces of history were at work and Yehuda had made a pragmatic decision of what to preserve and what to let go.

IT WAS A pleasant spring day. Yehuda was feeling chipper. Max Pinsker, owner of the textile mill, had had his first son born to him. Max was one of a half-dozen wealthy members of the community and a major benefactor of his fellow Jews. He supported the yeshiva among his other notable charitable causes and almost no one begrudged him his seat on the Eastern Wall.

There was a residue of bitterness when the union attempted to organize his factory. He stopped the attempt ruthlessly. Everyone knew the labor people were wild radicals and agitators filled with anarchist philosophies coming out of Russia. They were no damned good! Moreover, Max was humane to his employees, more or less.

One of Yehuda's positions was that of the *mohel*, the circumciser. It was an honorary job but no one failed to slip the *mohel* a couple of rubles for his services. There were always a few slices of cake from the celebration for him to take home to his family.

From a man so esteemed as Max Pinsker came a ten-ruble gratuity for the circumcision. This was a week's earnings. Yehuda was feeling a bit tipsy and expansive from a tad too much wine at the celebration. What was more, the Sabbath was coming and already people were passing him and bowing.

"Good *shabbas*, Rev Zadok."

"Good *shabbas*, good *shabbas*."

Mordechai was at his father's side, hands clasped piously behind him, imitating his gestures. Of course, the title of "Rev" was also honorary, to denote Yehuda as a learned man. Mordechai would become a true rabbi, a real Reb.

Sophie grabbed her husband as he entered the cottage and with a special urgency that suddenly dampened the spring day.

"Mordechai, look after your brothers and sisters and get them ready for *shul*," she ordered. "Yehuda, come with me."

She led him across the yard to the woodshed. Nathan sat shriveled in a corner, his nose streaked with dried blood, his shirt torn and his cheeks bruised.

"Will someone kindly inform me what is going on?"

"He tried to run away. He took three rubles from my thimble box. The police brought him back, looking like this."

"Stand up, Nathan," his father demanded sharply.

The boy struggled to his feet warily, sniffling.

"What happened?"

"*Goyim* caught him on the road. They took his money from him," his mother said.

"You little *goniff!*" Yehuda cried, raising his hand to deliver a clout. On further note, he decided that his son didn't need another *klop*. "So where did you think you were going with three rubles, to China? Speak up!"

"Bialystok," he answered in a quivering voice. "I was going to take the exam to enter the gymnasium."

"Gymnasium! Not even yeshiva, but gymnasium. Such fancy ideas! The blood is still flowing in the streets of Bialystok and you have a head filled with notions of grandeur. You'll go to gymnasium when onions grow in the palm of my hand. Get into the house and stay in your room. You will not come to *shul* tonight."

Nathan limped off. His father had not even asked about his injuries. Late that night, with the pain from the blows fully settled in, Nathan groaned close to the wall, put a glass against it, and listened to his mother and father.

"That boy is like a board with a hole in it," his mother said. "We are lucky not to be having a funeral."

"We can't spit on the truth," Yehuda said.

"And what is the truth?"

"Mordechai is the one who must go to yeshiva. It would be a waste to send Nathan. I don't know where he got the crazy business in his head of gymnasium. I'll talk to the savings and loan and maybe they will give him a full-time job."

"Now who's talking crazy? He'll run away again."

"Maybe you can tell me how we are going to support his elegant ideas?"

Sophie, as usual, was slightly ahead of her husband. "If Nathan goes to Bialystok, his bed here will become available and we can take in an out-of-town yeshiva student and charge the family two rubles, which, in turn, we will use to pay for Nathan's room and board in Bialystok. So, what's the loss?"

"What about the ruble a week we will lose from Nathan's salary at the savings and loan? And Mordechai will have expenses at yeshiva on top of it."

"So, you'll have to ask your brother, Sam."

"I can't *shnorr* him. Sam is not a well man and he hasn't had such a good year in business. Besides, he's supporting our mother and God knows how many relatives."

"He wouldn't turn you down, Yehuda, not when it comes to education."

"It gives me such a lump in my chest to have to ask him."

"I know what Mordechai means to you," Sophie said after a long time, "but Nathan will have to be on his own sooner or later. Even emigrate. We are duty-bound to give him the best education he can get. We'll manage, we'll manage."

Bialystok, 1906

KALONYMUS WISSOTZKY, the "Tea King of Russia," was among those elite Jews given dispensation to live in Moscow. The fortune he amassed as an international merchant was given away to charity nearly as fast as he earned it.

After the pogroms of the 1880s, it was apparent that there must be an alternative to the misery his fellow Jews endured in Russia. Along with the Baron Rothschild and a number of other Jewish philanthropists, Wissotzky helped found and support the new movements to Palestine.

Wissotzky died just about the time of the renewed pogroms of 1903, but with the knowledge that Zionism had taken root and a door of escape was now opened out of Russia.

His entire fortune was left to a foundation which dispensed moneys to innumerable charities throughout the Pale. One of these was the gymnasium in Bialystok that bore his name and to which Nathan Zadok came in 1906.

Nathan found living quarters in the home of Esther Ginsburg, the widow of a leather worker in the impoverished Channakes district. Over the years she housed a number of students from Wolkowysk. Her rate of two rubles, fifty kopeks a week was the cheapest to be found. For this she provided a bed and four meals a week, and washed and mended the boys' clothing.

Nathan was faced with a new problem, hunger. No matter how bad things had been at home, there had always been some part of a chicken to eat. Here it was a luxury.

Fortunately there were designated "eat" days for the poorer students, a dubious distinction for which Nathan qualified. On Mondays, Wednesdays, and the Sabbath, different families alternated in feeding the students an evening meal. It was mostly lentils, cabbage dishes, potatoes, and a concoction with a carp base called gefilte fish. Few and far between were whiffs of even the stringiest meat.

On the Sabbath, the students fared a little better because this day brought out the pious instincts of some of the more affluent families. But the gnawing edge of hunger never left Nathan's belly.

During his first year, when Nathan had no seniority in Mrs. Ginsburg's home, his bed was a lumpy couch in the living room where his single blanket had to be augmented for warmth by newspapers he piled on himself.

Otherwise Bialystok was a revelation to Nathan, a city burgeoning with culture and surging with currents and countercurrents of ideologies.

The smaller towns of the *shtetl* generally wore a uniform coat of drabness. What distinguished one from another was the degree of orthodoxy and the domination by one of a number of religious sects.

Bialystok was dramatically different. Located at a crossroads between Russia, Poland, and Prussia, the Jews originally settled at the invitation of the Polish nobility, where they became purveyors to the advancing, retreating, and occupying armies. Bialystok grew into a major textile center. By the turn of the twentieth century, over three hundred and fifty mills were in operation and these were almost entirely Jewish-owned.

This brought a strong trade union movement with heavy socialist leanings. Largely because of Wissotzky's personal interest in Bialystok, equally strong Zionist organizations took early root. When these diverse groups were added to the traditional *shtetl* religious sects, a Yiddish press and theater, capitalists, czarists, and an assortment of intellectuals, freethinkers, and mystics, Bialystok was a lively mix.

All these philosophies found their way into the Wissotzky Gymnasium, which proved to be liberal and modern with courses in Russian, Polish, and German, along with math and the sciences. There was training in business and several of the skilled trades. For the first time, Nathan was exposed to the history of nations beyond the Jewish Pale and a first peek at the world outside.

Nathan broke out of the cave of Talmud in which he had been locked and drifted naturally toward languages. In a matter of six months, he had mastered enough Russian for the entirely new world of Russian literature to be open to him.

Nathan, the loner, had found the loner's paradise through books. Books not only stoked his world of fantasy, they proved a practical tool in working himself into group life.

Not many of the students were so captivated by literature. This afforded Nathan a special status, a subtle form of snobbery and a forum to draw attention to himself. So, he read and read and read. Nathan's book reports became a salable item, particularly to students whose parents were able to afford fresh fruit.

Nathan wasn't particularly sought after. His personal popularity was close to nil. He didn't play sports, lust after girls, or indulge in the general mischief befitting gymnasium students. He remained shy and often nasty in response to civil conversation.

But Nathan now had a commodity. Reading gave him his first true social opening, a way to enter and dominate conversation which he could bend around to his sphere of knowledge. By being able to hold court he grew larger in his own eyes, and he played it for all it was worth.

Nathan discovered that his loneliness could be alleviated by lecturing or arguing in the debating club about the books he was reading. As few other students had read the books and knew nothing about the authors, Nathan had an uncontested platform.

"Do you know?" he would ask many times during a talk. Of course the audience didn't know and that made Nathan smarter than his listeners. This opening gambit of putting them down worked famously. And it led to an invitation for him to join the labor Zionists, who courted intellectuals. This group had their own defense committee with a hidden stash of lethal weapons, pikes, clubs, and petrol bottles. On obscure outings, Nathan usually got himself scheduled to lecture. The more he spoke, the more fiery an orator he became. He could hardly wait to return to Wolkowysk and ram all his knowledge down Mordechai's throat.

Nathan's first trip home was for his bar mitzvah. Yehuda was thoroughly confused by the mishmash of philosophies Nathan now espoused. To his father, the boy represented the curses, confusion, and secular heresy of the big city. His ideas, when one could clearly define them, were close to godless. Why, the boy was not even wearing a prayer shawl anymore.

Nathan felt he had outgrown Wolkowysk, a perennial *shtetl* town which had doomed itself to live in the past. Moreover there was another mouth to feed, a new baby sister, Bessie.

Nathan returned to Bialystok and remained for two more years. His situation at Mrs. Ginsburg's boardinghouse improved when Nathan was able to find work during the vacation months as a clerk in a food warehouse, which purveyed to the nearby army camp. Nathan endured ruthless harassment and was sometimes roughed up by the soldiers, but the food and the money to be earned were too powerful an incentive to quit.

He graduated from the living-room couch into a room with three other students, and his "eat days" now offered more substantial meals.

IN WOLKOWYSK, a sudden disaster all but turned the family into wards of charity. Yehuda suffered a minor stroke and would not be able to work for an indefinite period.

To make matters more distressing, Uncle Sam in America had fallen on hard times. America went off the silver standard and this brought the mining industry in Colorado to the brink of collapse. Sam carried large amounts of credit on his books, mostly staking miners, and those debts were now uncollectable.

Yehuda and Sophie came to the wrenching decision to send as many children off to live with relatives as they could place. Mordechai, naturally, was to be afforded the best piece of the chicken. Yehuda got him to Vilna first, where he was safely tucked away in the yeshiva and fully supported.

On the day of his fifteenth birthday, Nathan received an urgent letter to return home.

NATHAN

Wolkowysk and Kiev, 1911

I, THE OLDEST SON, Nathan Zadok, came to my father's bedside. His beard hung outside the sheet halfway to his stomach and his eyes drooped with world-weariness. He shrugged as he recounted to me the gravity of the family problems. Groaning with despair, Father told me I had to leave the gymnasium.

Homes had been found for two of my brothers and two of my sisters. As for my own fate, I had to help support the family. Had my father and mother found a situation for me? My mother's sister, Tante Sonia, was married to a well-off coal merchant in Mariupol and had offered to take me in and give me a job. Mariupol? Mariupol! So why didn't they send me to Mongolia?

I hid in the woodshed and wept all night. I considered running away, but really there was no choice but to obey.

My father at least showed a twinge of guilt. While preparing me for this trip to the end of the earth, he showed me more kindness than he ever had before. You can be sure the magic name of Mordechai was missing. I said goodbyes to Reuben, Matthias, Rifka, and Sarah as they went in all directions to live with *mishpocha*.

Soon my own ticket arrived. If proverbs could be sold in the open marketplace, the Jews would have all the wealth in Russia. My father sent me off with the great wisdom:

"If fortune calls, offer him a seat."

To which my mother added, "If rich people could pay poor people to die for them, the poor would make a fine living."

Mariupol, a port city on the Sea of Azov, was over three thousand miles away. By train it meant five days and nights, during which seven changes had to be made. My belongings easily fit in one straw suitcase, which was sent ahead by baggage mail. I carried a package of dried food, because there wasn't always something to eat at the stations. In many cities along the route, Jews were not allowed to leave the train station area and enter town. I had five rubles to see me to Mariupol and the first memory of Momma crying over me.

Always on the trains, hoodlums and soldiers looked for Jews to victimize. My shabby coat would give me away. I climbed upon the wide slab like a shelf in third class, balled up in a corner, and kept a newspaper in front of my face.

Things did not go too badly until I arrived at Kiev. There was to be an eight-hour layover until the next train, which would take me as far as Poltava. So, what to do for eight hours? Kiev was forbidden for Jews in its sacred streets. Even Jewish tourists in transit were confined to the station where they were easy picking for the hoodlums.

I was very curious because Kiev was the home of my father. There was a suburb called Podol where Jews were permitted. Hoodlums around the station were making me very nervous, so I decided to take a risk. If I got to the Podol district, I could remain in a synagogue until train time. The streetcar was a wonderment! An astonishing piece of machinery, which was able to drive without horses pulling it.

For fifteen kopeks I ate a meal in a kosher restaurant. All of the conversation around concerned the trial of Mendel Beiliss, which had been taking place in Kiev. You ask me who is Mendel Beiliss? I'll tell you. He is the Jewish victim of a frame-up, accused of killing a gentile boy for ritual purposes. For Jews, Kiev has always been the shithouse of Russia. No matter how bad things were for us, it was worse in Kiev. Mendel Beiliss was the victim of an organization of *goyim* pigs, who were called the Black Hundred.

I couldn't resist taking the chance to go to the courthouse where the trial was being held. I got directions to the center city, but with warnings to stay away. I couldn't help myself. I was drawn immediately to a large crowd waiting outside the courthouse, hoping to maybe catch a glimpse of Beiliss, so I could lecture about it someday. Suddenly everyone pointed beyond the police lines to a droshky that had just pulled up.

A priest emerged and made for the courthouse.

"Pranaites!" everyone screamed.

The name of this animal was well known among us. Pranaites the priest claimed to be an expert on Talmud and was a key witness for the prosecution. His "scientific" testimony was that the murder had all the characteristics of a ritual murder allegedly practiced secretly by the Jews. It was known that Pranaites had a long criminal record, but nevertheless the fine people of Kiev cheered him as he entered the building.

I turned away in anger—directly into the largest man I had ever seen, a gendarme with a red face and drunken eyes. His enormous hand clamped on my shoulder.

Propelled by fear, I broke loose and ran over the street with the whiskey policeman and a half-dozen others after me. I ran right down a dead-end alley, leaped and tried to scale a wall. First stones hit me, then hands grabbed my legs and pulled me smashing to the ground.

I crouched like a turtle and felt kicks to my ribs and head. The policeman finally took control.

"Yid! Let me see your passport."

"Please, sir. I was only passing through Kiev. I went to the Jewish section for a meal because there was nothing to eat . . . please, sir, let me go!"

The crowd screamed and spit on me, urging the cop to take me to jail. He handcuffed me and dragged me to a police van on the main street. As we drove off, the crowd cheered.

I was so terrified I shook all over and could barely speak. Everyone was rough to me at the police station, as if they had caught the biggest criminal in the Ukraine. After being photographed and fingerprinted, I was put into a holding cell which had no bench or seat, only room to stand. This becomes very painful after a few hours.

I had done a dumb, stupid, idiotic thing by going into Kiev. The punishment for Jews caught outside the Pale was to send them to the place of their birth and leave them there until they died. I was born in a village called Novogrudok and to return there forever was worse than a death sentence.

The building, fear of the policemen, fear of terrible punishment, all closed in on me. I must have fainted because when I revived, I was in a different place.

"The Jew boy has woken up."

"The Chief wants to see him."

I was dragged into an office obviously belonging to a high-ranking authority and was seated before his desk with a huge guard on either side of me.

The Chief did not appear as though he had gotten his position through kindness. His face spoke of too much vodka and his heavy hands appeared to be the recipient of many bribes.

"Sir," I pleaded and tried to repeat my case, but was silenced by his fist banging on the desk. He looked me over to determine how much I could spend for a bribe. He didn't like what he saw.

"Did you look in the lining of his coat?" the Chief asked.

"Yes, nothing hidden."

"Shit. Little turd bastard. All right, Jew boy, do you know anyone in Kiev who can pay your fine?"

"No, sir."

"You are in serious trouble. Take him away."

That night was the most horrible I ever spent. I was tossed into a huge cage of a cell that held a dozen drunks. There was only the wet cement floor to lie down on and no toilet. Drunks were urinating and vomiting all over the cell, which was already covered with bugs.

As soon as it turned dark, I felt the hands of a very powerful man on me. He reached between my legs and tried to fondle my private parts. His smell was something which I will never forget. I managed to run to the other side of the cell screaming.

"Murder! Rape! Help!"

A guard removed the pervert to another cage. I was almost dead with fear. Nor could I eat the slosh they slipped in under the door with a slice of bread.

One of the prisoners decided he would be my protector for the night and I eventually calmed down, but I could not sleep for a single instant. Every little move startled me.

As the darkness came on, I shivered throughout the night in a tiny corner. I blamed my father for this. Why should I be sent so many thousands of miles away, while Mordechai was safe in one of the finest yeshivas in Russia? It was not fair. It had never been fair. God forgive me, but during the night I personally hoped my father would die from his stroke. It would serve him right. But he should not die until my body was shipped home for him to see.

At last morning came.

"Jew boy!" a guard called at me.

I was taken again to the Chief's office.

There was a very well-dressed Jewish-looking gentleman with a Van Dyke beard. My passport was returned. I was given to the custody of the gentleman, Mr. Lapidis, who I understood paid my fine. I found out from his carriage driver that Mr. Lapidis was a wealthy merchant with special permission to live in Kiev. The Chief had a thriving business in catching stray Jews, for whom Mr. Lapidis always paid the fines. This kindly gentleman had saved me from a terrible fate. He drove me to the station and admonished me to stay put. You can bet I wasn't looking for more adventures in Kiev.

Mariupol, 1911

I HAVE NEVER BEEN in such a house as belonged to the Borokovs in Mariupol. There were seven rooms if you can imagine such a thing. The parlor and a separate eating room were filled with silver and cut-glass crystal and figurines. The furniture was upholstered with velvet, like a rich bride would wear, and the curtains were made of fancy lace. Rugs were beneath your feet wherever you walked.

Tante Sonia was a tall woman who dressed every day like it was the Sabbath. Her fingers were filled with rings and she never had a hair out of place. She was a pinched, tight woman who tried to smile, but when she did her mouth went crooked, and when she reached to pat you all you could see were her long, bony fingers and those rings. She ran the house like it was a museum. You walked around, I guarantee you, on tiptoes.

Uncle Boris likewise didn't have a shabby thread on his coats and jackets, which were numerous. He spent as much time away from Tante Sonia as he was able, withdrawing to his personal library to read and work on accounts. Their meals were wordless.

Let me tell you something, that even with all the high-and-mighty business the food was delicious. Tante Sonia had a woman who did nothing but cook for them and there was meat three, maybe four times a week.

"The first thing you must learn, Nathan, is how to eat properly," I was informed. For such food I could take a little torture with her meat slicing and napkins and hands in the lap and eating soup without making noise. I also saw, for myself, for the first time in my life, oranges.

So Mariupol was heaven? Not exactly.

The Borokovs had two sons, both older than me and both of them in Palestine studying at the famous Herzlia Gymnasium. I therefore not only had a bedroom to myself, I had a closet filled with clothing the sons had outgrown. Tante Sonia had burned the clothing I arrived in, particularly my coat.

Because Uncle Boris had sons in Eretz Israel, he was a self-proclaimed Zionist. He bragged endlessly of the great sacrifice he had made for the redemption of Palestine.

The third child was a daughter, Tilly, who was a year younger than myself. To be quite frank about it, Tilly was a real *mishkeit*, an ugly. She was about twice my size to start with, and from there it got worse.

When I was told I would receive a salary of twelve rubles a week, I should have become immediately suspicious. Nobody pays anybody so much money for nothing. Tante Sonia announced she would send eight rubles a week directly to my family. The other four rubles would go for my room and board. Somehow, it didn't seem quite right, but here it was and here I was.

For this enormous salary, of which I received nothing, I worked sixty-two hours a week. If there is anything filthier than killing chickens, it is the coal business. Despite my mounting disillusions, there was the knowledge I was keeping my family alive, although after a day's work shoveling coal it gave me very little satisfaction.

Uncle Boris had an office on the docks. Every day he promised that I would work myself into the office to a nice desk job, but until then I had to learn the coal business from the ground up.

My first job required little genius. I worked in the coal packaging yard. This was for smaller sales. So I shoveled from the bins into burlap sacks, sewed the sacks, and stacked them on wagons. Then I went into coal delivery, another profession that didn't require a university education.

Later I graduated to a checker. When a shipload came to the docks, I had to see to it that the correct tonnage was delivered to the yard and oversee the transfer to coal trains. After ten to twelve hours of work and another two hours to clean myself up, I was often too tired to eat, despite the fantastic meals. The only day off was the Sabbath and I could scarcely drag myself out of bed to go to synagogue.

MARIUPOL HAD problems for me other than the Borokovs. We were a small number of Jews living among a large number of Ukrainians, a formula for catastrophe. There was no real Jewish communal life—we only went through the motions. There was neither a Jewish marketplace nor schools. Cultural affairs, such as Zionist meetings, were frowned upon even by the rabbis and had to be held in secret. The Borokovs admonished me not to use Yiddish. They spoke Russian at all times, even in synagogue.

The Jews of Mariupol had learned their place, to shut up. With Russia boiling from one end to the other with massive discontent, the Borokovs pretended nothing was happening. Nonetheless, as invisible as the Jews tried to make themselves, the Ukrainians reminded us regularly that we were dirty Jews. For me it was a very miserable existence, without a friend, to say nothing of—that "God should strike them all dead"—the coal business.

There was another matter that was not the least of my problems— namely, Tilly. She let me know in not so subtle ways that she didn't object to having a cousin living under the same roof.

Each night I would have to scrub in the yard for over an hour and as soon as my shirt and pants came off, Tilly appeared like magic. A few times I scalded myself jumping into the hot tub to avoid letting her see me naked.

Tilly found the oddest times, both day and night, to come into my room for incomplete reasons. Maybe I needed something? Did I get my laundry back? Would I like to smell this new perfume all the way from Paris? She had it down to a science, making me squirm.

I, in turn, tried to be friendly and enrich her with the vast knowledge I had gained by reading literature and becoming a lecturer of some note in Bialystok. But all she would do was giggle. She rarely put six words together without ending with a shrill giggle. Despite the sophistication I had gained in gymnasium, I still remained innocent regarding matters of girls. Even though Tilly was a genuine ugly, there were certain parts of her which might become interesting if I so inquired.

I thought all the time of running away. Not such an easy matter. I was a prisoner in golden handcuffs. Despite Tante Sonia's beautiful home and the food, I had no railroad ticket, no money in my pocket, and Uncle Boris kept my passport in the safe in his office.

Fate stepped in.

After almost two years and the passing of my seventeenth birthday, I developed a cough. Probably I had breathed in half the coal dust in southern Russia. Within a week, the cough became so bad I was unable to report for work. After another week, Tante Sonia finally took me to a doctor, but he failed to share with me the results.

For the Borokovs to stop sending my parents the eight rubles a week because the son is being worked into an early grave presented for the Borokovs a delicate problem. It all unfolded at a Sabbath dinner.

"The time has come," Uncle Boris said with great aplomb. "Nathan, you will move into the office and learn the books."

Tilly giggled.

"To be utterly candid," I replied, "I am not finding the coal business as enriching an experience as I had hoped."

"From the outside, coming to the inside, you will find things much different," he assured me.

"God forbid I should sound ungrateful for your generosity, but there are other problems as well," I said.

"What possible problems could you have?" Tante Sonia interjected indignantly. "We are feeding you like a dog, maybe? Your room is not spotless? Your clothing is rags?"

"It's just that . . ."

"What?" they demanded jointly.

"I don't have any time off, not to read or anything. I haven't even been to the library."

"But this is a promotion, Nathan. Going to work in the office is automatic shorter hours."

Tilly giggled.

"I don't feel so good about being a Jew here," I finally blurted out.

"And who understands that better than I do?" Uncle Boris intoned, slipping into a profound mood. "You cannot say that your Uncle Boris is not a Jew. I have given sons to Palestine, gladly. However, Nathan, you will learn that living quietly, away from all the problems of the *shtetl,* is not such a difficult adjustment. For those of us smart enough to get along, we make for ourselves a very comfortable life."

I didn't argue back, but in a million years I could not feel at ease in a jungle of Ukrainians. "I don't have a kopek in my pocket to spend," I croaked.

"Uncle Boris and I have talked it over and decided to give you a pay raise of two rubles a week," Tante Sonia said. "One ruble, I insist, should go into savings. The other ruble, mad money. Put it in your pocket, go to the cinema, do with it what you want. Make merry!"

So, why are they behaving this way to me now? Are they sorry for how they have worked me? Did an angel come in the middle of the night and threaten them to be good to Nathan, or else? All I could say of the moment, it was not typical Borokov.

A few nights later it occurred to me exactly what was unfolding. I was taking a pish in the thunderbowl, which was kept under my bed, when all of a sudden I heard that giggle. It was muffled, but unmistakable. I had never given much thought to it, in my innocence, but Tilly's room was connected to mine and there was a transom between us. It was covered with special paper, but on close examination I found that some of it was scratched away and so, standing on a chair, she could look directly into my room. God only knows, she may have been watching me sit on the pot for weeks, even months.

What a stupid I'd been.

My beloved mother, Sophie, and Tante Sonia had made a *shiddach* for me with—GOD SAVE ME—Tilly Borokov. A plot hatched over three thousand miles. I needed some kind of confirmation.

There was an old yard hand I had befriended by the name of Gregor. He was not a bad fellow, as Ukrainians go. Gregor was afflicted with the usual Ukrainian disease of alcoholism. When I had saved up three rubles, I took him one evening to the tavern. Information flowed after the first drink.

"So, Boris Borokov is telling you that shit about what a great Zionist he is. His sons ran away to Palestine, because they hated equally that house and the coal business. He has no heirs except Tilly, and Mariupol is not big enough for finding a husband for that one. You are a marked man, Nathan."

What to do?

I went back to bed and coughed and coughed. I coughed in their faces. I coughed at the dining-room table, spraying everyone's food. I spit and missed the spittoon, landing my wad on Tante Sonia's most precious Turkoman carpet. I tracked coal over the parlor and got dirty marks all over her doilies. I lost the documents on a coal shipment, which cost Uncle Boris double taxation.

God must have heard me coughing, because the war broke out between Russia and Germany. For the next several months the coal business was in a bad state. All winter long I remained useless to Uncle Boris because my cough continued until springtime. All of us, by this time, wanted to get rid of one another.

Mail was slow with the war on, but by March I received a letter that a job was waiting for me in the city of Minsk in the jewelry store of another uncle, Bernie Zadok.

Minsk, 1915

THE TRAIN TRIP from Mariupol to Minsk, likewise almost three thousand miles, was a certified nightmare. The Russians, from the Czar on down, blamed the Jews for getting them into the war. Their logic escapes me, but every empty wall, particularly in the railroad stations, was filled with anti-Semitic slogans: KILL A JEW AND SAVE RUSSIA.

Before the war it was difficult for a Jew to make a long train ride without having a bad experience. Now it was completely impossible. Soldiers heading for the front prowled for Jews as though it were a blood sport.

From the minute I left Mariupol, I could not escape from the Jew-baiting, from the slogans on the walls to the newspapers to the gossip on everyone's lips.

Every car I boarded, they would be looking for me. I was easy to pick out and easier to pick on. First came the dirty remarks and the pushing around. Then came the humiliation of having my pants pulled down to see if I was circumcised, and it ended with a slapping around or a beating. Once it was established that you were Jewish, at a whim of the Russians you were not permitted to sit down, even on the floor. The soldiers made all of us—men, women, and children—stand from station to station. After a few hours people would start collapsing. Sometimes I stood for so many hours I crawled off the train in a state of exhaustion. Food had to be eaten carefully. For example, bread could not be gobbled so you hid in the latrine and ate it slowly. If you had potatoes or cucumbers, you gobbled it down fast.

The worst was during the final leg, when the train was boarded by a company of Cossack soldiers returning from the front, where they had taken a terrible beating from the German Army. My overcoat was ripped apart to see if I was hiding money and when they found none, I was beaten unconscious. This is the condition my Uncle Bernie found me in at the Minsk station. I was in the hospital for over a week, with cracked ribs and a broken nose. One more train ride and the story of Nathan Zadok would have been over.

MINSK, I AM happy to say, was a change for the better. Uncle Bernie had become a man of means. He owned a small jewelry manufacturing business with a retail outlet on the elegant Gubnartorsky Street. Along comes the war and his business is booming. Minsk was a major staging area for the Army and its streets were filled with soldiers and many officers had their women. No one seemed to want to go off to war without buying a trinket or two. Uncle Bernie's was filled from opening to closing.

Despite his new wealth, Bernie Zadok was a real mensch. He and Aunt Sarah remained earthy people with no fancy-shmancy ideas like the Borokovs. Decent and generous, especially to orphans, Uncle Bernie had a seat on the Eastern Wall. Because of the war there was a shortage of workers, so I fit right in and in no time whatsoever I am jack of all trades.

At home in Wolkowysk, the family situation changed for the better when my father was again able to resume his profession as *shohet*. With the war on, his wholesalers had contracts with the Army and he was butchering chickens around the clock. My father was a good *shohet*, but nobody would appreciate that except, in a strange way, the chickens. The birds he slaughtered were not kosher of course, but good enough for the Russians.

TONIGHT OPENING MEETING OF THE POALE ZIONIST ORGANIZATION OF RUS-SIA REGIONAL CONFERENCE. KEYNOTE SPEAKER, NATHAN ZADOK WHO WILL RECOUNT HOW HE SECRETLY COVERED THE MENDEL BEILISS TRIAL IN KIEV. A daring account of one young Poale Zionist and how he secretly interviewed the evil Pranaites.

Perhaps I made a slight exaggeration about my participation in the Beiliss trial, but people were coming halfway over the city to hear me speak and there were delegates from all over the eastern part of the country. What's the sin? What's the crime if I make them feel proud?

I cannot hardly describe the sensation of approaching the rostrum after thunderous applause. Thousands out there and me, little Nathan Zadok of Wolkowysk, the youngest delegate to the entire convention.

"Comrades! Fellow workers! Fellow Zionists! Before I speak to you about the Mendel Beiliss trial, I should like to touch on the point that all Poale Zionists should be concerned about. Today, all over Russia, we see unfolding a sinister plot of Lenin's agents infiltrating into one Poale Zion chapter after another, trying to take over the leadership or wreck the structure of the only organization that spells liberty for the Jews. When I speak of labor and socialism and Zionism, one organization alone holds aloft our banner. Poale Zion! Lenin would have you believe that overnight a thousand years of terror against the Jewish people is over. Lenin is a liar. Lenin tells us of a land where White Russians and Ukrainians and Lithuanians are going to reverse the course of their history and embrace us with open arms, after bashing our skulls for centuries. Lenin is a liar. [Now the crowd was chanting "Lenin is a liar" on cue.] Lenin says there will be freedom and equality for the Jewish people. I say that will happen when I grow onions in the palm of my hand! The only path for the Jewish people is the path out of Russia to join our people in the redemption of our homeland—Eretz Israel! Zion! Palestine! [On mention of any of these three names, the people go berserk, so I made certain I spoke all three words in the opening of the address.] Our feet must follow the dictates of our souls and we must blaze a path to our promised land now and we must make settlements so that when this war is over, hundreds of thousands of Jews will follow our example, yours and mine."

To say that my address was received enthusiastically is to be overly modest.

I CONFESS that I was still extremely bashful and inexperienced when it came to the opposite sex. Whenever I was sitting like a cripple in a living room, I could only wish I had the same dynamics as I had at the rostrum. I got many invitations for dinners and, I must admit, many flirtatious glances were cast in my direction, even though most of the girls were taller than me.

In the girl business, I had a break. My Uncle Bernie also owned the cinema in Minsk and I had free admission at all times.

If things were looking bright for me in Minsk, they weren't looking so bright for the Russian Army. By late 1915 they were retreating with heavy losses. Much of Poland and the Baltic states was already under control of the German Army.

We could tell that casualties were heavy by the number of bloody uniforms being sent to the various tailor shops to be cleaned, patched, and reissued.

Just how heavy were Russia's losses came crashing into my life like a thunderbolt on a Saturday morning late in the summer. On the front page of the *Minski Golos,* the daily paper, was a special order that all men born in 1896 were to report for military duty. This was my year. I thought I would be safe because the service age had been twenty-one. Uncle Bernie and I both agreed I had better get back to Wolkowysk and make a decision with my father.

WHITE RUSSIA

Wolkowysk–Bialystok, 1916–1919

THERE HAD NEVER been what might be termed a stampede by the Jews to rally around the flag of Mother Russia. Forced into conscription at an early age, many Jewish boys were sent off to Siberian duty and were not heard from for years. Once the Jews were in the Army, the authorities used fair means or foul to get them to convert to Christianity.

Avoiding service in the Russian Army was considered an honorable pursuit by the Jews in the Pale. False documents were a standard commodity and no one in the Jewish community considered it ethical to profit from their traffic.

As soon as the Czar's new edict calling up eighteen-year-olds was published, Yehuda Zadok traveled immediately to the nearby town of Lida where a close rabbi friend had excellent connections for obtaining false papers.

One of the common methods was not to report the death of young men to the authorities, but keep their documents and pass them on to someone who needed a set.

Yehuda was able to acquire the papers of a seventeen-year-old youth who had died of pneumonia. On Nathan's arrival home from Minsk, his father presented him with his new identity, that of one Pinchas Hirsch.

Nathan's reunion with his family was rather pleasant. He was welcomed with an affection he had never known before from his father. Right was right. The boy had worked very hard to keep the family fed and was always prompt in sending money home. He deserved some respect. Not exactly the respect one would afford a scholar like Mordechai, but respect nonetheless.

Since he recovered from his stroke, Yehuda Zadok had also changed many of his attitudes. Mainly, he became a supporter of the Zionist movement. Yehuda's sentiments favored the religious elements, but he no longer disdained the socialist labor movement of Poale Zion which had captured the imagination of the younger people.

Their family reunion was limited to only one meal, hardly enough time to get caught up, but it didn't matter to Nathan. He almost completely ignored the fact that his older sisters were blossoming—not raving beauties, but nice solid girls in a plain and wholesome way. He showed equal disinterest in the progress of his younger brothers. He made a perfunctory inquiry about his father's health and, of course, never mentioned Mordechai.

What was most important to Nathan was that he had won the right to hold court at the table, now that he was respected. He used the opportunity, speaking nonstop of his accomplishment as a Poale leader in Minsk, his mastery of languages, and some of the more palatable experiences in his journeys. With only a passing comment on the outstanding meal Sophie had scraped together for the occasion, the occasion was over.

Nathan was scheduled to register for the Army in a few days, so an urgent meeting was called at the rabbi's home. Aram Hornstein was the local leader of the Poale Zion chapter and the main mover of young men trying to avoid army conscription. The general plan was to move the escapees as far west as they could get by train. Once into Polish territory they would be beyond the reach of the Russian authorities. It was a dangerous business. In order to get to Poland, one had to pass through the battle lines. There were a number of safe houses in the *shtetl* villages forming an underground route. The ultimate object was to reach Warsaw where Poale was strongly organized.

Hornstein reckoned it would be best to move Nathan out of Wolkowysk that same night. He was to board a train when he reached Bialystok, which still had rail traffic moving west.

For fear of being spotted by the local police, Nathan left Wolkowysk without so much as a farewell to his mother. The next morning he reached Bialystok by foot and found a train heading for Siedlce, which was halfway to Warsaw but also very close to the front lines. In Siedlce Nathan was to find a Poale Zion guide named Perchik, who would take him to the German side.

The scene at the Bialystok terminal was chaos beyond chaos. Not only was the station filled with thousands of young men of military service age, but tens of thousands of Jews from the entire scope of society, escaping from pogroms which had rent the fabric of the whole country.

Along with these there were gentile boys fleeing service, as well as a huge sprinkling of Russian deserters. Everyone was suspicious of everyone else. Fortunately the Russian Army was in retreat and the civilian train no longer carried its full complement of military inspectors, so documents were scarcely checked.

Toward the end of a stop-and-go day, the bulging train pulled to a halt at a siding. It was too dangerous to continue west and soon came a terse announcement that they had reached the end of the line.

As everyone milled about wondering what to do, some of the suspicion eased as people began to identify themselves to find people of their own organizations.

"Say," someone called to Nathan, "aren't you Nathan Zadok?"

Nathan balked. "You've got the wrong person. My name is Pinchas Hirsch."

The young man persisted; he took Nathan aside and whispered in his ear. "I heard you give the keynote speech at the Poale Regional Conference in Minsk. I am Yossi Dubnow. I was a delegate from Kaunas— Lithuania."

Nathan looked over the tall, striking young man. He seemed like a good person to have along in such a situation. Nathan shook Yossi's hand. Together they hunted for more Poale people and found Daniel and Avni Finkel from Slonim. The four of them decided they had just the right size group to move around quickly and they teamed up.

Although the train had dumped them some distance away, Siedlce was still their first objective. It was there they had to find Perchik, the guide to take them into Poland.

They pooled their resources and bought a ride on a farm wagon, moved through the forest by night, edged evasively during the day, stayed under cover in populated areas, and some days managed to advance only several hundred yards.

It was torturous, hungry, and dangerous going, but survival was a strong motivation. Warsaw loomed in their imaginations as some sort of nirvana—the golden city.

Yossi Dubnow proved to be clever, resourceful, and strong. In five days of cautious movement they worked themselves to the outer fields beyond Siedlce. By then, Yossi was in full and unquestioned command, although Nathan, through his speech at the Poale Conference in Minsk, had earned a great deal of respect.

As they approached Siedlce they heard the sound of gunfire. They surveyed their area for the best cover and came upon an abandoned brick factory that had several deep clay pits around it. Yossi reckoned they could hide themselves there as well as anyplace.

"What do you think?" Avni said. "Shouldn't we go into Siedlce and look for Perchik?"

"I don't like it," Yossi answered. "We all can't just go marching in. First of all, we'll be recognized as strangers and second of all, they may be fighting for Siedlce."

"Yeah, we don't want to get caught in a street battle," Daniel said.

"I say we stay here and lie low until the firing stops, at least," Nathan said.

"One of us has a better chance than the four of us," Yossi said. "I've had some military training in school. I'll go, you stay put."

The others agreed and found a narrow rail tunnel, large enough to pull carts of clay from the pits to the kilns. The tunnel was deep, sturdy, and would provide good cover.

Yossi set out for the nearby village of Chodow to gather information. This had to be done with extreme prudence because all sides—the Germans, Poles, and Russians—could very well turn them in. Yossi's first objective was to see if the village had a synagogue and if so, find the rabbi or a Jewish family. As he approached Chodow from a hillside, he could make out large numbers of Russian troops deployed along the Liwiec River. They were digging in hard to stop the Germans from fording the river.

Yossi returned to the brick factory just as the day came to an end. He drew a map in the dirt. "The Germans are deployed over the river both north and south of the city. They may well try to cross anyplace along a four-mile stretch. In fact, they may even come right over the top of us here."

"So maybe we'd better head north," Nathan said.

"No," Yossi answered. "We've got excellent cover here. I say we get into the tunnel as far as we can and ride it out."

"Suppose the Germans send a patrol in? If they see us, they'll either shoot us or take us prisoner," Nathan protested.

"I say we ride it out," Yossi repeated.

Avni and Daniel supported Yossi. As the last words left their mouths, they heard the swish of an incoming artillery shell. A few seconds later it shattered just beyond them.

"Let's move it!" Yossi commanded. They needed no further prodding as the air was suddenly racked with a barrage. The boys huddled together, cowering as the pounding above became murderous.

Nathan suddenly gagged with fear, wept softly, and curled up in a ball, his hands over his face. Throughout the darkness he felt the reassuring touch of Yossi Dubnow.

After three hours the bombardment seemed to advance beyond them. Yossi crawled from the tunnel, up the side of the pit, and tried to make sense of what had happened. Streaks of tracer bullets arched in the direction of the little village. Yossi strained to hear. Perhaps he actually did hear the sounds of men screaming as though they were charging. Perhaps it was an illusion. The bombardment had played tricks on his ears. During the next hours, the racket grew dimmer and seemed to move away from them.

Yossi staggered back down into the tunnel and risked lighting a candle. Nathan and the Finkel brothers were glassy-eyed and sat the rest of the night with their backs propped against the cold, dripping wall. They were too disoriented from the shelling to speak or take much more than a sip of water.

As the first slant of light probed a hill behind the factory, Yossi went up again and called for them to follow. A thick, low, still cloud wove through hillocks and gulleys over a windless field. The field was pocked with hundreds of craters created by the violent artillery fire, and the smell of it was like fireworks on the Czar's birthday.

They lay on their bellies in a hole and remained still until they were sure no one was in the area.

"We're luckier than hell," Yossi said. He pointed down toward the river. "The Germans must have crossed over to the north. They swept right past us."

"Look, the ridge is burning," Avni said.

"They must have concentrated their attack on the ridge," Yossi reckoned. "Yesterday there were Russians digging in a defense. It's possible the battle may be past us."

"On the other hand," Daniel Finkel said, "German advance units may be pushing forward, but most of their troops are probably still on the other side of the river."

"The question is, who now holds Siedlce?" Yossi said.

They looked from one to another in puzzlement. "We can't all go marching into Siedlce," Avni said.

"You guys stay here. I'll go in and try to find Perchik," Yossi said. "If

I'm not back by tomorrow morning, you're on your own in getting to
Warsaw."

With that, Yossi picked a route through the field of shellholes and
darted off as his frightened comrades watched.

SIEDLCE WAS in a state of anxiety, the townspeople not knowing if
they had been benevolently liberated or brutally conquered. The Poles
disliked the Germans and Russians equally and were equally despised by
both sides.

Although Yossi didn't look particularly Jewish, he was a stranger in
town, speaking mostly Russian and therefore given a wide berth. He was
mistaken for one of the Russian stragglers who had dumped their uniforms, sold their weapons, and retreated.

By listening keenly, Yossi was able to gather that the main Russian
force had collapsed and was in full retreat. Siedlce had been officially
surrendered and would be occupied by the Germans before the end of
the day.

In late morning, a few people dared to go out into the streets and,
seeing things peaceful, started doing their daily chores. Others soon
followed. Refilling the larders was the first order of business. Stocks
were close to bare because of the prolonged fighting and there was fear
that fighting might break out again. Yossi worked carefully around the
Jewish marketplace and finally selected a pushcart peddler to approach.

"So, where are you from?" the peddler asked.

"Kaunas."

"That far?"

"I was running away to escape military service. The train dumped us
without warning in the middle of the countryside."

"Listen, this happens every day with the trains, now. It's like we
don't already have enough mouths to feed. So, you're looking for the
shul. There's a soup kitchen. The rabbi's name is Bitterman."

"I'm not looking for a rabbi," Yossi answered in measured tones that
afforded the two a quick eye-to-eye exchange.

"Sorry," the peddler said.

"I'd like to see somebody from Poale Zion," Yossi said.

"I don't know any Zionist people," the peddler snapped quickly and
gave a motion that his hands were clean.

"Thanks anyhow," Yossi said and turned away.

"Hey, boy, come back," the peddler said. He studied Yossi up and
down several times, then asked a number of questions in Yiddish that

only a Jew could answer. Satisfied, he closed his stall and ordered Yossi to follow him at a distance.

LATE IN THE afternoon, Yossi Dubnow returned to the brick factory with the man called Perchik. Stubby and fiftyish, he had the deep markings of having been a lifelong worker. He was a single-minded Zionist, with his commitments dead centered.

"You boys can't stay here long," Perchik told them. "By tomorrow the Germans will have moved into the entire district in strength. They'll have roadblocks up and they'll be dragging the woods for stragglers and deserters."

"Actually," Nathan said, "we aren't technically in violation of anything against the Germans."

"Four Jewish boys on false documents," Perchik responded. "Don't be ridiculous. They don't need to give any reason whatsoever to do anything they want with you."

"Just what will they do?"

"Put you in a labor battalion," Perchik answered. "Some survive, most don't."

"Well . . . that's plain enough," Yossi Dubnow said.

"There's only one choice. Get through the German lines as fast as you can, right now."

"Gevalt," Nathan mumbled.

The Finkel brothers, followers by nature, shrugged in reluctant assent.

Yossi nodded in agreement as Perchik spread a crude hand-drawn map and marked their location at the brickyard. "There's a gap in the German lines south of the town. I can get you through if we hit the river right away. The rest of the way to Warsaw is fairly routine."

"And when we get to Warsaw?"

"Trading the Russians for the Germans and Poles in Warsaw is no bargain, but at least in Warsaw we have thousands of our own people and plenty of options."

Yossi looked to the Finkel brothers who nodded in the affirmative.

"Nathan?"

"Include me out," Nathan replied.

They looked at him puzzled.

"Perchik," Nathan said, "maybe you'll find for me here a hiding place for a few days. Someplace where I can get maybe a piece of bread."

"You mean you're not coming with us?" Yossi asked.

"Look, we're all only trying to survive the best we can. As soon as the Germans capture my home town, Wolkowysk, I'll go back. Believe me, I will escape from service in a German labor battalion."

"What about Palestine?" Avni asked.

"So, what about Palestine," Nathan answered. "You think maybe God will mount you up on wings of eagles in the middle of a war and fly you to Palestine?"

"I don't believe this!" Yossi shouted.

"What's not to believe?" Nathan retorted. "All we were trying to do was escape service in the Russian Army. Now is not the time for Palestine. Believe me, it will still be there when we're ready."

"Wait a minute!" Yossi cried. "You, Nathan Zadok, were my inspiration. You remember the Poale Zion Conference in Minsk? I, Yossi Dubnow, sat in the back row of the auditorium listening to you. Lenin is a liar, you said. And the crowd began chanting Lenin is a liar. The only path for the Jewish people is the path out of Russia to join our people in the redemption of our homeland. We must blaze a path to our promised land now and we must make settlements, so that when this war is over, hundreds of thousands of Jews will follow our example, yours and mine. You see, I remembered every God-damned word you said—"

"Listen, Minsk was Minsk. At this moment my family needs me more than Eretz Israel."

"You're a coward and a liar," Yossi said, slapping Nathan across the face.

Perchik stepped between them and pushed Yossi away.

"Oh, you can't imagine how courageous he was shouting down at us from the platform in Minsk."

"Shut up, Yossi!" Perchik demanded. "Or I'll make chicken soup from you."

"Are you angry with me, Perchik?" Nathan sputtered.

"Why do you think I risk my life running our boys through the battlefields? You'll never be anything but a *shtetl* yid. You'll live groveling and spouting out every phony street-corner philosophy and you don't deserve any better."

Nathan was more than willing to explain, to argue that his decision was motivated by his overpowering love for his family. But he had no one to argue with. They left him standing there in the clay pit, ankle deep in water in his shabby, ill-fitting coat, and lost themselves quickly in the lingering smoke and fog that had come up from the river.

WITH YOSSI GONE, the way became difficult for Nathan. He was frightened all of the time, indecisive a good part of the time, and lost a great deal of the time. Somehow he made it to the outskirts of Bialystok before he collapsed from hunger and fatigue in the barn of a peasant. Nathan had not been too crafty in his moves. A farmer and his son had watched him cross their fields and crawl up into the hayloft. He had barely dozed off when he was awakened by a hard kick in the sole of his shoe and ordered in Polish to stand up.

Nathan wobbled to his feet and grimaced as the prongs of a pair of pitchforks pinned him against the wall.

"Russian deserter," the farmer ventured to his son.

"No, I am Nathan Zadok. I am a Russian, but I am not in the Army. I was traveling west and the train stopped out in the middle of nowhere. I am only trying to get home to Wolkowysk."

The farmer and his son digested this suspiciously.

"So, I can be going on my way now?" Nathan said.

The farmer's eyes opened wide as something occurred to him. "Yid?"

"Pull down your pants!" the son ordered.

"I'm a Jew," Nathan whispered dejectedly.

Smelling the extra reward the Germans had put out on stray Jews, the farmers trussed Nathan up, threw him into a cart, and drove him to a barracks the Germans occupied at the freight depot of the railyard. The peasant was paid a bounty, enough for a bottle of vodka, and Nathan was dragged off by a pair of guards to the office of the commanding officer.

"Russian stray, Jew boy," one guard said. "He told a couple of Poles his name was Nathan something, but his papers say Pinchas Hirsch."

"So, who are you?" the officer demanded.

"I am truly Nathan Zadok of Wolkowysk, only trying to get home," he answered in German.

The officer studied Nathan's smallness, calculated his worthlessness. He wouldn't last two weeks in a labor battalion. What's the difference? Every day, a hundred more, a thousand more. Jews were fleeing all over the landscape, clogging the roads, cramming the rails. The German shook his head and laughed aloud—everyone's trying to chop off their tails with a carving knife. . . .

Nathan trembled but remained wordless. The German detested Nathan's silence. Why didn't the Jew boy at least plead for his life? Why didn't he argue? Was the acceptance of inevitable death so easy for him? As he picked up his pen to sign an order, the guard leaned over the desk.

"Begging your pardon, sir, but Major Mühldorf is having some trouble getting organized in the marshaling yards. He badly needs someone who can translate from German into Polish and Russian."

"How good is your German? I don't mean Yiddish. I mean German."

"I read Schiller and Heine," Nathan managed through dry lips.

"Polish?"

"I have lived on the border most of my life. My Polish is fluent."

The German drummed his fingers on the desk a moment. "Take the yid to Major Mühldorf. If he can use him, all right. If not, bring him back for transfer."

Major Rudi Mühldorf, the yardmaster, had arrived on the scene only a few days earlier. He was a hoary old civilian railroad man who had been pressed into military service.

His immediate problem was to get the yard and roundhouse into functioning order, the difficulty of the task being compounded by the need to use three languages. Nathan assured him of his value. Mühldorf neither liked nor disliked Jews. He liked trains and only trains.

Bialystok was now a key junction in the German advance into White Russia, the Baltic, and the Ukraine. Troops and artillery supplies would be pouring through to the fronts, but Mühldorf was faced with the chaos of war as well as an antiquated rail system. He was determined to make Bialystok at least a smooth operation, even if not by Germanic standards of perfection.

Thus Nathan earned himself a cot in the yardmaster's building, German enlisted men's rations, and a distinctive cap and armband to denote he was a protected worker.

Nathan thanked God he was not one of those hundreds passing through the yard in locked freight cars for the labor gangs, to repair rails and bridges. The death rate among them was fearsome.

Nathan spent most of his time at a desk translating manifests, repair orders, parts requisitions, regulations, and schedules. He was on call several times a day to straighten out foul-ups due to language. The major benefit of his situation was that he could help his family.

The German occupation was conducted with merciless disregard for civilians. With all the meat and poultry markets out of operation, Yehuda Zadok was again without a means of making a living. Everything usable from the land was confiscated by the Germans, leaving the population to fend for themselves.

The desperate food situation was made more devastating by a massive epidemic of typhus.

Material poured into the Bialystok depot for transshipment to the front, and a predictable black market evolved and flourished. Most of the rail system was operated by German civilians whose patriotism could easily be compromised.

Major Mühldorf knew the drill well. A little thievery always accompanied the romance of freight yards. Once in a while, when a black market gang became too greedy he would have them strung up or shot, to cool the fervor.

Nathan made himself an inconspicuous "honest broker" between buyer and seller for a small and reasonable piece of the transaction. It was a simple matter for him to hitch a ride to Wolkowysk, a few hours away, at least once a week with a package of food for the family.

Wolkowysk, 1920

YEHUDA ZADOK was back at his old stand, slitting the necks of chickens.

For years there had been a broil of armies—Reds, Whites, Ukrainians, Lithuanians, and Polish, all bashing at one another to snatch off pieces of the Czar's fallen empire. While they slaughtered one another, they all shared a common enemy, the Jews. But the postwar, post-revolution pogroms paled even the worst of them a half century before.

"If you're a Jew," Yehuda told Sophie, "it seems you have to face the history of the world all over again, every day." Yehuda's forays into religious ecstasy at the chopping block eased his pain, but his thoughts were also invaded by the future of his family.

The saddest of days was the Sabbath and visits to the cemetery. The two youngest Zadok children, Reuben and Bessie, died in one of the typhus scourges before the end of the war.

The cemetery sat in a grove of leafless silver-bark birches, their bony top limbs pointing upward like fingers twisted in anguished prayer. Tombstones had been overturned and graves robbed during the pogroms. Desecration was perpetual.

Yehuda would wait at the cemetery gate so that Sophie could have her time alone with her two dead children. She had long mastered the art of muffling grief, but the loss of Bessie and Reuben had inflicted permanent pain.

Yehuda's mind was always on the family. All but Bessie and Reuben had survived the war, but now he had to face the business of dissolving the family and scattering them forever.

For him and Sophie there would be no move. Palestine? Out of the question. Palestine was for young people. The matchmakers were chirping around to find suitable mates for his three girls, Rifka, Sarah, and Ida. They weren't exactly raving beauties and the daughters of a *shohet* were not likely to catch a prince. Moreover, Rifka was too late for a really desirable marriage because of the war.

Yehuda hoped they would marry perhaps a carpenter, perhaps a leather worker, and if God smiled, a butcher, a merchant. For the daughters he did not worry so much, not that he wasn't an affectionate and loving father. In his daily prayers he beseeched that at least one of them would remain in Wolkowysk and have children and maybe the pain in Sophie's eyes might go away in time.

The fate of the boys disturbed him the most. The three oldest had all strayed from what he had envisioned for them. Yehuda couldn't bring himself to say it out loud, but Mordechai was a bitter disappointment. By the time he was ready to graduate from yeshiva in Vilna, Mordechai had drifted away from the religious life his father had so carefully guided him into. Not exactly a rebellion, not exactly a rejection, but a definite decision not to go into the rabbinate. Mordechai had chosen instead to become a teacher and writer, of sorts.

Vilna was one of the heartland cities of the *shtetl*, a little Warsaw abounding with Jewish heritage and culture. Mordechai was appointed to an instructor's position in a secular gymnasium; he wrote a weekly column in one of the local newspapers and was otherwise immersed in the scholarly activities of Vilna's Jewish community.

Vilna was particularly bad for the Jews these days. The city had been ceded by treaty to the Poles and this set off vicious fighting between Poland and Lithuania, with both armies exercising their ritual of murdering Jews who were blamed by both sides for their troubles.

The final realization of Mordechai's independence came with letters that he was interested in a girl from an affluent but nonobservant family. What had it come to when a father could no longer arrange his child's marriage?

Yehuda concluded that times had changed. Perhaps his efforts to have Mordechai remain a *shtetl* boy would come to nothing. So, what did it matter as long as his son was happy? If he would take a bride without Poppa's personal stamp of approval the sun wouldn't fall from the sky.

THERE WAS ANOTHER surprise in the Zadok family. Matthias, who had just turned seventeen, had been an enigma in the family—quiet, intense, the dreamer. He was also a different Zadok physically—taller, stronger, very steady and reliable. At the end of the war when Nathan failed to pick up the banner of Poale Zion, which was starting up chapters again all over the Pale, Matthias, to everyone's surprise, became the Zionist of the family. He organized thirty young people in Wolkowysk and undertook the arduous task of raising funds, obtaining visas, and cutting through red tape which was essential for the trip to Palestine. It was Matthias who was now being asked to speak in the regional conferences and Matthias who was the delegate to the major congress in Warsaw.

One day when Yehuda and Sophie returned from the cemetery, Matthias was waiting for them. The boy dreaded those hours after their graveside visits but what was happening needed an immediate decision.

"Good *shabbas*, Poppa, Momma."

"Good *shabbas*, Matti. I thought you were overnight at a meeting in Slonim. You didn't travel home by train on the Sabbath?"

"Of course not. I got home last evening before sundown. I'm sorry I didn't go to *shul* last night. There was an urgent meeting at Lufka's house."

"So tell me what's on your mind before you jump out of your skin."

"I'll make first a glass tea," Sophie said. The fire in the stove was down to a whisper. She stirred it and reached into the wood basket for a small log.

"Woman! It is still the Sabbath. Since when do you cook on the Sabbath?"

"I need a glass tea," she repeated. "You can pray for my soul all week; I'm having a glass tea."

"So, I'll have a glass tea too," Yehuda agreed. "*Nu*, Matti, what world-shaking decisions required a meeting last night at Lufka's?"

"The district received a special grant from Baron von Epstein in Geneva to send another of our members to Palestine. I was voted the one to go."

"Nathan was at the meeting?"

"Yes. He doesn't attend often, but he was at this meeting."

"He likewise voted in favor of you?"

"No, Poppa. He screamed at us that the decision was unfair. He raged out of Lufka's. When I ran him down he called me ten thousand dirty names. Poppa, I swear to you, I had no idea Nathan even wanted to go to Palestine anymore."

Yehuda Zadok emitted a groan that had taken the Jews of the Pale a thousand years to develop. Matthias leaned against the window frame and touched the curtains, very fragile from age and too many washings.

"It's all right," Matti said. "Nathan deserves to go first. So what if it takes me a little more time? I'll get to Eretz Israel."

"You are certain you want to give Nathan your place?"

"Yes, I'm sure."

Yehuda patted his son's shoulder affectionately.

"I told the comrades we'd meet again tonight. I'm sure they'll honor my wishes and send Nathan."

Sophie peered into the boys' bedroom. Nathan's bed had not been slept in. "I wonder where he is?" she said.

"In the woodshed," Matthias said.

"In the woodshed," his father repeated with an ironic laugh. "Nathan is in the woodshed."

"I'll try to talk to him again," Matthias said.

"No, no, Matti, take for a walk your girlfriend. I'll talk to him."

When Matthias left, Sophie and Yehuda stared at their untouched glasses of tea. "You see what happens when you cook on the Sabbath," Yehuda managed to say.

"For me personally," Sophie said, "I'm glad he's going if only to make him stop listening to this Bolshevik *dreck*. More and more he listens."

"Lenin has decreed that there is no longer a Pale of Settlement for Jews. We can travel anywhere in Russia, even Moscow. Who knows, times may be changing."

"Yehuda, you're a first-rate crazy. Do you think one scratch of the pen will change a thousand years of Russian history? Russia will be a good place for the Jews to live when it stops snowing in Siberia. Lenin may be able to convince the Ukrainians they're Russian, but he'll never convince the Jews."

"So what do you want, woman?"

"I want you should encourage Nathan to go to Palestine before he gets too mixed up in this Bolshevik business. What does he think? If he goes to Moscow they'll throw flowers at his feet? The Russians are the biggest liars in the world."

"So what are you breaking your head on, Sophie?"

"What? What? Look in every direction, Yehuda. Everyone wants the honor to destroy us. This place will end up being one big graveyard. The sooner the children leave, the better."

"Sophie, you don't understand nothing at all."

"I understand what I understand and I understand it perfectly."

"You're speaking cows, I'm speaking horses. Sophie, our son Nathan doesn't know what he wants. He never has. He probably never will. If he goes to Palestine, I tell you he is going to fail. If he goes to America, he will fail."

She blinked at him, not understanding.

"I say the following with a stone in my heart," Yehuda continued, "but Nathan is a *shtetl* Jew. He knows how to survive in this atmosphere, but put him in another place and he'll create a misery. Some people are meant to be born, live, and die in the *shtetl*, just like you and me."

Tears came to Sophie Zadok's eyes. "Let him go to Palestine. I cannot go on living if another of my children is in the Wolkowysk cemetery."

TO PALESTINE

Warsaw, 1920

THE NEWLY RE-CREATED state of Poland was actively and openly anti-Semitic by national policy, a policy endorsed by the vast majority of its citizenry and its Roman Catholic Church. But Warsaw held nearly four hundred thousand Jews and mere numbers afforded an illusion of safety.

In Warsaw, Judaism was vibrantly alive in a variety of forms. There were dynasties of black-bearded Hasidim in long black coats. There were street-corner philosophers of every stripe and pushcart vendors of every product. Every philosophical branch of Zionism had its publications, speakers, cultural venues. There were socialists, now locking horns with Communists. There was Yiddish and Hebrew publishing and a vibrant theater. There was an aggressive labor movement, courting tens of thousands of nonunion workers. There were a few wealthy Jews, but mostly they were a population on the edges of poverty. There was a smattering of Jewish gangsters and prostitutes.

Warsaw had swelled to its current Jewish population by a constant influx of refugees from around the former Pale and Poland. Thousands came on the heels of every new pogrom.

Nathan Zadok liked Warsaw. Here he could be swallowed up in a sea of his own people all speaking Yiddish. Over three hundred synagogues, ranging from one-room affairs to the great Tlomotskie Temple, held a constant flow of worshippers; the stages of forty theaters rang with restless prose; a dozen newspapers cried their protests, and a hundred schools bulged with students of every subject.

The Poale Zion staging center was an old building, a former leather factory on Mila Street in the poorest section of the town. Poale Zion conducted a bare-bones operation in a cavernous main hall, a communal kitchen, and some small side offices. The influx of youngsters making the aliyah to Palestine had swamped their facilities.

Those who had friends or relatives in Warsaw or enough money for a hotel room were in luck. The majority slept on tables, benches, and the floor and ate the worst meals of their lives.

When a group of three hundred had assembled and been processed, a train was organized to take them to Bratislava on the Czech border. They sang all the way. Even Nathan sang. It was his first train ride without fear.

Nathan, also, for the first time, set eyes on Rosie Gittleman. There were only forty girls among the three hundred pioneers. With all of the boys bigger and better-looking than he was, Nathan was certain he could not possibly form a personal friendship with a girl.

Rosie Gittleman would not turn anybody's head. She was not precisely an ugly, but somewhat beyond plain. Her appearance was thin and drab. How could such a girl be a pioneer? Nathan wondered.

At first, Rosie and Nathan exchanged a few glances. Nathan could not believe he was being singled out. With a bit of foxy maneuvering, he arranged to sit next to her.

Nathan had the skill to dazzle anyone for the first few hours of an acquaintance. Rosie didn't know much about literature, so there was his opening. She was definitely impressed.

He was surprised to learn that a year and a half earlier she had been sent to the TB resort of Zakopane in the Carpathian Mountains. Being a Jewess, she was unable to get a room in a regular sanatorium and had to stay in a pension for six months.

Her strict Orthodox family was certain they had a spinster on their hands for the rest of their lives. She first surprised them by surviving her illness and being declared healthy. Having won that battle, she found the wherewithal to stand up to a tyrannical father and declare her intentions of making aliyah to Palestine.

By the time the train had left Krakow and wormed through the passes of the Little Carpathian Mountains, Nathan and Rosie had become adept at brushing against each other and otherwise touching, while pretending not to.

Bratislava

MOST EVERYONE had dozed off when a sudden electricity of excitement flashed through the cars. They had crossed the border out of Poland! Cheering was mixed with farewell curses. Yet, there had to be sorrow as the image of a mother or brother passed through their minds. Nathan felt a twinge of hurt he had not expected.

Lord only knew what was up ahead. Perhaps he should have stayed in Warsaw. No matter how bad things would get, Warsaw always offered a measure of safety. Perhaps if he had met Rosie earlier, they could have talked about it and stayed together. Perhaps . . . perhaps . . .

The train sped across Czechoslovakia, another of those states put together at the end of the war, this one from the defunct Austro-Hungarian Empire.

Toward morning, the train halted on the Danube River at Bratislava, a gateway city between three nations and now the capital of Slovakia. The pioneers disembarked to stretch and milled about until a new train arrived to take them across the river.

The early arriving yard workers were in a state of half-awakeness, certainly angry over their cup of watery coffee and loading up with resentment over another "Jew train."

"Dirty yid" remarks grew louder and more profane. The pioneers, warned to stay out of trouble, huddled together in a tight circle. This encouraged the rail workers and some pushing and shoving began.

Among the pioneers were a few dozen husky young men not so inclined to grovel. Misha Polokov, who had been gaining leadership since Warsaw, grabbed the shovel from the hands of the Slav ringleader and nearly tore his head off with it.

In the melee that followed, the Slavs took an unusual beating. Nathan made himself scarce, going through the motions of setting up a defense picket around the girls. He had never seen a Jew hit a *goy* before, much less knock one down and even kick him on the ground. It was a nice thing to watch, but also quite terrifying. What would happen if word reached the city and a mob came out and massacred them? He was numb with fear when troops arrived.

The pioneers were quickly hustled aboard a line of cars and soldiers were deployed to protect them as the cars rolled onto a train ferry and scooted over the Danube.

Nathan sulked. He should have done better during the fight. He now wanted very much to earn the respect of Rosie Gittleman.

Vienna

VIENNA, once a mecca for the best in mankind, lay gasping in the backwash of war. The city of dreams was boarded up and hunger gnawed at its people.

The pioneers were put up in a public bathhouse and deloused, as a precaution against the typhus epidemic. Clothing was boiled in a cauldron of carbolic acid and came out wrinkled, discolored, and foul-smelling.

Rations consisted of a single slice of bread and a bowl of suspicious-looking dark liquid, with a few leaves floating on the top, three times a day. By the end of the third day, everyone had become lightheaded with hunger. Nathan made a sacrificial gesture of giving Rosie most of his ration.

Misha Polokov, whose accordion had scarcely stopped playing since they left Warsaw, had emerged as their uncontested leader when he covered himself with glory in the brawl in Bratislava. Misha got a group together, including his sister Bertha and Nathan, and scouted the city for some kind of pickings. He located a thriving black market in a corner of Prater Park, where peasants gouged the less fortunate city people out of everything from jewelry to antiques. Money, in currency form, was worthless.

After discussing the situation with his gang, Misha felt it would be impossible to make a snatch and run in Prater Park. He turned to studying the various stretches of road in and out of the city. Highway robbery was the answer.

Bureaucratic red tape and railroad inefficiency forced the pioneers to remain a fifth day. Things at the bathhouse had reached a low point when Misha and a half dozen of his merry folk, including Bertha and Nathan, pulled up in a cart with a hog large enough to feed a small army. The cart also contained a barrel of home-brewed schnapps.

When pressed by the other comrades, Misha confessed he had set up a careful ambush. The unfortunate farmer was caught on a lonely section of back road, bound up, gagged, taken to a nearby village church, hauled up to the steeple top, and left to dangle without his trousers some fifty feet over the ground.

Now came an ethical question of severe gravity. Namely; can a pig be made kosher? A sort of ad hoc rabbinical council was formed to debate the matter.

Nathan Zadok, dizzy from hunger and almost blotto from a glass of schnapps, played devil's advocate brilliantly to convince the comrades that this was not the time to stand on ancient ceremonies.

"God often disguises His mysteries and works in riddles. When we captured this pig, it was a cow. Before our very eyes, it changed. Why is the Lord testing us? To see if we have the courage to get to Palestine, which might not happen if we don't eat this cow. We cannot let God down after coming this far."

As the comrades emptied the barrel of schnapps, it began to make a lot of sense, what Nathan was saying. The fact was, the animal was beginning to resemble a cow more by the minute.

A vote was taken and, indeed, it was overwhelmingly agreed that this animal was truly a cow in disguise. All the pioneers asked silent forgiveness of their parents and their rabbis. The animal was respectfully named Nicholas, after the late Czar, and in a ritual unique in the annals of Vienna became the only hog ever butchered and roasted in a municipal bathhouse.

Misha's accordion went into action and those who were still able danced. Many of the pioneers, not used to the taste or notion of forbidden food, delicately repaired to the toilets and vomited.

As the party reached a peak, officials from Poale Zion arrived to let them know that a train for Trieste had been found and was waiting for them at the Bahnhof.

"Nathan, you were wonderful tonight," Rosie Gittleman said boldly, laying her head on his shoulder. He summoned up the courage to put his arm about her, and after a time she slipped down so her head was on his lap and she fell asleep as he stroked her hair till far into the night.

Trieste

THE PIONEERS broke into song the moment the train left Vienna. Their bellies were full and the scenery was grand. The train snaked through sweet-smelling high meadows and the overpowering visual opulence of the Alps, picking its way to Trieste, the port of embarkation.

During the twenty hours of the train ride, Nathan became increasingly worried about Rosie. She was fragile to begin with and now she was not bearing up well. She felt feverish and looked extremely pale.

"You shouldn't worry, Nathan. It is probably this up-and-down business with the mountains. I remember when I first went up to Zakopane with the trouble with my lungs. The mountains made me dizzy. It will go away."

By the time they passed through Ljubljana, Nathan was quite fearful. "I think you should maybe see a doctor in Trieste."

Rosie was adamant. "No, and don't you go babbling to the others. I've come this far. Nothing is going to keep me off our ship."

"But, Rosie, you look like the color of paste."

"If you mention so much as a single word to the others, I wouldn't speak to you ever again."

Nathan tried to bury his concern. Such a brave girl, he thought. For the first time in his life he allowed his mind to stray in a certain forbidden direction. With a woman like her at his side, Palestine would be far less forbidding. Maybe, miracle of miracles, she could possibly want and need him as well. Together, they could get through the hard times ahead. He chastised himself. It was total nonsense to think such grand ideas.

Trieste was a volatile piece of turf, an ancient prize, the rule of which periodically transferred from one winning empire to another. Since the war, Trieste had been ceded with a strip of land to the victorious Italians. But as a consequence, the port lost its natural hinterland of Slovenia. Trieste was the lifeblood of the province, but now operated at a sluggish pace.

Economic fright always brought on political bombastics. The pioneer train entered a city which was once again playing out a familiar turmoil. The long arm of the Bolshevik Revolution had reached the Balkans. Communist slogans defaced every wall, and leaflets covered the streets like newly fallen snow in the wake of perpetual demonstrations. Ships' crews, generally supporting the Communists, staged debilitating strikes. All of this chaos was carried out with bravado.

Nonetheless, the Zionists were well organized and general conditions were better. The city had become the major port of departure for some forty thousand Russian and Polish Jews of the third "rising" to Palestine.

Misha and Bertha Polokov, as well as some of the other comrades,

also spotted Rosie's condition. She sloughed them off, and after a few
days in Trieste and some decent food she seemed to be faring better.

At the end of a week an Italian freighter, the *Padua*, entered the port
to take the pioneers to Palestine. They were put up on the open top
deck. Their rations were an issue of dried food, with no provisions for
cooked meals. Toilets were temporary shacks which accessed directly to
the sea. Their beds, thin mats with blue sky above.

Captain Gionelli and his crew were friendly. Through Misha Polokov,
the captain loaned them all the extra canvas aboard so they could put
up a tent city to protect them from the elements.

She was far from being a luxury liner, but nothing could hold down
the bursting enthusiasm of the pioneers as the *Padua* eased out of her
berth and proceeded down the Adriatic. Although they never lost sight
of land, they could not help but feel that the tie with the *shtetl* and all
the Jew hating was cut forever.

The pioneers broke into small groups and studied and argued and
sang and danced. Nathan was in his glory, going from audience to audience giving lectures on anything anyone would listen to.

On the third day out, seasonal meltemi winds from the north roughed
up the *Padua* and climaxed in a nasty blow through the Strait of
Otranto. Activities halted as the pioneers huddled together tightly and
queasily. Finally a blessed calm befell and the skies put on a show of
star showers as they sailed smoothly down the Greek coast.

The great debate between crew and passengers was the merits of
communism over Zionism. The price for joining Lenin's Communist
International was to renounce all ethnic groups.

"It is not possible," Nathan argued. "A Jew is a Jew and an Italian is
an Italian. You cannot simply eliminate an entire ethnic people without
destroying the culture itself. Lenin is crazy."

And so it went, as the battle for the minds of the Europeans now
raged between socialism and the new communism out of Russia. These
discussions had little interest for the lovers who paired off. The gregari-
ous Captain Gionelli granted them use of the lifeboats to sleep together.

"I have come to an important decision," Rosie said to Nathan one
night. "I have concluded that you can be just as true a Zionist if you
choose not to go out and redeem the land. We must have cities and
factories and hospitals as well as farms."

"Yes, but everything we have been taught centers on the land," Nathan answered.

"I must admit that it may be too difficult for me to live on a kibbutz," she said. "I may apply for work in Jerusalem."

"I am in accord with your decision one hundred percent," he answered. "I suppose for myself, I should be a farmer."

"So what's wrong with Jerusalem?"

"From what I understand, it is filled with Hasidim. It would be like moving to another *shtetl.*"

"Then what about Tel Aviv? There are already ten thousand Jews living there."

Suddenly it occurred to Nathan that what Rosie might be suggesting was in line with his own secret thoughts. "Tel Aviv is an idea of merit. It should be given some thought," he said.

"You'll pardon my boldness, Nathan, but two people together in such a strange place might be better than one person alone."

Nathan blushed and looked at her quizzically. She lowered her eyes modestly.

"No one says you can't be a good Zionist in a city," he declared at last.

"So, maybe we'll talk about it a little more?"

She nodded and his heart almost leaped out of his throat. She reached over and pecked his cheek and he moved back slowly.

"It's all right, Nathan. All the comrades know I hold you in high regard. You'll pardon my shamelessness, but Captain Gionelli said we could have the last lifeboat."

That night was the most wonderful of Nathan's life. They snuggled up together, but with great respect, and held each other until daybreak.

As the *Padua* plowed along through the Sea of Crete, the meltemi blow faded altogether and the sea dished up another fright from its endless bag of tricks. Zephyrs from the inland deserts of Arabia called "khamsin" drifted out to the sea, flattening it mirror-smooth. The air turned into a furnace. The canvas afforded no relief as temperatures flared over a hundred and ten degrees. The crew hosed down the pioneers regularly with salt water, but after a few minutes it was little better than nothing.

Their songs melted into drones of agony. The steel deck became too hot to walk on. It took two harrowing days to reach Cyprus. The weakest among the pioneers were breaking down fast. A doctor came aboard to examine them and urged that two of the girls and one of the boys be taken to a hospital for sunstroke. During the examinations, Rosie had hidden.

At Famagusta, while the *Padua* took on a cargo of winter potatoes, the pioneers were able to renew themselves ashore with fresh water, a shower, a day in the shade, and a decent meal. They returned to the *Padua* in high spirits, knowing that Jaffa was less than a two-day sail.

Once under way, the ferocious heat of the khamsin returned. By nightfall Rosie had passed out from heat prostration and Nathan could no longer cover for her. He went to Misha weeping. Captain Gionelli fixed her a berth next to his own cabin, and as a half dozen more fell ill, radioed ahead to Jaffa for emergency medical help to be on standby.

Nathan continually bathed her face and sweat-soaked body to try to cool her down, but she broke into a raging fever followed by chills and spent the rest of the journey in a state of delirium.

The battered members of the Third Aliyah lined the rail of the *Padua*, most of them crying openly as specks on the horizon enlarged into a flat coastline. A wave of white buildings could be made out along a ridge, and now a minaret poked through. As they eased toward Jaffa, the joy of seeing Zion was tempered by concern over seven fallen comrades. Rosie in particular was on everyone's mind.

There was also an unmistakable feeling of hostility in the stillness of the air that one could sense from out at sea. The heat and dreariness and flatness and lethargy did not conform with their lifelong visions of Palestine. When it came into view, what they saw was a weary old place baking and rotting under a cruel sun.

A stunned silence was broken by the sound of the anchor chain rattling down and smashing into the water. The port, such as it was, consisted of little more than a breakwater pier and a few warehouses.

First out to greet them was the harbor master's launch, with a medical team and a proper British Government authority. After a quick examination of the sunstroke victims, landing formalities were waived to get them ashore quickly.

Captain Gionelli and Misha took the British major aside and appealed to him to allow Nathan to go ashore with Rosie. The Englishman huffed and puffed for a moment, then nodded approval.

They were removed to Neve Shalom, a sector of Jaffa that had been purchased by the Zionist Settlement Department from the Arabs. The hospital was actually a large old Arab house, recently bought by an organization of American Jewish women called Hadassah, which had undertaken to provide medical care for the Jews in Palestine. The hospital held ten beds and was staffed by a pair of American doctors and five nurses.

One by one, the other pioneers came around, but Rosie Gittleman

remained in critical condition. She rallied on the second night long
enough to recognize Nathan.

"We made it, Rosie," Nathan said. "We're here, in Eretz Israel."
Rosie managed a small smile and then she died.

TO PALESTINE

1920–1921

IT WAS NO LAND of milk and honey. In truth, Palestine was a weary and neglected place, eroded by sun and infested by swamp. Feudal Arab overlords fought any progress the newly arriving Jews might bring, preferring to continue to suck dry their own lethargic and defeated people.

The British, now ruling under an international mandate, were overtly sympathetic to the Arabs and permitted their gangs to prey on the Jewish community with impunity. The mufti of Jerusalem, a rabid Moslem clergyman, fomented hatred and riots erupted continually throughout the country.

The older Jewish settlers had transplanted much of the *shtetl* mentality to Palestine. They owned the large private farms, vineyards, and factories and were content to go on using cheap Arab labor.

A Jewish land agency was buying up acreage as fast as it could be acquired from absentee Arab landowners, but there was already a long waiting list of immigrants ready to start up new settlements.

To Nathan it seemed like the horrors of the *shtetl* all over again. What he had come to was a small, impoverished Jewish community unable to absorb the rush of new young idealists.

What Nathan Zadok saw was Jews walled in to defend themselves, roads impassable by night, and heat of unbearable intensity by day. Tel Aviv was a sorry town with little cultural life or entertainment. The hatred shown to Jews by the Pole, Cossack, Russian, and Ukrainian was amply replaced by that of the Arab. There was neither land to go to nor a living to be made.

"I'VE GOT A JOB as a guard," Misha told Nathan a month after their arrival. "Bertha is coming along with me as a cook. There's an opening for you as well."

"What are you guarding?"

"A Jewish-owned orange grove during the picking and crating season. We're protecting against Arab theft in the fields and marauders from the outside."

"So what do I know from guns? I'll go with you if they'll let me at least pick oranges."

"The pickers are all Arab."

"No Jewish pickers on a Jewish farm?"

"There were Jews last year, but the Labor Federation tried to organize them."

Nathan shook his head. "For this we came to Palestine, to be exploited by Jews?"

"We've only been here a month, Nathan. Conditions are going to change. We knew it would be rough at first."

"I don't need from you a Zionist lecture," Nathan answered. "Palestine is filled with Jewish exploiters, Arab exploiters, and British reactionaries. None of them give a damn for us. They're sucking our blood to line their pockets."

"So don't you give me a Bolshevik lecture," Misha shot back.

"And even if a union comes, does that mean we will automatically start having a love affair with the Arabs?"

"We can't go back, Nathan. Poland, White Russia, and the Ukraine are covered with Jewish blood. The pogroms are worse than 1880, worse than 1905."

"No, we can't go back. You take the guard job, Misha."

"And you?"

"I have relatives here somewhere. I'll *shnorr* them and see what happens."

Nathan had the addresses of his first cousins, the Borokov brothers from Mariupol, who had made the Second Aliyah to Palestine before the war. Cousin Sidney was a teacher at the highly regarded Herzlia Gymnasium in Jaffa, where some of the more affluent Jews of the *shtetl* sent their children. Like everything in Palestine, the gymnasium was struggling for funds.

Sidney Borokov was a decent sort, with a houseful of kids, a low wage, and no authority. Nathan had no qualifications to work at such an institution, which was already overstaffed with underpaid scholars and intellectuals. After a week of listening to Nathan's recounting of the tragic affair with Rosie Gittleman, Sidney took him to see his brother, Morris.

Morris Borokov was one of a small number of Jewish businessmen who had succeeded. He owned a villa in the upper-middle-class German colony on the edge of Tel Aviv. The coolness between Sidney and Morris and Morris and Nathan was mutual. Morris's main operation was importing coal. *Gevalt!* Nathan thought. It was Mariupol all over again, only worse.

Being first cousins imposed certain obligations, so Morris housed Nathan, in the servants' quarters with the Arabs, and complained constantly about how bad business was. He had all the unpleasant characteristics of his father, Boris, and was a notorious exploiter of his workers. After a few uncomfortable days, Nathan came to a decision. Cousin Morris was only too glad to pay for a train ticket for Nathan to go to Jerusalem and toss in a few pounds of living money.

As THE TRAIN WENDED through the great ravines and vales of the Judean hills, Nathan's spirits lifted as the sense of Jerusalem and its mystical powers began to overtake him.

Jerusalem! Jerusalem of gold! Why had it taken him so long to come to it? He wondered. A lot of Yiddish was spoken in the city and there was certain to be work.

But Nathan's euphoria was short-lived. Jerusalem was a line of barren hills swept by ominous winds, a city of glaring stones and dust. It had not recovered from losing a third of its population to hunger and disease during the war. It was the poorest of cities, lonely and remote, a place reserved for only those with the most powerful faith.

Jerusalem of gold was tarnished from too many sackings over too many centuries and its resurrection was a long way off, if ever. Nathan found a cot at a hostel in the Jewish Quarter of the Old City. This square mile within Ottoman walls contained the wildest potpourri of religious ferment on earth. It was a short walk to the Wailing Wall, but the route was safe because it was traveled by sufficient numbers.

Within the walled city lived the poorest of the poor, existing from hand to mouth. Streams of Hasidim and ultra-Orthodox men pounded the stone pavements to and from the Wall in their severe long black coats, bobbing in prayerful motions as they went, their earlocks flopping beneath black broad-brimmed beaver hats. Supported largely by world Jewish charities, they spent their lives in study and prayer.

It was a tight, suspicious place, where one trod cautiously on the filthy streets, always aware of the dark, hostile eyes probing the back of one's neck.

Beyond the wall were cliques: scores of Jews from different lands, Bukharians, Yemenites, Moroccans, Syrians, Poles, each in their own fortress neighborhood.

Nathan found no comfort in his wanderings. It was a place where one could exist if one wanted to drown in false religious promises, Nathan thought. At best, it was a place to come to die.

Obviously, there was no work for him. The religious groups were impenetrable, their schools staffed with their own, their living conditions dismal.

He beat a retreat from Jerusalem after a fortnight of disenchantment.

In the next months he worked as a common laborer on rail and road gangs, carrying sand to mix with mortar for public buildings, whitewashing houses, laying water pipe, and splitting rocks with a sledgehammer. Workers were underfed and underpaid and labor trouble was always brewing.

Seven months after their aliyah to Eretz Israel, Misha found Nathan digging ditches near Hadera.

Misha related that his sister, Bertha, had fallen in love with a *Kibbutznik* and joined his settlement. Miracle of miracles, a place for both Misha and Nathan had been found at the kibbutz.

"You didn't bring this news a minute too soon. Where are we off to?"

"The northern Galilee. A kibbutz called Hermon."

"Hermon!" Nathan cried. "My God, Misha, that's only a few kilometers from the Tel Hai massacre," he continued in reference to a recent battle between Jew and Arab. "I think we'd better wait until some new land opens. Hermon is in the jaws of the tiger."

"Maybe we'd better wait for the messiah," Misha retorted. "I'm tired of all this shit here. At least at Hermon we can begin to be Zionists and do what we came here to do."

Outside Nathan's tent was an endless ditch to be dug. "Include me in," he said at last. "I will go with you to Hermon."

THE ZIONIST SETTLEMENT Department provided Nathan and Misha each with a bedroll and a rucksack of rations and essentials. The way north was from kibbutz to kibbutz. What Nathan and Misha saw, for the most part, was a group of new settlements popping up in the Jezreel Valley. Pioneers were battling centuries of swampland resulting from Arab neglect. The settlers existed on thin man's diets in primitive conditions. A few of the older kibbutzim had made marked progress and there was some greenery to contrast with the naked brown of the landscape.

At the northern end of the Sea of Galilee they came to a kibbutz named Degania, which was lush and filled with date palms and banana groves. Degania lay below sea level in a natural hothouse. This was the "mother" of Palestine's kibbutzim, now thriving in its twelfth year. Here was the Garden of Eden, the kind of settlement the pioneers had fantasized about back in the *shtetl*, one of the few tangible fruits of Zionism thus far.

North of Degania was wild country, a dangerous place. A convoy formed to take Misha and Nathan and supplies to the last settlement, known as Kibbutz Hermon. Past Huleh Lake and a nasty swamp, Kibbutz Hermon was the end of the line.

MOUNT HERMON, a small but mighty mountain of nine thousand feet, laid her skirts down at a convergence of three separate districts, Palestine, the Lebanon, and Syria. Mount Hermon's foothills held an assortment of impoverished Shi'ite Moslem and Druze villages, built into the steep terrain for protection. After the turn of the century the Jews had established an elite mounted guard called the Shomer, or Watchmen, who protected the distant settlements. They traveled by horseback, spoke Arabic, and dressed in Bedouin robes. Their skills in dealing with raiders and marauders became legendary. A group of Watchmen established Zionist settlements at Tel Hai and Kfar Giladi. These outposts came under heavy Arab attack and after sustaining severe casualties, the Watchmen were forced to abandon them.

A few miles beyond Tel Hai and Kfar Giladi sat Kibbutz Hermon, which had successfully fought off the attacks and remained the farthermost Jewish settlement in Palestine. Beyond its perimeters lay Baniyas, a magnificent grotto and oasis where mountain streams flowed down to form one of the headwaters of the Jordan River. Once the land of the biblical tribe of Dan, this was now a no-man's-land. Ruins of Dan and Baniyas and an ancient mountainside fortress that had held against the Romans were all within walking distance of the kibbutz.

Although it was a mere fifteen miles from the Sea of Galilee to the foothills of Mount Hermon, the climate underwent a drastic change, going from the below sea level semitropical to the moderate climate of the mountains, with cool nights and a snowfall in the winter.

Nathan had heard of the leader of Kibbutz Hermon, a heroic figure named Ami Dan who had arrived during the World War, had become a roving Watchman for a short time, and then established the kibbutz in 1917 with ten men and two women. Kibbutz Hermon was able to hang on because of Ami Dan's personal leadership after Tel Hai and Kfar Giladi had been abandoned.

Ami Dan, it appeared, had earned his reputation when he gathered a group of Watchmen and crossed into the Lebanon just before the harvest and torched the entire Arab Marjioun Valley, then afterward went back and discussed peace with the local mukhtars and chieftains. His message had gotten through loud and clear. Kibbutz Hermon was never attacked in force again, but was constantly being sniped at and raided by small parties of marauding Bedouins. Although it was relatively safe, precautions were always in effect.

Kibbutz Hermon had grown to sixty members, a third of them women who now included Bertha Polokov. Their greatest pride was the children's house where a half-dozen babies had been born.

Despite the abundance of water, the variety of crops was limited because the ground was of porous limestone. Because of the altitude and coolness, apple and fruit orchards flourished and bore standard crops along with a centuries-old olive grove.

The convoy stopped at an outer stockade wall rimmed with guard towers. They entered a compact village center built of native black basalt rock that held a men's and women's barracks, a building of private rooms for married couples, the children's house, farm buildings and offices, and an all-purpose recreation/dining hall, library, and clinic.

"Misha! Nathan!" Bertha Polokov cried, racing over the compound to welcome them. Kibbutz members surrounded the convoy to greet the newcomers and bombard them with questions.

The crowd suddenly opened an aisle as they felt a presence. The kibbutz leader, Ami Dan, came toward them. He was not all that large a man, but his unkempt beard gave him a look of power and he had the unmistakable manner of a leader.

Ami Dan embraced Misha. "Welcome to Hermon, comrade." He turned to Nathan who stared at him for ever so long and then came remembrance.

"Yossi Dubnow?" Nathan asked.

"That is right. I was once Yossi Dubnow. The last time I saw you was in Poland, at an abandoned brick factory outside Siedlce. We'll talk about it later."

Ami Dan turned to the others. "All right, comrades, your questions will have to wait. We will have a meeting after dinner and get caught up on the news of the outside."

As they were shown around this roughhewn stockade, Nathan suddenly realized there were no electricity, phone, or telegraph wires entering the kibbutz, and he did not share Misha's elation.

THE KIBBUTZ OFFICE was a spartan room attached to the end of the men's barracks. As Nathan entered, Ami Dan was seated at a crystal radio set writing down dots and dashes of an incoming message. When the transmission ended, he doffed his earphones and waved to Nathan to take a chair.

"When Bertha Polokov submitted your name, I was really taken by surprise," Ami Dan said. "I could have sworn I'd never see you in Palestine."

Nathan Zadok had, over the years, developed a near total capacity to forget any past incident in which he had been at fault, or tuck away into a far corner in his mind an unpleasantness. Ami Dan's opening remark passed over him without striking a chord.

"Bertha assures me that you have changed and you'll be an asset to the kibbutz. I understand you've paid your dues here in Palestine. Well, I'm willing to forget what happened between us."

Nathan was unresponsive. "You'll be so kind to tell me," he said, "what's by this Ami Dan?"

"My Hebrew name," Ami Dan answered. "Yossi Dubnow was left in the *shtetl*. Most of us here have chosen to take new names."

"I am aware of this business of changing names," Nathan said.

"You might want to take a Hebrew name as well."

"Never," Nathan shot back. "My father would never understand such a thing. Something is wrong with Zadok? Zadok was one of our most revered Jewish dynasties."

"There's nothing wrong with Nathan Zadok," Ami Dan said.

"It's a Jewish name, a true Jewish name."

Ami Dan smiled and changed the subject. "Misha and Bertha told me that the three of you have had a difficult time."

"An understatement."

"I promise you that it is not going to be easy here either, but turning a spade in our own soil is a lot different from breaking rocks for a

British road. We have made a tremendous start for the future. In five years this place will be like Degania."

Ami Dan painted an upbeat picture. The Syrians in the villages in the foothills had been unable to dislodge them. Marauding, a way of life among the Bedouin, had almost been curbed. Jewish settlers would soon be returning to Tel Hai and Kfar Giladi, so they would again have close neighbors.

Kibbutz life? It was simple and hard but no one left the table hungry. The hours were long, but never a night ended without singing and dancing and debates and storytelling. Most of all, their efforts had been blessed by the six infants in the nursery, and another three were on the way.

Nathan's mind flashed back to his Uncle Bernie's cinema in Minsk. He remembered what a great favorite the American cowboy films had been. The covered wagons, the Indian attacks, the privation. At the time he couldn't possibly have equated Americans crossing the prairie with Zionism, but now there seemed to be amazing similarities between Kansas and the northern Galilee, except that the earth of Kansas showed more promise. The rest of it—the constant peril, the isolation, and the enemies—was the same. Only here there would be no U.S. Cavalry to save them.

"I should like a job," Nathan said, "to do clerical work at which I have had considerable experience."

"That's not how we operate," Ami Dan answered. "Unless you come in with a special skill like a carpenter or a blacksmith, we all rotate positions. In that way each of us learns every job on the kibbutz. After a year, when you are voted in as a full member, you can petition for a semi-permanent position."

The rest of it was a portrait of spartan life and nearly total communal existence. Clothing, time off, a few pounds a year spending money, medical care—all necessities came out of a common pool. All decisions were made collectively.

NATHAN'S FIRST assignment was as assistant custodian of the barn, which housed a small dairy herd and the workhorses and mules. It was the simplest of jobs, however unpleasant. Nathan likened it to the coalyard in Mariupol, with manure replacing coal as the object of his loathing. Manure, he learned, was a useful commodity to nourish the orchards.

The rest of the work was simple. Mending harnesses and other leather work he had learned from his father. Shoveling hay into stalls, pumping bellows for the farrier, and whitewashing did not require a higher education. Nor did watchtower duty, a nightly obligation. The future held little promise.

Nathan could not understand the mentality of Comrade Amos, who was in charge of the barn and herd and spent his days singing and extolling the glories of Zionism. It seemed that Comrade Amos got a spiritual uplift out of merely smelling manure.

Once he had mastered milking the cows, Nathan felt he would be able to petition to move on to more promising work. The cows proved uncooperative. "Kicking the bucket" took on new meaning. Nathan did not listen too well to Comrade Amos's instructions and it took him a week to realize that the cows expected to be milked from the right side instead of the left. Nathan was kicked repeatedly, stomped on, developed milker's elbow, and wore his hands raw.

On the other hand, Comrade Amos loved the cows. And they loved him. On those icy mornings when Comrade Amos laid his head against the cow for warmth, the animal responded. Nathan realized they talked to each other. Comrade Amos and the cows actually held discussions.

Nathan struggled on with swollen hands, overturned pails, barked shins, as he learned deft moves to get out of their way. The most unpleasant part of it was when the cow did a large wet flop that streaked down its tail, then swished it quickly, banging it into the side of Nathan's face. The milk production fell so low that the children were going without. Comrade Amos finally asked that Nathan be assigned elsewhere.

EACH MORNING at five o'clock, when the kibbutz came to life in earnest, Nathan wondered if this was truly where he wanted to spend the rest of his life.

Many things came to Nathan's attention that bordered on the shocking. Since his arrival in Palestine, he had become hardened to the fact that the women did not practice traditional modesty. One could certainly overlook short sleeves and no head kerchief because of the type of work, although his mother always wore long sleeves, even during heat waves. He had seen a number of women expose their legs, wearing brief pants that were rolled up to *there*, since his arrival in Palestine. He had never before seen a female in public exposed up to *there*. At Kibbutz Hermon all of them, married or single, dressed immodestly.

This lack of demureness, an affront to Jewish life, carried over to other things in daily kibbutz life. Nathan had a problem with the showers. In Wolkowysk there were no showers. A tub in the yard had greeted him at the end of the day, the water heated to a pleasant warmth. Here the showers were icy, particularly at five o'clock in the morning.

The men's and women's showers were separated by a flimsy partition that was partly open. If one wanted to catch a glimpse, it was no problem.

The worst of it was that this perpetual condition of nakedness didn't seem to annoy anyone but him. After all, these were all *shtetl*-born people, traditionally observant Jews who were cautioned about such exposures. He began seriously to ponder to what extent Zionism itself might be the corrupting influence.

Moreover, Nathan wondered, what kind of a Jewish farm was it without a proper synagogue? Also, the kibbutz raised hogs in secret. Furthermore, it was known that when the girls went to the Arab market in the villages, they would barter the kibbutz produce for camel meat, another forbidden food.

There was a building on the kibbutz that no one spoke of. Misha, who had had a year of military training, went into it immediately. When Misha told him casually that they were manufacturing guns and bombs, Nathan almost choked. There were constant comings and goings of groups of young people from settlements farther south. He learned they were members of the newly formed Jewish Defense Force, the Haganah, and Kibbutz Hermon was a training base for them.

Such disillusionments continued to pile up.

NATHAN BLUSHED when he was assigned to Malka, a very plump girl who likewise wore her shorts up to *there,* for rifle training. He had never held a gun before, and the very concept of it staggered his imagination. Guns were for *goyim.* His hands sweated whenever he touched a weapon. For three days Malka taught him to take the rifle apart, clean it, put it together, and squeeze the trigger without ammunition.

To conclude the instruction, he had to shoot ten rounds of live ammunition which was manufactured at the kibbutz. As he sighted in on the target, Malka stood over him with her big bare legs and he got so flustered he forgot his instructions. He jerked the trigger instead of giving it a slow clean pull, and he also forgot to keep his thumb tucked down. The rifle butt slammed into his shoulder, causing him to see stars, and at the same instant he jammed his thumb into his eye. He missed the target.

THE WEEKLY kibbutz meeting took place on Wednesday after dinner.
"Do we have any new business?" Ami Dan asked.

Nathan popped up.

"I have a matter which I would like to present for serious consideration," he said.

"It is not customary for a comrade to participate if he is not a full member of the kibbutz, but we will make an exception. What is on your mind, Nathan?"

Nathan paced, stared like a righteous rabbi to set the frame of mind, then shook his index finger at them.

"I am thinking, comrades, what is the big *megillah* about the name Hermon? Why does such a mountain, belonging almost entirely to Arabs, have the distinction of having a kibbutz named after it?"

Most of the members gaped in disbelief. "The mountain has great biblical significance," Ami Dan answered. "And it also happens to be where we are located."

"Just how many Hermons will be enough?" Nathan went on without listening to Ami Dan. "What is it? A sacred mountain? Does God send down special blessings from Hermon?"

"Speak in Hebrew," Ami Dan said testily; "it is a kibbutz rule."

Nathan continued his harangue against the mountain in Yiddish.

"Would you kindly get to the point, Comrade Zadok."

"I am thinking and with deep feelings, with which I am certain the comrades will be in agreement, that a kibbutz, to properly commemorate, should be named, instead, for a real person. I have in mind a martyr of Zionism. I am proposing that we change the name of the kibbutz to Kfar Gittleman, in memory of one who sacrificed her life to reach Eretz Israel. . . ."

"You are out of order, Comrade Zadok."

"What could be a more magnificent name and so simple a gesture? Kfar Gittleman," Nathan continued. . . .

"You are out of order."

AFTER ROTATING Nathan to a dozen different jobs, none of which he performed successfully, Ami Dan realized it would only be a matter of time until Nathan would leave, voluntarily or otherwise. The members were growing impatient with him, even Bertha and Misha. Nathan was not a communal being. Some people simply weren't cut out for kibbutz life, but no one ever showed less of a capacity to accept instruction or acknowledge criticism.

Ami Dan decided to press the issue by assigning Nathan to the most dangerous job on the kibbutz, and ordered him a month's duty as a perimeter guard. They went out in two-man teams, leaving the stockade after sunset, sleeping in the field, and roving the outer boundaries on watch against Bedouin marauders.

Ami Dan had made a serious mistake. On the fourth night there were some stirrings near Nathan's position. His partner, a lad named Levi, went out to investigate. Alone and terrified, Nathan forgot the password and just about everything else and shot at Levi as he returned. Fortunately, Nathan's aim was not a thing of beauty and Levi escaped unscathed.

"Do WE HAVE any new business?" Ami Dan asked.

Nathan popped up.

"I have a matter which I would like to present for serious consideration," he said.

"You are out of order," Ami Dan snapped and his sentiment was echoed about the room.

"I am certain, when the comrades hear what I have to propose, they will find me very much in order."

"Very well, Comrade Zadok, but make it brief."

"Today I again visited the library, as I often do, for I read several languages and have a background in literature. I find to my dismay that there are books in English, in Hebrew, in German, and in French, but not so much as a single volume in Yiddish. I cannot alone reverse the mentality in Palestine that says the tongue of Eretz Israel must be Hebrew—a language, as you all know, reserved exclusively for prayer. So, I accept what I cannot do nothing about. However, it is a disgraceful criminal matter that Yiddish has been abandoned. And I tell you that in the end, the Jewish community in Palestine will return to Yiddish, because Hebrew is not usable as a modern language."

Ami Dan quickly quieted the members down. "You are way out of line, Zadok!" he retorted angrily. "We did not come to Palestine to transpose the *shtetl* but to build a new country. Spanish-born Jews do not speak Yiddish. American-born Jews do not speak Yiddish. African-born Jews do not speak Yiddish, nor do they speak it in any of the Moslem countries, where half the entire world's Jewish population lives.

Yiddish is not the universal language of the Jews. It is the language of
the *shtetl* and the ghetto!"

Nathan ignored the applause at the end of Ami Dan's words.

"I propose the following," Nathan continued. "Each of us should
write home and have Yiddish books sent to our library. I, personally,
will take the responsibility of teaching Yiddish to the children of the
kibbutz, who should not forget they are Jews."

"WHAT DO WE do with Nathan?" a frustrated Ami Dan asked Misha
and Bertha.

"I know I made a terrible mistake by vouching for him," Bertha said,
"but I still don't want to see him have to undergo the humiliation of
being voted out of the kibbutz."

Misha fingered his accordion. "He sits alone at night and reads. He
never bothers to come and join us. I've never seen him sing or dance."

"I didn't tell you the story of when we met in Poland," Ami Dan
said. "I should have. This place is not for him. He's driving everybody
crazy."

"I'd talk to him," Misha said, "but he has no listening apparatus."

"So what do we do?" Bertha said, repeating Ami Dan's frustrated
question.

"I have an idea," Ami Dan said suddenly. "It's a bit of dirty business,
but it could work. The land fund has assigned us two thousand dunams
of new land on the Huleh Lake."

"But it's all swamp," Misha said.

"Exactly," Ami Dan answered.

THE PLAN to develop Huleh Lake was a joint venture with Tel Hai
and Kfar Giladi. An expert from the Far East had been sent to Palestine
to study the feasibility of building ponds to seed, grow, and harvest
fresh-water fish. It was the dicey business of rebalancing nature.

First a portion of the swamp had to be drained. No human physical
labor matched it for filth, sweat, and danger. Six volunteers and Nathan
were sent down as part of the team from Kibbutz Hermon.

All told, twenty men and four girls from the three settlements went
at the swamp. They were short on machinery, but long on spirit. They
hacked away with machetes at the papyrus reeds that hovered high over
their heads, working in waist-high muck, and hand-dug a labyrinth of

channels to drain off the waters. Every slimy creature and every biting
insect in Palestine had relatives in the Huleh swamp.

Over a period of years, most of the pioneers had developed a measure
of immunity to malaria. Newer members hit for the first time often
went down hard. Nathan lasted for three weeks in the swamp and was
on the verge of quitting and running away when the decision was made
for him by an unfriendly mosquito.

His temperature shot up so high he became delirious. When the fever
failed to break, it was decided to move him to the small Hadassah
hospital in Tiberias.

Chills and fever raged for several days. The quinine treatment added
to his hallucinations and left his head ringing constantly.

When the malaria subsided, Nathan was so debilitated he was
scarcely able to walk. He opened his eyes on the sixth morning to see
Misha and Bertha sitting at his bedside. Misha handed him a letter from
his father. Nathan set it aside to read later.

"I have come to a decision," Nathan said weakly. "Namely, I am
leaving Kibbutz Hermon. No, no, no, don't try to talk me out of it."

Bertha and Misha somehow managed to register dismay.

When they had gone, Nathan sat up and opened the letter from his
father.

My son, Nathan,

    . . . it was good to get from you, your last letter, and hear
firsthand what a great success you are making in Palestine, particularly after your terrible tragedy with Rosie Gittleman.

    I write to you wonderful news, namely, your brother Matthias
is going to make aliyah in a few months. Such joy for a father.
Two sons in Eretz Israel!

    . . . beyond all expectations, the *shiddachs* have been made for
Ida and Sarah, which only goes to prove that sometimes charm is
better than beauty. Ida is to marry soon, Modele the baker, whom
I'm certain you recall. He's a bit older, no Greek God, but a good
provider and even from peculiar matches can come beautiful children. And Sarah soon afterwards is to go to the *chuppa* with
Manny Dinkle, a teamster who works steady.

    . . . but the biggest surprise is Rifka, who we thought was
beyond marrying age. Who should she get, no less than the respected widower Rabbi Silverstone.

    . . . your brother, Mordechai, has become one of the most important intellectuals in Vilna and his wife is expecting a second child. We pray, hopefully, for a boy this time.

. . . as for ourselves, what can I say? A young tree bends, an old tree breaks. We are creaking, but so long as there is such pleasure from the children, we bear up.

My son, my son, I hate to close with bad news, but the pogroms by the Poles are worse than anything the Czar could have dreamed up, worse than 1880. They say a hundred thousand Jews have been slaughtered so far. We are relatively safe here in Wolkowysk, but who knows.

The Ukraine, they say, is even worse than Poland. Over a hundred separate pogroms have taken place. It is not like the Cossacks riding through town and leaving. This is organized. Entire villages are being burned down. They even kill by hand to save bullets and no known torture has been spared. . . .

Nathan trudged into the office of Mrs. Cohen of the Zionist Settlement Department, took off his cap, set down his rucksack, and sat opposite her desk.

"Are you absolutely certain about this?" she asked.

"Yes."

Mrs. Cohen, a portly, motherly woman, shook her head sadly. "My husband and I came to Palestine in the Second Aliyah. I know it's difficult to believe, but things were much harder in those days."

"I don't want from you a talking-to," Nathan said.

"I'm entitled," Mrs. Cohen answered. "I put a child into the grave here during the war. She died of malnutrition. My husband was tortured by the Turks for spying for the British. He was crippled and also died of his injuries."

"So, with such horrible memories, how can you go on living in Palestine?" Nathan asked.

"How can I not go on living here? Can I tell my husband and daughter it was all in vain? From yesterday to today and from today to tomorrow, I see things change. Give us a year or two, Nathan. The Labor Federation is really beginning to change conditions. The Haganah has stopped the Arab outrages cold. And the best news of all is that a large land purchase for the entire Jezreel Valley has gone through. We are going to form at least a dozen new settlements, immediately. I can get you assigned to one of them."

Nathan shook his head. "No."

"Where do you intend to go? The pogroms in Russia and Poland are worse than anything Europe has seen since the Middle Ages."

"America," he answered.

"Very well. Do you have relatives in America who will pay your passage and vouch for you?"

"Yes."

She took some forms from her desk and shoved them over to him. Nathan began to cry, softly.

"It's all right," she said. "You're not the only one leaving Palestine."

"Zionism has failed me," he wept.

PART THREE

AMERICA! AMERICA!

GIDEON

IT IS DIFFICULT to know when my flight of ecstasy segued into a horrifying awareness. I was buzzing along merrily in my morphine haze when the *zzzz* turned from pleasant to hostile and became louder and louder, then switched to a shrill, ear-splitting scream.

I fought my eyes open at the same instant that angry puffs of earth and stone erupted all about me like little geysers and sharp little bits of stone sprayed into me like hornet stings. Machine-gun bullets!

I caught a glance of Shlomo as he pounced on top of me and covered me with his body. "Don't move!" he yelled.

No sooner had Shlomo pinned me down than the shooting stopped and the screams tailed off quickly. We were being attacked by low-flying jet aircraft. Shlomo rolled off me.

"You all right?" he asked.

"Where the hell are we?"

Then I began to recall: Lydda Airport . . . Val and my daughters taking off in flying boxcars . . . the beach . . . Natasha . . . Grover Vandover . . . the slow agonizing flight of the Dakotas into the Sinai . . . the parachute jump. The parachute jump! Jesus! Hadn't I been injured on the landing?

The screaming sounds returned . . . louder . . . louder . . . louder! This time the earth bounced from the impact of bullets as Egyptian MiGs, engines shrieking, flashed over at what seemed touching distance, the noise nearly splitting my skull. Ugly bastards! Shlomo smothered me once more.

"Get off me, you goddam ape," I shouted at him and lifted my head to catch a glimpse of the plumes of a pair of jets streaking away. I propped myself up on my elbows and watched our guards firing at them futilely.

"Medic! Medic!"

A paratrooper was shot up only a few yards away. He was a damned mess, his entire upper body gushing blood.

"Stay put!" Shlomo ordered. "They're coming back."

I watched the MiGs appear over the horizon, a couple of specks, banking, then growing larger and larger as they zeroed in for another pass.

Suddenly the Egyptians pulled out of their dive and zipped skyward. Shlomo had his field glasses on them.

"Yahoo!" he cried. "Yahoo! Yahoo! Gideon! Our boys are after them!"

Another pair of specks tore after the MiGs, which hightailed it for the Canal and safety. Cheering erupted from the ground, and then a massive sigh of relief. Attention turned to the wounded soldier.

During the night, while I was unconscious, the injured had been moved from the exposed open ground into a small wadi to afford us a measure of protection. There wasn't too much cover anywhere, but it's amazing how you can burrow into the smallest crack.

The balance of the Lion's Battalion had made a forced march to the mouth of Mitla Pass, had found some good elevated ground, and were digging in to halt any attempt by the Egyptians to break out and reinforce their troops in the Sinai.

During the night, supplies, artillery, and jeeps had been dropped by parachute. Of the dozen jeeps, nearly all were damaged. A number of tires burst on impact, and other vehicles hit the ground engine first. Working in near-total darkness, so as not to draw fire from inside the Pass, they cannibalized six of the jeeps for spare parts to get the other six into working order.

Dr. Schwartz got the wounded lad quieted down and his bleeding under control. About this time I was reminded of my own pain, which was again becoming considerable as the morphine wore off.

"Let me try this bugger out," I said.

Shlomo pulled me to my feet very slowly and held my hand for balance. I saw my hip through torn trousers. It looked like a rotten banana and was still swollen to almost the size of a basketball. I gingerly set some weight on the leg, took a step, and fell onto Shlomo, then pulled back from him carefully. I could bear my own weight, but my balance was tentative. I hobbled a few crooked steps, probably looking like the Hunchback of Notre Dame. Well, at least I could move somewhat on my own.

"How is it?" Shlomo asked.

"Shit city."

A few more steps, each a bit better, but it was hurting. I sank to the ground. "Afraid you're going to have to scratch me from the hundred-yard-dash competition," I said.

"Not so bad," Shlomo said. "Dr. Schwartz says that in three or four days you should have pretty good movement again, so take it easy."

"We got anything to eat?"

As Shlomo opened a can of rations, I allowed myself a few mouthfuls of water to rinse out the grit and unpleasantness.

"Take yourself a good drink," Shlomo said; "the Egyptians left us a full water tanker lorry near the monument."

I guzzled. Water in the desert! Lord, it was among the greatest of all sensations. However, the rations fought back at me angrily.

"How in the hell can those sons of bitches in your kitchens go out of their way to make anything taste so gruesome? Jesus H. Christ, this is worse than Marine Corps C rations, and nothing is worse than Marine Corps C rations."

"Kosher," Shlomo answered, "we've got to keep kosher."

"It's what makes the Israeli Army so mean, these mother rations."

Shlomo pacified me with an orange from his knapsack. If you travel with Shlomo, you never go hungry. A cloud of dust rose from the desert floor in the distance, heralding the arrival of a convoy consisting of the six working jeeps. The wounded para was loaded first and was rushed away. The rest of us "walking wounded" piled aboard the other jeeps for a twenty-minute sprint to battalion headquarters, which was situated on a rise halfway between the Parker Monument and Mitla Pass.

Activity now carried an air of urgency as the paras hacked away at the hard-baked soil and rock to dig in before nightfall. Four recoilless rifles and a pair of heavy mortars dropped during the night were now being entrenched and zoning in on the Pass.

A phone line was hooked up between Major Ben Asher at the command post and the forward observation post. Canvas panels were being laid out to indicate a landing strip on a flat stretch of track below.

Only minutes after the panels were staked down, a little Piper Cub glided in like a toy and sputtered to a halt. While the wounded soldier and a medic were being squeezed aboard, the pilot handed a packet of communications to the major. Shlomo and I, who were privy to discussions with the officers, went to the edge of their circle and listened.

The balance of the Para Brigade, which had to cross a hundred and fifty–odd miles of desert track through the middle of the Sinai in order to link up with us, had apparently run into stiff opposition from fortified Egyptian positions. The desert itself was ravaging their vehicles and armor.

The commander of Para 202 Brigade was a semi-legendary figure, Colonel Zechariah. We took some comfort in the conviction that if anyone would break through to us, it would be Zechariah. Yet, with the day only beginning, the hours would be long and filled with tension and, perhaps, battle.

About forty minutes after the first Piper Cub flew off, a second one found its way in, and the two paras with broken legs were boarded. The pilot brought further disconcerting news that an Egyptian column had been spotted on the road from the Canal moving into the opposite entrance of Mitla Pass, some sixteen miles away.

Ben Asher ordered the balance of the walking wounded to assemble and went into a consultation with Dr. Schwartz. As they broke up their meeting, the major came directly toward me.

"You will go back on the next plane, Zadok," he said to me tersely, his hands on his hips. Why is it that all friggin' officers have to authoritate with their hands on their hips?

"I've come too far for you to do this to me," I pleaded.

"Either go peacefully, or I'll have you tied up."

"Major, hey, old buddy, I've come halfway around the world to find this place. I have to stay."

He glanced at my leg, shook his head, and turned to leave.

I grabbed him instinctively and this drew a crowd. Everyone gawked as Ben Asher took my hands off him. He seemed on the verge of ordering me put under restraint.

"The wounded will be evacuated," he said. He continued to stare at me and his stare was frightening. The major was a concrete block of a man, who could do away with me with a single backhand blow. I was going dry and I knew he could see me grow pale and faint. He reached down, picked up a rock, and turned and threw it. It landed over a hundred feet away.

"If you are not wounded, you should have no trouble retrieving that stone and bringing it back here inside one minute," he said and immediately started time by looking at his watch.

"There's a difference between a wound and an injury," I pleaded. "Anyone knows that!"

"You have wasted ten seconds," he said.

"But . . . God dammit—I have to stay!"

I don't know what possessed me, except that I knew I had to do something flamboyant and do it quickly. For some odd reason, I have always been able to stand on my head, even as a little kid. I loved to sucker guys into head-standing contests in the Marines, especially when we had a half case of beer in us. I could also have challenged him to an arm wrestle, but the size of his arm discouraged me.

So I stood on my head. God, let me tell you, I thought my bloody leg would fall off. I was determined to maintain balance, no matter how.

The move caught Ben Asher by surprise. I could see that upside down. His grizzly arms dropped from his hips and he gaped. Suddenly cheers began to break out from the paras. The major looked around at everyone threateningly.

I remained in this ridiculous position, even though every square inch of my body began to ache. Ben Asher was going to see how long I could take it.

It was no longer a game. I could feel the veins in my neck bulging and sweat erupted all over my body. I felt myself swooning, on the verge of passing out.

"You're a real pain in the ass, Zadok," he said. "All right, you dumb son of a bitch, get off your head. You can stay."

Shlomo grabbed me as a rousing cheer went up from the men. Ben Asher whipped around and snarled everyone into instant silence, then cracked the meagerest of smiles.

The business of war interrupted in the form of a half-dozen mortar shells landing on our perimeter. God, if there's anything I really hate, it's mortars. They're on you before you have a chance to react and their blast can leave you reeling, punchy, and half dead.

Ben Asher was at the field phone to the forward observation post, and in a minute our own mortars and recoilless rifles responded. The Egyptian shelling stopped. Ben Asher ordered the Recon platoon to move forward and take the position away from the Egyptians.

Fortunately, it was a typical Arab hit-and-run attack. Coffeehouse fighters. They abandoned the position and fled into the Pass without further ado. That didn't mean they wouldn't try to sneak back under cover of darkness and give us a miserable night.

After the Recon platoon secured the position, Ben Asher decided to move into it with more men and use it as our own forward post. A heavy machine-gun and rifle squad deployed and dug in. We were, in effect, inching up to the Pass against our orders.

The major was concerned about nightfall. The Pass was over fourteen miles long. On the other side of Mitla, beyond our reach, the Egyptians could cross the Canal by rubber raft and put God knew how many troops into the Pass.

I watched through a pair of field glasses as the phone line was being run to the new observation post. Mitla Pass was beginning to take on a weird fascination. The warrior's blood said, "Go in and take the son of a bitch." But that was tempered by common sense. It had to be a death trap in there.

"God help us if we ever have to go in and try to take it," Shlomo said. I agreed.

It was only nine in the morning. In the distance, we could hear activity. Whose planes were they? Was it the Israelis going after the Egyptian convoy on the other side of the Pass? Or were the Egyptians taking to the air en masse to challenge us from the other side of the Canal? Maybe, just maybe, it was the British and French coming in to neutralize the Egyptian air bases.

Shlomo and I found our crevice.

"Great show you put on," he said.

"Ben Asher's really pissed at me."

"Naw, he loves you. He's always had this trouble with smiling."

A sudden jolt of pain sent me into little spasms. I unlaced my boot. The whole leg was beginning to turn purple . . . and blue . . . and a pale yellow . . . right down to the sole of my foot. Having won my skirmish with the major, I couldn't quit now, but I was wondering if I could bear up under the pain.

"Do you think you can talk Dr. Schwartz into seeing me? I might need another shot. Just a little one."

The doc came over and probed. "Hmmmmmm, getting nice and mushy," he said. "That was quite an exhibition you put on for Major Ben Asher," he continued. "Do something like that again and you have an excellent chance of going into shock."

The probe was painful.

"Stay off the leg, absolutely," the doctor ordered.

"How about another of those delicious morphine shots?"

"Don't start enjoying them too much," he warned.

For the first time in my life, I was really happy when someone stuck a needle in my ass. "Thanks, Doctor," I said.

And away we go! I lay back, shaded my eyes, and watched the mean desert sun grow higher and hotter. Our shade was minimal . . . water situation good. I helped myself to some wet rags for the back of my neck.

. . . Come on, baby, put me out of my misery, let's get that Sinai glow . . . all distant horizons are filled with sounds of airplanes . . . theirs . . . ours . . . who knows? . . . So anyhow, I kissed my mom goodbye and headed back to the Coast after a furlough. . . . Mom, I'm going to be fine . . . aren't you proud of your gyrene?

. . . Oh, Mom . . . I wish I could tell you . . . you're not to worry about that telegram from the Marines . . . I wasn't really wounded all that badly, just caught a little shrapnel in the shoulder . . . it's going to be okay. . . . Wish I could tell you that we're safe now, in New Zealand. . . . You see, Mom, it still hurts me when I remember opening that door and you in bed with that guy . . . like, who the hell was he?

. . . Mom saw my reflection in the dresser mirror and screamed and threw a towel about herself and slapped me and slammed the door in my face. . . . Later she told me she was sorry . . . but . . . I had come to realize . . . you know . . . it hurts when you're a nine-year-old kid. . . .

. . . Something always makes me want to put women down . . . like they're a disease. I go after them, conquer them, then dump them . . . but I always do it in a nice way . . . with class. . . .

. . . Hey, man! . . . Things don't feel too bad on the old hip . . . wow . . . floaty, floaty . . . wheee . . .

Just before the battle, Mother, . . .
I am thinking most of you, . . .
While upon the field we're watching, . . .
With the enemy in view. . . .
Comrades brave are 'round me lying, . . .
Filled with thoughts of home and God; . . .
For well they know that on the morrow, . . .
Some will sleep beneath the sod. . . .

Hark! I hear the bugles sounding, . . .
'Tis the signal for the fight, . . .
Now, may God protect us, Mother, . . .
As He ever does the right, . . .
Hear the "Battle Cry of Freedom," . . .
How it swells upon the air, . . .

Oh, yes, we'll rally 'round the standard, . . .
Or we'll perish nobly there. . . .

Farewell, Mother, you may never . . .
Press me to your breast again, . . .
But, Oh, you'll not forget me, Mother, . . .
If I'm numbered with the slain. . . .

IRELAND TO AMERICA

Queenstown, the Port of Cork, Ireland, 1887

THE AMERICAN CONSUL GENERAL was waiting at dockside with sealed envelopes as the USS *Quinnebaug* tied up. He was piped aboard and welcomed by the ship's skipper, Captain Percy Holifield. After exchanging pleasantries and making a dinner engagement ashore, Captain Holifield repaired to his cabin and opened the envelopes, one by one.

The contents of the first caused his face to widen into a vast, satisfied grin. Here was his long-delayed promotion to the rank of Commodore and an assignment to a new post, one he had coveted for years.

He allowed himself a glass of port wine, stood before the mirror, and toasted, after a long period of self-indulgent admiration, "To Commodore Percy Poindexter Holifield, the next superintendent of the United States Naval Academy."

Returning to his desk, he studied the balance of his communications. After a week's layover for necessary repairs in Cork, the *Quinnebaug* was to proceed with all deliberate speed to Portsmouth, England. There she would join an international flotilla of naval vessels, as America's representative at Queen Victoria's Golden Jubilee.

Thereafter, he would be relieved of his command and was to return forthwith to the United States, to the Academy.

The *Quinnebaug*, a sail-and-screw corvette of nineteen hundred tons, with a complement of two hundred officers and crew, was part of a two-ship squadron that constituted the European Station. For three years

Percy Holifield had sailed her on a round of endless ports of call to "show the flag." Her route had taken her to such unlikely places as Samos, Zante, Villefranche, and Latakia and the steamy route down the west coast of Africa to the likes of Monrovia, Junk River, and Libreville. A graveyard of a career had just been redeemed.

He scrawled his signature on an order for shore leave. The Irish members of his crew, who constituted almost half of his men, would receive five days' liberty, while the others would make do with three days ashore.

Holifield ran down a list of what would be needed to spiff up his ship, to make certain she would proudly represent America, and wrote out detailed repair and maintenance orders.

He went to his sea chest and dug down to the bottom, where he had carefully stowed a bolt of blue Navy cloth, several rolls of gold braid, and packets of buttons. From these he would have crafted a new commodore's uniform.

There was endless socializing with the ships' captains of the various European navies. Despite America's great strides in naval warfare during the Civil War, the Europeans continued to look with disdain at the Yankees, particularly at their spartan uniforms. Well, he'd make them eat their epaulets, by thunder!

Having attended to his ship and men, he ordered a carriage and made for Cork with his bolt and buttons and braid and a number of photographs of the commodore's uniform. The carriage stopped at Callaghan and O'Brien, the city's finest men's haberdasher on the Grand Parade, Cork's main shopping thoroughfare.

Devastating news was delivered to him by Mr. Callaghan himself. "Terribly sorry, Yer Excellency, but there's absolutely no way such an elaborate furnishing can be done in under a month, and we're badly backlogged."

"You understand, of course, that this is for the Queen's flotilla."

Callaghan tilted his head, bit his lip, and sighed in sympathy. "Aw, I'd be after lying to you, sir, if you were an Englishman, but I'd not do such a thing to the skipper of an American vessel such as yourself. I have many relatives in America, sir, and I wouldn't be treating you that way."

"But Lord, man, look at these rags I'm wearing. They're all but rotted out from the west coast of Africa."

"Pity, sir, pity. Hold on just one moment," Callaghan said and consulted sincerely with his partner, then returned to the disconsolate commodore.

"There is a chance, just a chance, mind you, but there is a Jewish tailor in Queenstown, where your ship is tied up. He specializes in naval uniforms, enlisted men, mainly, but why don't you give it a go?" and with that he wrote the name and address of one Moses Balaban on a slip of paper.

The commodore drove back to Queenstown and pulled to a halt on the quay, just a few blocks from where the *Quinnebaug* was tied up. Holifield emerged from the carriage before a tiny storefront with the inconspicuous lettering reading M. BALABAN—TAILOR. His heart sank to see that the shades were drawn. He jiggled the door latch vigorously, then thumped on the window. "I say! Anyone in there?"

"Can I be helping you, Admiral?" a voice behind him said.

He turned and looked at a disreputable personage, whose breath reeked of rum, a man of the lowly type who hung around the wharfs in every port in the world.

"Do you know where the proprietor lives?"

"Try the back of the shop, Yer Worship."

At that, Percy Holifield banged and shouted again.

"Ah sure, that will do you no good at all. It's the Sabbath to old Moses, and he won't be coming out till sunset. He's a quare sort, a Hebrew, you know."

The commodore fumed, then gave the informant tuppence, for which he was voraciously thanked. He took out his pocket watch. Two hours until sunset. After another unsuccessful round of door thumping, he drew in a deep breath, clasped his hands behind his back, and paced before the shop with one eye on the sun.

As twilight at last overcame the quay, he knocked again, but this time respectfully. The door opened a crack and there stood Moses Balaban, a slight Jew, mostly likely in his late twenties, with a straggly goatee and wearing a black cuplike cap on his head and a shawl over his shoulders. He could well have been Shylock from *The Merchant of Venice.*

"Why are you making all that noise?" he demanded. To Holifield's surprise, the man spoke with an obvious twinge of an Irish accent. "You desecrated my Sabbath."

The commodore, not used to being reprimanded, ground his teeth, mumbled beneath his breath, but held back his pride, for he needed this chap, urgently. "Kindly accept my apologies. I am somewhat desperate for a tailor. You are Mr. Balaban?"

The Jew looked him up and down, then opened the door. "Come in," he said tersely.

The shop was shockingly unkempt, something that would obviously grate upon a naval officer who ran a shipshape vessel. Bolts of cloth were askew without rhyme or reason. Tailor's dummies were fitted with half-sewn uniforms being made for men at sea to collect when they returned. The shop had a foul, stale aroma, and from the rear the commodore could hear the voices of two young squabbling children.

"Shut up back there," Moses shouted, "or you'll get a lump on your noggins." He turned to Holifield. "Just what is it you want that is so important as to interrupt my prayers?"

"Sir, my ship has been ordered to sail to England to join a celebration in honor of Her Majesty Queen Victoria. My uniforms are threadbare from months at sea. I have, outside in the carriage, cloth and everything else needed, as well as photographs for a new uniform. I am willing to pay a handsome bonus for the job. I do realize that this will be more ornate . . ."

Moses held up his hand for silence. "I am Romanian. Have you ever seen all the junk on a Romanian admiral's uniform? You are an American?"

"I am indeed, sir."

The tailor looked pensively out of the door to the quay. "I have watched a thousand ships sail to America from here, filled with half-starved Irishmen and -women. This is a port of tears, of misery," he said as though speaking to himself. "Your name?"

"Excuse me. I am Percy Holifield, newly promoted from captain to commodore. My ship is laid up here for repairs."

"When do you sail for England?"

Holifield closed his eyes and prayed beneath his breath. "Next Friday."

Moses Balaban studied the configuration of the commodore, encircling him slowly. He had a difficult body to enhance. He was stubby, potbellied, and swaybacked, a challenging combination to overcome in so short a time. Percy Holifield's eyes watered with silent pleading.

"You have not kept yourself in very good shape," the Jew said.

The commodore smarted but held his tongue.

Moses Balaban walked around him again, then threw up his hands. "All right, it can be done."

"Oh, thank you, sir, thank you," Holifield erupted, shaking the little tailor's hand. "Let me say again, your time will be well rewarded."

Ignoring the commodore's effusions, Moses already had the measuring tape out. "We must start without delay."

IN THE ENSUING week, the commodore and the Romanian/Irish/ Jewish tailor were thrown together for hours on end and evolved a friendship of sorts. Balaban's two little boys were adorable, about the age of Holifield's own sons. But Moses Balaban was a difficult man to know. He snipped out his words and was always cavalier in manner.

Holifield would enter the shop and invariably see the slender Moses sitting cross-legged on a pillow atop his cutting table, stitching away meticulously by hand. Balaban would greet him with a mere nod.

He learned that Moses had been born in the Romanian Black Sea port of Constanta, where his father and grandfather had established a paltry means of livelihood with a tailoring business specializing in naval uniforms. Most of their work consisted of repairing enlisted men's clothing, with a few odd commissions for uniforms for low-ranking officers. The captains and admirals had theirs made in Bucharest or Paris.

The Balabans were a typically large family of a dozen children, eight boys and four girls. Only one of the sons, the oldest, could take over the family business. The others had to look to emigrate. Three of the Balaban males went to England and Scotland, where tailors were in demand.

One of them, Herman Balaban, a confirmed bachelor, signed up for a British transatlantic passenger liner, as ship's tailor. After a couple of rough crossings, he decided that life at sea was not his cup of tea and he jumped ship in Queenstown, where he eventually opened a shop on the quay.

"And your three other brothers, Moses?"

"In Savannah, Georgia. They are out of the tailoring business entirely, and for the best."

What he did not tell the commodore, of course, was of his lifelong reputation as a disagreeable, even nasty, person. His family in Constanta did not want him, nor did his brothers in Scotland and Savannah.

It boiled down to brother Herman, toiling in the remote colony of Ireland, who finally sent for Moses to assist in the shop. Moses was fifteen when he arrived in 1875, and in a matter of five years took over the shop when Herman died in a cholera epidemic.

The Jewish community of Ireland consisted of a few hundred families, mainly in Dublin and Belfast, with but a handful in Cork. Life was generally peaceful for the Jews, although there was a terrible sense of isolation. Cork had one synagogue and one kosher butcher, but there was little in the way of traditional communal life: no Hebrew school, no

Yiddish newspaper, no debating societies, dramatic clubs, or ritual baths.

This did not seem to bother Moses, who existed as a loner. He'd go to Cork to synagogue during the holidays, or for special occasions, but his little shop in Queenstown was a personal bastion of his orthodoxy. Moses was largely friendless, a dour, stingy man who seemed to do little else but sew, pray, and play checkers with an old pensioner.

A few years after obtaining the business, he entered into a marriage contract with the daughter of a poor Belfast cabinetmaker, who bore him two sons, Saul and Lazar. The mother died in childbirth, with the new infant.

As a widower, Moses continued along, raising his sons in the small flat in back of the shop, with the help of an aged Irish nanny.

Moses had put out feelers to make an arrangement for a new wife, but he found the doors closed to him in the Jewish community in Ireland because he had earned a well-deserved reputation for meanness. Moses was known to burst out of his deep shell with sudden violent fits of temper that often included wife and child beating.

With no Jewish girl available to him in Ireland, his alternative would be to work out a costly arrangement with a matchmaker to have a girl in the old country sent over to be wed. But who would come to Ireland, to Cork? Some third-rate ugly who couldn't find herself a husband in Romania.

From time to time Moses cast an eye toward America, but he hesitated. His brothers in Savannah, knowing of Moses' irritable temper from childhood, were not all that anxious to bring him over.

In addition, Moses lived on the waterfront. He knew about too many voyages to America where unscrupulous agents had crammed emigrants on death ships. There were terrible tales of epidemics and deaths at sea, almost as bad as during the slave-trading and famine days. Moreover, there would be further privation in the promised land itself. He knew that most Jews landed in New York, where an enormous hellhole of a ghetto emerged on the Lower East Side, which was already overflowing with tailors.

So he continued to sew and pray and save his pennies and yell at his sons, while holding a high opinion of himself for his unwavering piousness.

LATE FRIDAY afternoon, Commodore Percy Poindexter Holifield buckled on an ornate belt holding a gleaming saber as Moses affixed the commodore's hat on his head.

He stood before the three-way mirror, stunned by his dazzling appearance and steeped in self-admiration. Moses Balaban had created a miracle! What was more, the masterpiece was completed with three hours to spare before the Jewish Sabbath began. He turned and pumped the little tailor's hand with gusto. "Moses, how can I ever thank you!"

Moses offered his small version of a smile. The kids yelled in the back room.

"Now let us settle our account," Holifield said, thrusting forward a bag of gold coins. "I think you will find this quite generous."

To his utter surprise, he saw Moses hold up his hand.

"No charge," he said.

"I say, old fellow, you can't be serious."

"The Talmud says we must make one great gesture of this sort in our lifetime. You happened into my shop at precisely the right moment." Having performed few sincere acts of contrition in his lifetime, Moses was playing it safe.

"But . . . but," the commodore stammered.

"So go and be a jim-dandy for the Queen and knock her eyes out."

THE USS *QUINNEBAUG* slipped from her berth just before sunset. Moses Balaban and his two boys waved to the skipper, who waved back, choked with emotion.

In the next fortnight of celebrations in England, Commodore Percy Poindexter Holifield acquitted himself more than adequately to represent his country among the most elegant admirals of Europe.

Returning to America and assuming his post at the Naval Academy in Annapolis, he never forgot the little Jewish tailor, or his debt to him.

His new position involved him in a great deal of socializing, parties, dinners, trips to Washington, and the like. This required a higher standard of dress than that of an officer on sea duty. As superintendent, he was entitled to a number of privileges, among them the right to appoint a civilian as chief tailor. But alas, his new uniforms did not have the quality and flair of Moses Balaban's work. Several months later, Moses received a letter from the commodore.

My dear friend Moses,
    I have never forgotten your great kindness to me when I

needed you. What is more, my present chief tailor, who does the officers' uniforms, is simply not in your class.

If you are of a mind to immigrate to America, consider this letter to be an offer for you to assume the position of chief tailor at the Naval Academy. It will afford you a modest but steady income, good housing, and other benefits. I understand there is a large, thriving Jewish community in Baltimore, just a short train ride away.

If you are inclined to make this journey, simply take this letter to the American consul in Cork, who has instructions to arrange decent passage for yourself and your sons, in the first ship coming directly to Baltimore.

I hope you will consider this offer in a positive way and allow me to repay the gratitude I have felt all these months.

I look forward, hopefully, to a transatlantic cable informing me you are en route.

With kindest regards,
P. P. Holifield, Commodore, USN
Superintendent
U.S. Naval Academy
Annapolis, Maryland

Annapolis, 1888

AS PROMISED, Moses Balaban and his sons, Lazar and Saul, had a decent crossing. The change from the perpetual foul weather, grim destitution, and eternal sorrow of Cork to the gleaming little jewel of Annapolis forced a ray of light into Moses Balaban's life.

The Navy and its institutions were on the mend from a long decline that followed the Civil War. The Academy itself had become an orphan, lollygagging for appropriations and direction. Changes were in the wind with the Navy's transition from sail to steam, from primitive ironclads to steel battlewagons, from the old-salt sailors to sophisticated engineers and gunners. Under the direction of the previous superintendent, a legendary admiral, the Academy found its fortunes making a dramatic turnabout as he directed it toward becoming a first-class university.

The city of Annapolis nestled sweetly on the shores of the Severn River, near where it flowed into the mighty Chesapeake Bay. It was a place of many prerevolutionary buildings, of charm and quaintness, a pastoral setting to make its landfall, easy to abide in.

Moses Balaban found a small cottage a few minutes' walk from the campus and hired a negress mammy to take care of his boys and the home. Indeed, life had taken a turn for the better, and this was reflected in a change of the man's disposition. He was the house Jew, an oddity, but under the protection of the commodore. Moses was treated, not as a mysterious menace, but as a man with direct bloodlines to the Bible and therefore to be respected. He relished the status and now dressed snappily in one of his three handsome suits and tapped his cane and doffed his derby as he strolled, chatting it up with midshipman, officer, and civilian alike.

There were a few dozen Jewish families in Annapolis, mostly merchant families, but they were Reformed in their religious practice and were more Americanized than Jewish. He would have no truck with them whatsoever. In Ireland, he had felt little inclination to associate with his neighbors. It was the same in Annapolis, only better. The only place of worship was a tiny chapel on campus for the Jewish midshipmen, who rarely numbered more than one or two in a class. This didn't bother Moses, either. He was used to praying alone in a room.

Fifteen months after his appointment and six months after Moses' arrival, Commodore Percy Poindexter Holifield died peacefully in his sleep of a heart attack, after a raging session with the bureaucracy.

Moses prayed as he had never prayed before, as the new superintendent arrived on the scene. His prayers were not answered. Rear Admiral Adam Harper didn't particularly like Jews. However, he was a reasonable sort and offered Balaban what seemed a palatable demotion, at first.

Among the raft of new changes instituted was the manner in which uniforms were to be made, particularly those of the midshipmen. Previously they had been hand-tailored. Harper brought in a new-era tailor, who manufactured clothing on an assembly line, using mass-production methods. This was galling to Moses Balaban. Henceforth Moses was to supply only a variety of sizes of pants and vests and had to become a government employee, as well, on a fixed and meager salary. After a few months of this, he decided to resign.

But not foolishly.

Moses had been the epitome of frugality for over a decade in Ireland, stashing away a small but tidy sum of money. He traveled an hour and twelve minutes by train to Baltimore, which held a Jewish population numbering in the tens of thousands, and through the various agencies there made inquiries.

In a matter of weeks he heard of a tailoring business for sale in Havre de Grace, a town to the northeast of Baltimore. He went to see it.

Havre de Grace, 1889–1901

HAVRE DE GRACE, like Annapolis, sat on a river that flowed into Chesapeake Bay. By contrast, though, the Susquehanna River was a large body of water that ran deep into Pennsylvania and was partway navigable to commerce. The town had connections to the outside by both rail and ferry. There was a thriving canning industry for the farm produce from the Eastern Shore, a racetrack, a canal whose barges hauled coal and timber, and large fishing and oystering fleets.

The business for sale was a good-sized store, nearly three times as large as his shop in Queenstown. It was perfectly located on St. John's Street on the riverfront, with living quarters above the shop. With the help of a Jewish lawyer from Baltimore, he secured the deal. Twelve hundred dollars, cash, bought him the building, the inventory, and the goodwill of the late proprietor.

BALABAN MERCHANT TAILOR, the storefront window read. Thus Moses once again picked up his singular, semi-monastic life, a wandering Jew among the gentiles. It didn't bother him the least that there was no Jewish life in Havre de Grace. After all, Baltimore was only a short train ride away and it was grander than Constanta and Cork combined on the holidays.

Moses Balaban had long ago conditioned himself not to hear what he did not wish to hear or see what he did not wish to see. He personally crammed his sons with several hours of nightly instruction in Hebrew and the Talmud, to ensure they would grow up to be good Jews, but he did not look at the world in which they were existing.

Saul, now seven, and Lazar, now eight, were among five Jewish children in Havre de Grace of school age. For the first time in their lives they heard the words and learned the meaning of "kike" and "sheeny!" In such isolation, they either had to fight or drown.

Uncaring about their bloody noses, black eyes, cuts, and bruises, Moses was concerned only about their torn clothing, for which he slapped them about automatically, without listening to their explanations. The boys grew very tough and became accepted to some extent by the gentile children, but they were almost always singled out for punishment by the teachers. They received so many slaps of the ruler over their knuckles, their hands were constantly swollen. Living in this state of precarious balance, Saul and Lazar became painfully aware that they were different, and grew both wily and wild.

Moses sewed and prayed and stuffed the Talmud down his sons' throats. When the occasion required, usually weekly, he relieved himself, as he had done in Ireland, with a prostitute. Here it was a negro woman who lived with her six children in a shack on a small farm on the outskirts of town.

With the boys growing up rapidly and becoming more untamed by the day, Moses realized he had to make a drastic change. He needed a permanent woman, a wife to make him a home, cook his meals, take care of his sons, comfort him at night.

Each Friday morning he closed his shop, took the train to Baltimore well before the Sabbath started, and availed himself of the social circles that specialized in matchmaking.

One Friday evening after services, his eyes fell on Hannah Diamond as she came from the women's balcony of the synagogue. For the first time in his life, a spark of love flared in his dark soul.

HANNAH DIAMOND sat before the vanity mirror in the dressing room in the rear of her shop. Her expression was pensive, mostly sad. She pinched her cheeks to liven them up.

Hannah would soon be nineteen and remained a spinster by choice. This was America, dammit! Despite her having no dowry to bring into a marriage, there had never been a lack of suitable proposals. Moreover, both her parents were dead and she had only herself to please.

America had given her this choice, this freedom. Yes, it was difficult to retain her independence. Marriages were being made all around her. People were starting to point their fingers.

Whenever she tottered close to acceptance, she backed off, invoking the memory of her mother and the living example of her older sister, Sonia. Hannah rationalized this way and that. The basic truth was that she was terribly uncomfortable around men.

She became determined to avoid the life of struggle that her mother and sister had been condemned to. Back in the old country, Momma had ingrained into her the canon that all men, and her father in particular, were put on this earth for the purpose of making women suffer.

Make Momma suffer he did, every day of her married life, particularly during his outbreaks of violence that included physical beatings. Hannah rightfully blamed her father for her mother's early death, as well as her own wariness of men.

Her brother, Noah, attempted to chop off his thumb to avoid conscription into the Russian Army, but he botched the job. Noah was taken away and later transferred to Siberia, facing up to twenty-five years of imposed military service. It was a commonplace that those Jews drafted into Far Eastern duty were scarcely ever heard from again. Noah took the easy path out and converted to Christianity and later married a woman of Asian extraction.

Momma and Poppa were both dead when the pogroms of 1881 erupted. The Diamond sisters fled, along with hundreds of thousands of other Jews. They mostly landed in the wretched Lower East Side of Manhattan, two square miles of ghetto without a wall, the most thickly populated place on earth; a place of universal poverty and misery, roach- and rat-infested tenements, a breeding ground for TB, a hunting ground for exploiters to find herds of cheap labor, a place of broiling in the summer heat and numbing cold by winter.

After two years of it, a group of cousins and aunts and uncles collected enough to bring the girls to Baltimore. At least there one could breathe clean air and find some measure of relief from the foulness of New York.

On three hundred dollars borrowed from the Hebrew Free Loan Society, they opened the Diamond Sisters Wedding Gown and Wig Shop in the middle of poor Jewish Baltimore, on Lombard Street.

The sisters were good at what they did, so there was enough work but little profit. Each gown was fashioned from satin, velvet, or silk material and lavishly embossed with tiny beading, sequins, and paste jewelry. The headdress was covered with small pearls and crystals and the veil mostly made of antique lace. For the bride, it was a once-in-a-lifetime gown for which her family would spend its last penny. But making such a garment required hours upon hours of exacting hand labor.

But it was a living, and the Diamond sisters were industrious and fared decently until Jacob Rubenstein happened into the picture. Jake was a salesman, a good looker, a flashy article. He got Sonia pregnant and a quick marriage followed; then came three more children and a fourth was on the way.

Jake proved to be a no-goodnik, both as husband and provider. He fooled around with other women, even prostitutes, a fact Sonia was aware of, but remained silent about.

Jake? Jake was a dreamer, a door-to-door salesman. He failed to make a living no matter what line of merchandise he carried and he felt himself too good to be confined to selling inside a store. Every week, it seemed, Jake was chasing another get-rich-quick scheme. Every week another failure.

The goods he sold on his route were paid off by his customers at the rate of ten cents to a dollar a week. His customers were adept at not being at home on Sunday, which was the traditional collection day. Sunday night, when Jake would go through the ledger and bring the accounts up to date, there was usually barely enough to pay for his last shipments of goods. On those occasions when he collected a few dollars over his costs, he'd usually lose it in a pinochle game.

He always had his hand in the till of Sonia's dress shop, keeping the sisters buried in a hole out of which they never managed to climb. The relatives were constantly on Sonia. Why should she put up with this no-good bum?

Sonia stuck. Despite all of Jake's bad habits, he made her laugh. Always with the salesman's jokes and always with the kisses. He tried, after a fashion, to be a good daddy. He was very affectionate and the kids were still too young to know the awful truth.

At least Jake never laid a mean hand on Sonia or the children, and once in a while he'd hit it big at the card table. When he did *oy, oy, oy.* Jake didn't spare the horses. He'd lavish on Sonia jewelry, a fur, a millinery piece covered with stuffed birds. Sonia always had the bonanza gifts in reserve to take to the pawnbroker to hock, when it came down to meeting the shop's bills or putting food on the table.

So why had Hannah come to America? she asked herself. For a man like her father? Her brother? For Jake Rubenstein? There were a lot of Jews in Baltimore with stars in their eyes about America. Some, like her own cousins, were making for themselves a very fine-quality life. But what chance was there for a single, eighteen-year-old girl? Less than none.

Hannah was approaching the time she'd become too old to make a really fine marriage. What was her alternative? The life of an old maid, which was socially no life at all.

On the other hand, she longed to have her own children and become the *balabosta* of a Jewish home. If only she didn't have to take a husband in order to get it. Maybe yes? Maybe no? No prince charming had swept her off her feet, yet every time she went to a *bris*, she fantasized that the little boy was her own baby.

Sonia came to the rear of the shop where her sister was pondering, picked up a brush, and stroked Hannah's raven hair, which fell to the middle of her back. Hannah leaned back, resting her head on Sonia's belly, which was six months full.

"What should I tell Moses Balaban?" Sonia asked.

Hannah shrugged.

"He makes ends meet," her sister continued; "that's nothing to spit on."

"In Havre de Grace? Such a place is just like our brother, Noah, being shipped off to Siberia."

"Nonsense. It's only an hour from Baltimore."

"It might as well be a thousand miles. We would be the only Orthodox family there. It's an exile."

"So? This is America. You don't have to be surrounded by a million Jews. You won't have Cossacks smashing your windows. They won't rape you."

Hannah detached herself from Sonia, and came to her feet, and her voice showed alarm. "I'm afraid," Hannah said.

"Of Havre de Grace?"

"Yes, of Havre de Grace . . . and . . ."

"Moses Balaban?"

"I'm afraid of any man. You know that. Besides, he's nearly twice my age."

"That could be a blessing. With a boy your own age, you'd be asking for real *tsuris*, a real struggle. Also, what younger men don't know about women is everything. In the long run, a more mature man with experience could have a little more feeling, a little more understanding."

"Moses can be charming, but I think it's only an act he puts on on the Sabbath, to make himself feel holy. He's clever, but I also see things about him that make me worry." She suddenly went into a small spasm of shivering. "And what about those two sons of his, they're like wild animals."

"Hannahile, I've heard all this from you a dozen times before."

A long and difficult silence ensued until the front bell announced the arrival of a customer for a fitting. "I'll be right there!" Sonia called. "*Nu*, Moses will be arriving soon. He asked me to get an answer from you. What shall I tell him?"

THE EQUAL OF Hannah's wedding gown was not to be seen in Baltimore for the balance of the century. On the wedding day, late in 1894, she set aside her apprehensions and joined in the joyousness of the gathering. Moses' brothers traveled up from Savannah with a raft of nieces and nephews, while Hannah's *mishpocha* came from as far away as Cleveland. The catered affair was underwritten by her Uncle Hyman, who was on his way to achieving modest wealth as a drugstore owner.

The ancient ceremony took place in the Lloyd Street Synagogue, one of America's oldest. A lively music-and-dance-filled reception took place in China Hall, personally catered by the owner, Mr. Sheinbloom. This was a banquet room of note and they celebrated far into the night, damn the expense.

Because it was not the right time of the month, Hannah and Moses spent the wedding night in different homes, perhaps the only advantage a bride got. She felt it was a reprieve, an avoidance of the frightening moment of truth.

Hannah had not been to Havre de Grace, but had only seen photographs of the building on St. John's Street. She had met the sons in Baltimore. The size of the building, plus the elegant way Moses dressed, seemed to assure her that she was heading for a comfortable life.

Her hopes were soon dashed. The instant she opened his door she saw the effects of a miserly widower. Everything was wrong, indifferent, untidy, dirty. The kitchen in back of the shop was derelict, with squeaky, broken chairs and a table covered in peeling, greasy oilcloth. Pots and pans were caked in grime and the few unmatched dishes were chipped and worn.

Upstairs, in the living quarters, bedspreads, pillows, and towels were grungy and scraggly, and the mattress stained and lumpy. The windows were covered with torn shades and curtainless. Paint could scarcely be seen through layers of dust and dirt. Damp, musty odors permeated it all.

A major overhaul was called for. Linens, featherbeds, dishes, and the like were generally items that a wife brought into the marriage as part of her dowry. But Hannah had no dowry.

She'd make a thorough list, she thought, and put the place into sparkling shape. She'd set up a kosher kitchen with milk and meat flatware and dishes. This was her own first home and no amount of work would be too hard.

Despite her initial disappointment, Hannah did not despair. Work was no stranger to her. And look at the brighter side. This had a lot more promise than a tenement on the Lower East Side.

She had been clever also in making friends with the boys, Saul and Lazar. Anytime they came to Baltimore, there was a kitchen full of cookies. She'd get them to pitch in, getting the house in order. It would make them feel important. She'd bake for them and give the spoons and the pot to lick for rewards, and she'd get their wardrobes into spotless condition.

All of the housekeeping could wait for a few days. For now, there was the reality of the honeymoon night. Nothing had ever been mentioned about sex during their courtship. Foregone conclusions regarding the woman's role and duty had been part of her upbringing. Hannah did have the terrible legacy of her mother's tragedy and the fears that went along with sex. Crazy, but Sonia's marriage held out some hope. Although Jake was a sorry excuse for a husband, they did enjoy their sex together. Sonia had told her that many times.

Since Moses had the experience of a previous wife, they didn't have to be like a pair of frightened puppies, poking around clumsily at each other. She felt Moses would handle the delicate moments of the situation. If this were true, they could establish a pattern of tenderness, maybe even happiness. There was no putting it off now. The time had come and the mystery would soon be over.

As Hannah awaited him, the dinginess of the lantern-lit room overcame her. She ducked down deeper beneath the covers and soon was swept by sheer terror. The walls closed in on her, and when she heard the back stairs creaking out his arrival, she desperately wanted to run and hide.

"Lord, Hannah," she moaned, "don't make a fool of yourself," and overcame an impulse to cringe in the closet.

The door opened.

Moses returned from the outhouse, wearing an ankle-length nightshirt. He spoke nary a word, took off his yarmulke, turned down the lantern, invoking darkness, shuffled across the room, groaned down on the woebegone mattress, and fished around for her.

It was painful, thoughtless, bloody, and mercifully quick. He was soon asleep with his back to her, snoring, so he did not hear her stifled sobs. Hannah's fear had come home to roost, like a dire prophecy.

Hannah moved around in a daze for several days, shocked by the nightly onslaughts. There was no place for her to seek comfort or respite. There was no one to confide in. She called on her spunkiness to stave off a depression and told herself there were other things in life.

She could make a decent home. She would come to love Saul and Lazar. Perhaps she could have her own children. But, to look into the future coldly, there would be years of his sordid behavior to endure, perhaps the rest of her life.

"I've made a list of things we need," Hannah told him at the end of the first bitter fortnight. "If I make a trip to Baltimore to do the shopping, we can save a great deal of money."

Moses looked at the list and turned pale and angry. She wanted kitchen utensils, linens, towels, flatware, material for curtains, clothing for the boys, mattresses.

"You are furnishing the Dublin Castle?"

"This place is wretched. I am only trying to make a home for you and your sons."

"*Gevalt!* What is this business here?" he said with the paper trembling in his hand. "Suits for Saul and Lazar."

"They are shabby, like orphans. If you don't want to spend for them, at least you could sew them a few pairs of knickers. Buy me the wool and I'll knit them sweaters."

"What is this item? And this? And this? Eggbeaters, upholstery material, a knife sharpener, mattress pads, window shades. This is some kind of madness!"

"I won't live in such filth with your boys dressed in rags. And you might as well think about hiring a *shvartzer* to do some painting and paperhanging."

"Maybe," he cried, "if you had brought in a dowry like a proper wife!"

"My dowry has nothing to do with dirt. What is more, I am keeping kosher and I am going to sleep in a bed that doesn't have rocks in the mattress."

He glared at her list again, croaking incoherently. Hannah had had the gall to ask him to make an outlay of over a hundred dollars. And this would only be the beginning with such a woman!

"I don't have the money," he lied. "And I don't know where you get such royal ideas. Maybe you'd better go ask for some money from your Uncle Hyman. He spent a fortune for the reception in China Hall and what have we got to show for it?"

And so it went. Moses' stinginess went to war against Hannah's determination. Within a few months, permanent battle lines had been clearly drawn. He oozed, bled, and whined out a few dollars.

Hannah resorted to taking in sewing and advertised to make wedding gowns, but Havre de Grace was not Baltimore and the dimes and quarters came in grudgingly. By her deft management and scrimping, the place took on a new appearance by the end of the year and Saul and Lazar had lost most of their scruffiness.

What happened in the bedroom did not change. After fast, brutal, animal thrusts, he'd roll over, his back to her, and the snoring soon followed. At least, she reasoned, he didn't prolong the agony.

Saul and Lazar loved their stepmother as they had never loved anyone before. Although Hannah was only ten years the senior of Lazar, she was the light of their lives, their redemption from the loneliness and fear of being ignored and slapped, from a life of constant hurt. Hannah was bosom and hugs and kisses and pinches on the cheek . . . and laughter. Hannah was cookies and big plates of soup filled with matzo balls and clean shirts and trimmed hair and studying poems and churning ice cream and butter and the smell of bread baking and an *angel*, as she lit the candles on the Sabbath. She positioned herself between the boys and Moses to protect them whenever his vile spells consumed him.

"Momma, can I call you Momma?" Lazar asked. She beamed. Lazar was changing, accepting her affection, doing things to please her and make her proud. Almost like the first friend the boy ever had, certainly the first love of his life.

Saul remained wild and troubled, but some light had entered his life through her. Slowly, painfully, he responded to her, but opened up only a tiny crack at a time.

It was in the third month of her pregnancy when Moses plunged into the blackest of spells. Hannah had spent some money to start a layette for their expected child. In an outburst of rage, he demanded to know why she didn't sew the baby gowns herself.

"So don't worry, Moses," she retorted. "Expect to spend more. We'll need a crib, a carriage, diapers, bottles—"

"Borrow from Sonia! She has all those things. I'm not made of money."

"You're made of *dreck*," she told him in unvarnished Yiddish. He silenced her with a punch in the mouth. The next morning she was gone.

A very fine good riddance, Moses thought when he read her note. However, it was not very long before he began to miss her. So many things had changed while she was in the home. So many good things. Maybe . . . just maybe . . . he had been a little bit wrong, he thought. Maybe . . . just maybe . . . he would have to put up with a few of her fancy ideas. Of course, he'd never tell her where the money was hidden under the floorboards of the shop.

The house quickly fell from sparkling to drab. What was worse, the *shvartze* woman was an awful cook and the boys bellowed day and night for Hannah.

After a month, during which she did not crawl back, Moses caved in. He sucked in his pride, put his temper on hold, and went to Baltimore to reclaim her, hat in hand.

Hannah laid down a set of rules that covered everything from enough money to run the home properly to a limitation of once a week, on the Sabbath, for the carnal act. Finally she drew an absolute promise that he would never again strike her or the boys.

Moses reluctantly agreed to her terms and she agreed to return to Havre de Grace for a trial period.

Five months later, she returned to Baltimore again to deliver her baby. She held an infant girl, Leah, named for her mother, and wept bitterly as Sonia tried to comfort her.

"Moses is waiting outside," Sonia said.

"I hate him," Hannah wept. "I hate him!"

MOSES AND HANNAH Balaban had three daughters: Leah, Fanny, and the baby, Pearl, who was born just a few days into the new century.

Hannah had experienced a number of miscarriages, as well as three difficult full-term pregnancies and births. She was warned against having more children. Taking Saul and Lazar as her own sons, she was satisfied. The house was filled and lively and she was mother, homemaker, and protector.

Moses reduced himself to the role of star boarder in his own home, a semi-reclusive stranger. After a time, Moses stopped teaching Saul and Lazar Hebrew and the Talmud, further diminishing contact with his family. The boys matriculated into apprentice tailors and helped otherwise in the shop, sweeping, aiding the *shvartze* with the dry cleaning, doing some of the pressing, and making deliveries. As long as Hannah was there, they each played their roles without too much rebellion.

Moses did make his daily presence felt at dinner, invariably complaining, scolding, and Talmudizing. But make no mistake, Hannah was the *balabosta,* the one in control of the family.

As the years passed and the boys grew, it became apparent that they wanted out. They even concocted secret plans to run away. It was Hannah who picked up their drift, gained their confidence, and held them together. For love of her, the unit remained intact.

Moses Balaban was content to dull his way through life, sitting cross-legged on a pillow on his cutting table and sewing and praying. He overwhelmed himself with his sense of piety, always the good Jew, particularly on the Sabbath.

From outward appearances, Havre de Grace seemed a pleasant, quiet, pretty little Southern town. There were swimming holes and great open meadows and canal barges to hop and huge, gnarled oaks to climb and dogs to pet and frog-jumping contests and watermelons to gorge and that wonderful, soft-breezed Southern laziness.

But the Balaban boys did not enjoy an idyllic childhood. Life was continually ugly for Havre de Grace's only Orthodox Jewish family. The other three Jewish families were fully assimilated, not really openly admitting to or practicing the religion.

Inside the house, the Balabans spoke Yiddish, and insofar as their neighbors were concerned, they were foreign, strange, and even frightening. They were treated with suspicion. Gossip, however ridiculous, about weird rituals taking place was generally believed around town. Outside the classroom, the other children practiced children's cruelty.

Where they don't wear pants,
In the southern part of France,
But the things they do,
Are enough to kill a Jew.

Saul became the family defender. He was a tough, mean fighter. Life could have been intolerable had he not been able to retaliate on behalf of his brother and sisters. After Saul demolished the town bully, the word was out not to mess around with the Jew boys or their sisters.

But Saul couldn't whip the entire town, particularly when adults took up the banner of Jew-baiting with crude "Hymie" jokes. Moses had forbidden his children to play with the *goyim* and *shiksas*. However, they all had their secret gentile friends, but could never bring them home.

Although Moses ranted against it, the boys played the godless games of baseball, basketball, and football and became quite good at them. This opened a small passageway for them into the "other" world. For the most part, the Balaban children were isolated and clung together.

The house of the Balabans inevitably became permeated by the lovelessness between Hannah and Moses and between Moses and his children. It was especially hard for the daughters, who were growing up with a deeply etched loathing of their father. The Sabbath was a bad day that angered and saddened the girls, because they knew it was Hannah's duty to make sex with their father.

From their earliest memories, they watched their mother in pain afterward, oftentimes holding her back and grimacing. Although Hannah rarely spoke to them of it openly, they knew and they hated.

"Be careful of the boys," Hannah warned; "they will only bring you suffering." The legacy had reached a new generation.

Each year Hannah's pain grew more severe and the alienation of the daughters from Moses heightened. The prospect of becoming mature women was encased in fear.

The house divided began to molder. And Baltimore, with its large Jewish community and many caring relatives, expanded in their minds as a fantasy place, a nirvana, an end to the perpetual suffering.

The proposition of a move was always on the table and rarely did a month pass without Hannah's bringing it up.

"So what by you is the distinct honor of living in Havre de Grace, Maryland?" Hannah would demand.

"Do you have, in your noggin, any idea what it would cost to live in Baltimore?"

"You're a *meshugga*, Moses Balaban. You can't even earn a living here. Without me *shnorring* Uncle Hyman a couple of times a year, we would have had to close this miserable business years ago."

"How can you explain finances to a woman? Look at this kitchen. You bake for three armies. You think I don't know that the children give away enough cakes to supply a bakery to *goyim* friends they have made behind my back?"

"What has that got to do with moving to Baltimore? At least in Baltimore, I can start again making fancy gowns. Believe me, we'll make out much better. And in Baltimore—"

"Woman! You have Baltimore mixed up with Jerusalem."

"I have Baltimore mixed up with Baltimore. Your sons do not have a single Jewish friend here. Not one. They have no *shul* to pray in. They can't live a day without hearing dirty words following them."

"A Jew can live anywhere, so long as he keeps the laws. It says so in the Talmud."

"And where in the Talmud does it say the girls will find husbands in Havre de Grace? In a few years they will start becoming eligible for marriage. Husbands you expect will suddenly appear from the Susquehanna River?"

"We'll find, we'll find. Don't worry, we'll make for them good *shiddachs* when the time comes."

"How? This is America. You can't make matches like they were made in the old country. They must live in a place where they can meet Jewish boys."

The discussion always ended with Moses slamming the door to his shop and locking himself in. It was his sanctuary and he *davened* in prayer, asking forgiveness for his wife's stupidity.

After a decade of this, Hannah secretly plotted to leave with the girls. By scrimping and cutting corners, at which she had become a genius, and taking in alterations that kept her sewing far into the night, she was able to save a little money. It grew more urgent as the girls became older. Hannah knew in her heart what Moses feared most. The cheap bastard was quivering with fright that he might have to give them each a dowry.

She had her cache tucked away in a trunk that held a number of dresses she had sewn for the girls' trousseaus. Moses, who never revealed his true earnings, had his cache beneath the floorboards under the counter of the shop.

The Sabbath became particularly oppressive during the dog days. On a Sabbath in August, wet heat steamed off the river and the trees went limp and the grass browned and one could hear the cornfields crackling in agony. Rock the rocker and fan and dunk your head under the water pump. The house of Moses Balaban was shut tight, trapping the soggy stagnant air. Shades drawn . . . a dingy gray light . . . Moses at prayer.

Movement around the house. Every step ended with a long, whiny creak of the floorboards and steps. Hannah grunted torturously from her night of being plundered.

The children were locked in. They could neither sew, nor cook, nor read for pleasure, nor play loudly. A whispered game of checkers. Drowsiness and sweat. Oh God, where is thy blessed sunset?

Sore from sitting in one position, Moses emerged from the shop and trudged through the house, a martinet with his prayer book held before him in one hand and his other hand behind his back. Through the kitchen, he climbed the rear stairs, through each bedroom, glancing out of the corner of his eye to see that everyone was accounted for. He returned to the kitchen, where Hannah sat listlessly fanning herself.

"Where is Saul?" he demanded.

"Maybe he broke his chains and escaped. How should I know?"

"He's not here!"

His voice drew the other children into the kitchen, fearful as they entered.

"Where is he? Lazar, you are covering up for him."

Lazar shook his head.

"I will not tolerate the Sabbath to be desecrated under my roof!" He seized his cane from the coatrack and held it up like a bat, threateningly. "Saul will get the lesson of his life!"

Hannah came from her chair, slowly, wiping the perspiration from her face and neck. "You, Moses Balaban, desecrate the Sabbath every day of your life with your vile, rotten ways. You will not put a finger on that boy."

"Momma, please," Lazar said.

"Not a finger," she repeated.

Moses' eyes widened with shock at this sudden defiance. He made a gesture of anger toward her, which brought the girls around her to form a protective cordon. Then Lazar stepped between his father and Hannah. Moses shook the stick at them. Lazar jerked it from his hand and threw it into a corner.

"Go back to your praying," Hannah said. "You look like a mad dog. And what is more, this is the last Sabbath you lock us in like caged animals. There is nothing that says we cannot walk in the streets and the children cannot take a swim in the river."

Moses grasped his chest and staggered to a chair and slumped into it, glaring wildly at nothing. The sweat dripped off his beard and his black Sabbath coat became sticky with it.

A pounding at the shop door stabbed into the scene.

"Tell them to go away," Moses grunted. "It's the Sabbath."

The knocking persisted until Leah ran from the kitchen. In a moment she returned, screaming incoherently. Hannah knew at once when she saw them. The mayor, the chief of police, and a number of others stood before them and took off their hats.

"Saul!" she cried.

"It was an accident, Mrs. Balaban."

THE WHOLE TRUTH was never known, only suspected. A bunch of boys got up a baseball team and hopped a freight train to go over to the Eastern Shore for a pickup game. Saul, always the daredevil, climbed on top of the car. They said he fell. The family never ceased to believe he was pushed. His body dropped between two cars and was dragged over the tracks for over a mile before it shook loose.

Hannah Balaban's hair turned white overnight. A few days later, she left Havre de Grace with her daughters. She had known of Moses' secret hiding place for years and she departed with his money.

Moses went berserk when he found it missing and turned on Lazar. But Lazar was too big and too strong. Lazar also left for Baltimore, where he joined his sisters and his stepmother.

Moses remained. This time he had a new companion: a hideous nightmare of death and disfiguration that was to recur for the rest of his life.

BALTIMORE

1902–1913

"So, THANK your lucky stars, it's better starving here than sitting at the Queen's table in Havre de Grace," Hannah would say, "and we should likewise count our blessings we aren't living in the Lower East Side of New York. Such stories a person hears. *Kinder, kinder,* we are lucky to be alive."

Baltimore was borderline. Borderline hunger, borderline soles on the shoes. Whatever it was, it was borderline. Hannah's sister, Sonia, and her maligned husband, Jake Rubenstein, were in a perpetual state of struggle. Sonia's bridal shop had gone down the drain, sunk by Jake's gambling debts.

Uncle Hyman, the one success story in the family, owned a large pharmacy on Fayette Street, near the central post office, in downtown Baltimore. Hyman gave to the relatives in Baltimore, keeping them afloat, gave to the relatives in the old country, gave to relatives in Palestine, gave to the synagogue. He never stopped giving. Such a blessed man.

Uncle Hyman took in Lazar as an apprentice pharmacist and paid his tuition to study at night school at the Maryland College of Pharmacy. Hyman's gesture kept their heads above water.

From Moses Balaban, months would pass without so much as one thin dime of support money. Moses would meander into Baltimore on the holidays, spiffed up like the Prince of Wales, and honor his family with a visit. Once or twice a year he'd give each of the girls a new silver dollar. Otherwise, no wife, no support.

Hannah had to be beyond merely industrious. By day she sold a line of ladies' foundation garments on a door-to-door basis: corsets and bust bodices. She would pick up an occasional order for a wedding gown, always, it seemed, just in the nick of time to stave off a disaster, or to spare her from the humiliation of having to go to Uncle Hyman for money.

The girls ran the household. In the evenings, they helped Momma, enabling her to take in more alteration work. Hannah's foot was always at the treadle of the sewing machine until far into the night.

So they managed . . . barely.

After five years in Baltimore, Hannah was able to open a tiny shop on Gay Street, between the deli and a house no one talked about, except in whispers. It was an open secret what went on in "that" house, with its constant parade of men, particularly on payday. Her daughters, by the ages of eight, ten, and twelve, became deft at cutting patterns and even doing hand-beaded work.

After a year of apprenticing, studying, and cramming, Lazar became a certified pharmacist and things opened up a bit. They were able to move into a relatively decent apartment on the second floor above a bakery, where at least they always had that pleasant aroma drifting up. The baker, one of many charmed by Hannah, always gave her first crack at the day-old bread and cakes counter.

Lazar was a nice sort of fellow, not too bad-looking and quick with the smile and a joke. Someday, Hyman assured, he'd have a pharmacy of his own. Lazar had gone from boyhood to manhood unselfishly. In return for Hannah's early love and protection, he became entirely devoted to her needs and those of his sisters.

One would expect that Hannah and the girls would have held Lazar in special esteem for his sacrifices. After all, when he received his certification, he was earning enough to go out and live on his own and enjoy the fruits of bachelorhood. But Lazar remained in a cauldron of angry women. He was taken for granted, a semi-person within their walls. Lazar was Lazar . . . an all-right boy . . . an observant Jew . . . an altogether decent provider.

And with the passage of time the memory of the dead Saul expanded out of reality. They forgot how wild Saul had been, how irresponsible, how difficult to handle. How he had probably instigated his own death. Saul was remembered as the family defender, a sainted boy. Saul was credited like an Irish patriot for deeds he never did and songs he never sang. The *yahrzeit* of his death was observed with no less solemnity than Yom Kippur. Lazar lived beneath the shadow of his revered dead brother.

To be sure, Lazar was well served. He sat at the head of the table and his clothing was always spotless and mended. He had his own room, priority on the bathroom, first look at the newspaper. Yet, when Leah or Fanny or Pearl starched his dickey, or laundered his underwear, or when his shaving mug fought for space among their cosmetics, or when he smelled of bay rum, the iota of resentment was always there. After all, he was a man. A *living* man . . .

There was a strange counterpoint to this. When Lazar brought a girlfriend home or appeared to be more than casually interested, his mother and sisters suddenly elevated him onto a pedestal. No girl was good enough for "their" Lazar. Girlfriends were made to feel patently uncomfortable. The inference was always that they must be tramps. On the one occasion when the engagement was about to be officially announced to Zelda Meyers, the butcher's daughter, Hannah was stricken with a mysterious illness. Fainting spells, shooting pains, and insomnia led a parade of symptoms which miraculously disappeared when Lazar and Zelda broke up. After a time, Lazar stopped bringing girlfriends home. By his mid-twenties he seemed headed toward lifelong bachelorhood.

"Never mind, Lazar," Hannah would say, "if you like the girl, you have my blessings . . . go. And don't worry about us, we'll survive. Maybe you should first check a few things about her health. Some stories, probably idle gossip when she was younger . . . actually, who knows her real age . . . some certain disease . . . I wouldn't mention. Just be careful. You know what I mean. You're a druggist. You know what the little drawer near the register has in it. Just be careful."

So, Lazar hung out with the other bachelors, a little card game, a cinema, a lot of talk about poon, and all that manly stuff. Lazar's sole passion remained basketball, at which he was a wizard from childhood. He was star guard for the team of the Council of Young Men's Hebrew and Kindred Associations, the much respected CYMAKS, into which he channeled his excess energy.

WITH THE THREE Balaban sisters, the situation was amazingly similar, but slightly different. Hannah and her girls retained a tight little island for themselves in the riotous confines of poor Jewish Baltimore, a ghetto centered on a pair of aged synagogues on Lloyd Street.

Leah was not only the oldest, but the cleverest and best-looking. By her mid-teens she had grown taller than her mother and alluringly buxom and was crowned with a head of marcelled hair that flowed down to the middle of her back. She was the first to go out and skirmish in the world of young men. Her immense brown eyes knew how to flash out the signal that brought instant palpitations to the recipient.

Leah was both vain and passionate. She enjoyed the flirtations and became adept in the use of charm, allure, and manipulation. But the foundation for womanhood was shaky. The voice of her mother seemed to be always whispering in her ear. Womanhood was a place filled with traps and pitfalls. Beware.

Leah's suitors and, later, Fanny's and Pearl's were all poor boys with uncertain futures. After the initial kisses and embraces, the boys usually sensed something forbidding about the Balaban sisters.

The little flat above the bakery was a lively place. The kitchen also served as the living room, and Fanny played a secondhand upright piano well enough to convey the sentiments of the day, even though it was badly out of tune. The songs were about twilight and gloaming and strawberry blondes and men on flying trapezes and birds in gilded cages. The kitchen table was filled with baked goodies and lively discussions abounded about the organizing of the garment workers, or socialism, or news of the old country.

Beneath the gaiety, a sensitive man soon detected that Hannah and her daughters carried deep, hidden anger against the father, who was never mentioned, whose photograph was missing from the mantel. Disdain for males was never spoken of, or even admitted to directly, but many young men sensed it and never returned.

1914

HANNAH GOT UP from her sewing corner when Leah came home from work and, as she did each day, poured two glasses of tea from the always steaming kettle. It was 1914 and Europe was at war again, this time totally, from Russia to the Atlantic Ocean, from Africa to the Baltic Sea.

Leah had turned nineteen and was an operator in a small neighborhood beauty parlor. She was a chronic complainer, who seemed to be continually plagued by some exotic, unexplainable distress. Working on her feet all day was a perpetual curse. She mumbled to herself that she should go to secretarial school as her mother unhooked her shoes and massaged her feet.

"Where are Fanny and Pearl?"

"With boys, down at the penny arcade, where else?"

Lazar came in a few moments later, bussed his mother and sister dutifully, gave Hannah his pay envelope, and retired to the bathroom with a newspaper.

The women sipped. Leah knew immediately that her mother had that *shiddach* expression on her face. It was a subject Leah really hated to get into. She sighed and awaited the bad news.

"I have been spoken to," Hannah started, "about a match."

"No matches, Momma," Leah responded quickly. "You yourself have said a thousand times that this is America and we will make up our own minds."

"I know, darling, but this has some unique aspects."

"The lord mayor's son, or some German millionaire from uptown?" Leah mocked.

"I only want that my daughters should avoid a catastrophe such as befell me."

"So, who's the lucky suitor?"

"For one minute, listen to Momma. I am trying, with all my heart and soul, to steer you into a comfortable situation. First, I want that you shouldn't have to starve and scrape for every penny. I want for you a man of some little means, who can provide for you a nice home. And a man who, God forbid, is not a stingy dog like your father." Upon mention of Moses, Hannah made as if to spit on the floor. "Dowries are becoming a thing of the past. Here, in America, there is not only a freedom of choice, but there are also more eligible men than women to marry them. Here a man will even pay a pretty penny for a suitable wife."

"That's what you thought when you married Poppa."

"Believe me, Leah, I would not, for a single minute, consider a man who was not a kind and gentle person. . . . Do you think I would talk *shiddach* with someone as disgusting as Moses Balaban?" Again she made a spitting gesture.

"Not only a kind and gentle man," Hannah said, "but someone who is not out to conquer the world. These Socialists, these Communists, these street-corner agitators, I tell you, go home and make their wives and children miserable. What a woman needs, all things considered, is a nice, quiet, weak man, who can be controlled by his wife."

"Suppose I want someone with more spirit," Leah retorted.

"The bigger the spirit, the bigger the trouble, take my word."

"So you want I should marry a *nebish.*"

"A kind, gentle person who makes a living. Am I a criminal?"

The water pan on the wood stove came to a boil. Hannah took it to the water pump and mixed some cold water in to temper it. She placed the pan on the floor and added Epsom salts. Leah inched her feet into it and groaned with pleasure.

"What is it with Jewish men, Momma? What is it that makes our race produce so many miserly family abusers?"

"What is it? *Nu,* I'll tell you what it is. For two thousand years Jewish men have suffered nothing but humiliations and defeats. They must live through pogroms and massacres and watch helpless to even defend their families. And when there is no pogrom, the *goyim* never stop spitting down on them, not for a minute. In the old country it was impossible for a Jewish man to make a normal living. What they got was the *dreck* left over that the *goyim* didn't want. What does this do to a man, to his sense of manliness? It crushes it. So the Jewish man hides inside of his religion. He has no means to fight back, so he prays and justifies his cowardice from wisdoms in the Talmud. And when the world crashes down on his head, who can he strike out at? Where can he get rid of his frustrations? Only on his family. If you have no country to fight for, you have no heroes to copy. All you have is wife beaters."

Hannah sighed and contemplated for a moment to gather in her wisdoms. "In all conquered, beaten, subjugated people, the men behave the same way to their women and children. Look at the *shvartzers,* they are like animals to their women. And the Irishmen make ten babies and then flee the country."

"But this is America, Momma."

"It will take time, a generation, another generation, to shake off the shackles and mentality of the ghettos and the pogroms. It will take time before Jewish men, even in America, feel like full, real men. Meanwhile, Leah, my child, you must be extremely clever in the selection of a husband. That is why the proposition that came to me has some merit."

"Who is it already, Momma?"

"Here, let me dry your feet," Hannah said with obvious hesitation.

"Nu?" Leah asked after a time.

"A distant relative. You've seen him on numerous occasions, usually on holidays when they come to Baltimore to go to *shul.* In fact, he was in your very chair last Rosh Hashonah. You don't remember?"

"No, I can't think with you playing games. Is that why you went out of town last week like a spy on a secret mission? To look things over?"

"Yes," Hannah admitted.

"So tell me already."

"The one and only son of my second cousin . . . who, incidentally, owns a huge general merchandising store in Salisbury—"

"You mean Richard Schneider!"

"Listen for one minute, Leah, listen."

"Richard Schneider, oh my God!"

"Morris Schneider has one child, Richard, his only son. Richard will be twenty-five next year and Morris is not a well man. He longs to see his only son have a wife and children and take over the business. Entirely, take it over, lock, stock, and barrel, one hundred percent. Richard will be a wealthy man."

Leah came to her feet, slipped in the pan, grabbed the table for support as water spilled out of the basin. *"Oy vay iss mir.* Richard with the pimples! A pale nothing. He's as attractive as a boil about to be lanced."

"That was a year ago. Today, believe me, I saw him, he's taller, more sociable. His face is completely cleared up. He's always had a special crush on you. Leah, this is a very gentle person. You can train him like an animal. And let me tell you, their home is a mansion—"

"But Salisbury is on the Eastern Shore. Momma, it's worse than Havre de Grace."

"You wouldn't believe the size yard they have. As big as downtown Baltimore. And the silverware, and the carpets. Would you believe, an automobile, a Ford Model T. Who ever heard of such things?"

Leah clamped her hands over her ears.

"So what do you want!" Hannah cried. "We toil our fingers to the bone from birth to death, for what? You want a tailor? You want some hotsy-totsy street-corner agitator? Your cousin Morris is a generous man."

Leah put her hands to her face and wept, stepping carefully out of the pan, while Hannah dried her feet. Leah continued weeping at the table as Hannah busied herself sweeping up crumbs from around the cookie plate and removing the teacups. "Sorry I mentioned it," she said. "This is America. Nobody will force you."

At that, Hannah dropped into a chair and stared at the patterns on the wallpaper. "I was to go with you to Salisbury this Sabbath," Hannah mumbled after a time. "I'll tell them we aren't interested."

Momma's stone face told Leah that there was something else, more to it. They fenced in silence.

The mantel clock struck six. Hannah grunted about the room, cleaning away dust that wasn't there.

"What is it you're not telling me, Momma?"

"What possibly wouldn't I tell you?"

"Maybe something about Morris Schneider's generosity?" Leah suggested.

Hannah set down the feather duster and sighed, not once, but four times. "Morris offered me a settlement. One thousand dollars."

Leah swooned across the room and gripped the lace curtains and stared down on the pushcarts and bustle of the intersection. Women were lined up to get into the bakery to get at the day-old counter. A thousand dollars! It was beyond a fortune, staggering to the mind, so much money. Momma could lease the finest wedding gown shop in all of Baltimore. She'd get business from all the uptown German Jews with such a place. Her poverty would be over. Leah looked up to see Lazar standing in the bathroom doorway, staring at them curiously.

IT WAS TOUCH and go, but with a super effort Richard Schneider managed to carry Leah over the threshold of the bridal suite. Morris and his wife, Erma, applauded their son's feat as a pair of bellboys assaulted the stack of luggage in the hallway.

"These five pieces go down the hall to our suite," Erma pointed out.

The assistant manager, a fawning Austrian, drew the lead-weighted velvet drapes open to the view of the ocean and waited for the *ohs* and *ahs* that followed appropriately from Richard and his parents. The Austrian then pirouetted his way around the suite pointing out the cornucopia of amenities.

The bellboys were rewarded with twenty-five cents each, and the Austrian with a silver dollar, as he backed out bowing and closed the door behind the four of them.

"Well, *kinder,*" Erma said, "you wouldn't have need for us until dinner. Shall we meet in the dining room at eight, sharp?"

Richard glanced nervously at Leah as his mother awaited a reply. "Eight will be fine, Mother," he said.

Silence. Terrible, stone silence.

"I think I'm coming down with one of my migraines," Leah said.

Erma stiffened. "We didn't intend to be a bother," she said. "Elberon

is like a second home to us, isn't it, Morris? I've been coming here since
I was a child."

"Maybe the children would like to be alone," Morris ventured
meekly.

"Alone? Why, of course," Erma retorted.

"So, we'll see you tomorrow," Leah said; "after breakfast," she added
for good measure and opened the door to show them out. "We'll find
you on the boardwalk or the beach, maybe."

When they left, Richard was about to say "You shouldn't have" to
Leah, but didn't. She had already gone into the dressing room adjoining
the bedroom and was busy opening four new alligator Gladstone bags
holding her elegant new wardrobe, which had been part of the marriage
contract.

Leah had closed the drapes separating her from her husband and for
the next hour tried on one dress after another, before a full-length
three-way mirror.

Leah seated herself at the vanity table and leaned close to the mirror
and touched her clear soft cheeks with the tips of her fingers. She
looked deeply into her big, penetrating brown eyes, then felt her hair
sensuously and ran her fingernails over the shapes of her ears. She
puffed some perfume from the atomizer on her wrist, sniffed it, then
applied some to the cleavage of her bosom.

Leah was totally entranced with her own beauty. Ethereal! Beyond
beauty! Leah blew a kiss to herself, crossed her arms over her bosom,
and touched her own naked shoulders, thrilled at the feel of her own
flesh.

"God, you're ravishing," she said to her image, below her breath.

A light from the outside broke up Leah's narcissistic flight as Richard
entered and came up behind her. She rose from her seat and faced him.
Richard tried to speak, but was tongue-tied. Suddenly! He flung his
arms about her and lunged clumsily to kiss her, only to find her cheek
turned away.

"Leah," he croaked.

"Please, you're suffocating me," she said. "Everything in its own
good time."

After the same awkward spell he'd experienced all his life, Richard
backed up, mumbling that he needed some fresh air, and left the hotel.
He crossed over the boardwalk and took the steps to the beach, removed his shoes, rolled up his trouser legs, and sat in the sand close to
the water's edge, watching the bathers squealing in the breakers, glancing up time and again to the hotel suite. The shades remained drawn.

At teatime, Richard found a table alone in the outdoor courtyard. The hotel orchestra played a medley of Victor Herbert, the king of Broadway. Spotting his mother and father enter, he slipped away quickly and walked aimlessly up and down the boardwalk until daylight faded.

He returned to the empty parlor, then tiptoed into the bedroom, where Leah was asleep in shaded light on the chaise longue. Richard stood over her, adoring her beauty. His heart both throbbed and ached.

Soon all the uneasiness would be gone. She'd learn to love Mother. Mother would teach her proper taste and etiquette. Mother was widely traveled in Europe. She came from a fine old German family. The family home was near Central Park in New York. A mansion. Wait till Leah saw it. When Mother eloped to marry Father, there were a few years of ruckus. It was that damnable business of the German Jews looking down their noses at the Russian Jews. However, when Mother became pregnant, the family relented and established Morris in the mercantile business in Salisbury. At first they thought it an exile, but when he became very successful, the family let him in, inch by inch. Elberon was filled with wealthy German Jews, their answer to Newport. Oh, Leah, how lucky I am! We'll show them our marriage will be as good as Mother and Father's.

Leah stirred on the chaise longue.

"Leah," Richard said softly.

She blinked her eyes open.

"I'll order dinner," he said. "The first courses should be up in half an hour or so."

He left shyly for the parlor, rang for the butler, and ordered a magnificent banquet. Mother had taught him how: a cultivation he enjoyed. He adored ordering for his mother.

When he returned to the bedroom, Leah was dressed in a revealing petticoat and quickly held the lap quilt in front of her with modesty befitting an ante-bellum belle.

"We are married, you know," he said.

"Of course we are, Richard. I've just got to get used to—" She stopped. "Why don't I take a soak in the tub until the food arrives."

"Very well."

The table was set in a softly candlelit rounded alcove, which overlooked the courtyard. The butler lifted one silver cover after another and, to his own delight, described the dishes in French, a litany of gourmet appetizers.

"If this is a Jewish resort, he should learn to speak Yiddish," Leah said. "Who understands what he's saying?"

"Here," Richard said, filling a cracker with an unknown substance.

"What is it?" Leah asked.

"Caviar. We should have it with a pinch of dry sherry. Actually, I prefer iced vodka," he said to the butler.

"Caviar. I've heard of it," Leah said and nibbled. She grimaced. "My God, it's salty. What is it made out of?"

"Fish eggs. Sturgeon, imported from Iran."

"Sturgeon. From sturgeon we know," Leah said. "Momma used sturgeon sometimes to make gefilte fish, when we can't find carp. Sturgeon eggs? Well, no accounting for some people's taste."

Richard grinned sicklily. "To us," he proposed, handing her a thimble glass of sherry. She sipped and set it down quickly.

"I'm rather delicate. Too much alcohol makes me giddy. Oh, look, lox and liver."

"The liver is actually, well, a pâté. A very special blend called pâté de foie gras and truffle . . . goose liver with very rare mushrooms . . . and, er, the lox is salmon . . . from Scotland. . . ."

"Oh, my, my, my, fancy-shmancy."

As Richard went on and on about his mother, Leah's jaw clenched tighter and tighter. Successful they were, but not successful enough to find their precious son a high-class German Jewess for a wife, she thought. Who would want to go to Salisbury on the Eastern Shore but a poor Yiddish girl from the slums. That's why they settled on me. Look at him!

A few moments later, the butler revealed a pair of cold stuffed lobsters and uncorked the champagne.

"*Nu*, what is it now?"

"Why . . . why, it's lobster . . . uh . . ."

"Shellfish!"

"Yes . . . but . . ."

"So, what kind of a Jew are you, Richard Schneider? This is *traif*, forbidden food. Momma would have an apoplexy if she could see this."

"I'm sorry, Leah, but we don't keep a kosher home. It is impossible in Salisbury."

"That's not the half of it. You go to synagogues that have organs and mixed chorus and the men sit with the women and they don't even cover their heads. And you call yourself Jews. It was also impossible for Momma to keep kosher in Havre de Grace, but we'd never eat filth from the bay. Do you have any idea what these creatures feed on? They eat sewage and human you know what. It's very, very dangerous food. *Oy*, I can't even look at them. I'll have to talk to Erma about how we are going to share the kitchen."

Richard was on his feet and yanking on the butler's cord as though it were a fire alarm.

After the disastrous meal, made more so when Leah ordered liver and onions and there were none to be found, she made herself comfortable on a settee and turned the pages of the latest Jack London work, the novel *John Barleycorn*, with exacting slowness. Richard frowned when she lit a cigarette, but said nothing. He decided to let Leah have that one out with his mother, directly.

She looked over the top of the book to her badly disoriented husband. "Jack London," Leah said, "stands for socialism and the working class. How many people does your father employ?"

"Including the department store—and we sell farm equipment and supplies, and there are some orchards, which are share-cropped—and the traveling peddlers and vendors . . . I would say there are about fifty."

"I suppose the word 'union' is a dirty word by you?"

"We don't think about it too much on the Eastern Shore."

"To say the least. They don't even know the Civil War is over the way they treat the *shvartzers* on the Eastern Shore."

"Don't you think we ought to turn in, Leah. You know . . . turn in?"

"You take a snooze, Richard. This book has me absolutely enthralled."

Well past midnight, Richard Schneider still lay awake. When Leah had had her fill of Jack London, he could hear her move about, and this caused him to breathe audibly. He waited and waited, but she did not come to bed. Richard turned on the bedside lamp to see Leah sleeping on the chaise longue. He pulled himself together, flung off the quilt, and fell to his knees beside her.

"Leah," he cried, "Leah!"

She stirred, ever so slightly. "Richard. You woke me up. I was in a deep sleep. You don't wake someone up from a deep sleep shouting at them."

"I want you!" he croaked, stroking her hair clumsily.

"Oh, my dear Richard. I am so sorry. I'm having my menstrual period. I have terrible cramps and my back doesn't feel good, either. Why, Richard, your face is soaking wet with perspiration. You shouldn't have such a look in your eyes. You look like a madman."

By THE FIFTH NIGHT, Richard was exhausted from the lack of sleep. Erma remarked several times about how badly her son looked, but Morris knew what was what.

"They're honeymooners," Morris said; "a little too much nooky."

"Morris! Don't use that revolting word!"

"Lovemaking," he corrected.

Richard had a silent dinner with his parents. Leah was under the weather, again. When the meal was done, Richard stormed up to his suite, entered angrily, and slammed the bedroom door behind him. "I can't stand it any longer!" he shouted.

"You're so impetuous."

"I demand my husbandly rights!"

"Richard, I'm still not well."

"You are! I checked."

"You did what?"

"I checked the trash can in the bathroom."

"Oh my God, that's disgusting."

"Just which one of us is being disgusting?"

Leah wept very softly. "You have to understand, I'm quite delicate, Richard."

"I realize that. But . . . but after all, we're married. . . . Please don't cry, Leah, please don't."

When the bedroom was darkened, Leah slipped beneath the covers filled with determination now to get through this experience, not only without being hurt, but holding the upper hand. Leah removed her nightgown and waited.

Richard groped for her and, upon touching actual flesh, completely lost control. "Oh my God," he repeated, as his hands found breasts and buttocks, "oh my God!"

Leah strung it out. She waited . . . waited . . . encouraged a bit . . . then held him back. He was going completely wild. As suddenly as he had begun, he stopped, then started crying.

"Oh, Richard," she said, "you've made a mess all over the sheets. Oh, it's awful . . . awful . . . shame, shame, shame." She threw off the covers, ran into the bathroom, and slammed and bolted the door.

Richard rolled over in agony, grabbing the sheets and shaking with anger and mortification.

EACH NIGHT FOR the balance of the honeymoon, there was a varia-tion of the same theme: attempt without success. Leah fine-tuned each occasion to force him into an exterior ejaculation and then capitulation without actual consummation.

After each crushing setback for Richard, Leah felt a swell of victory. It came as a relief for him to know that the honeymoon would soon be over and he could return to the familiar surroundings of the store in Salisbury.

In the end, he no longer attempted to make love to her, but fell quickly asleep from an accumulation of weariness and medication. While he slept, Leah found contentment watching him thrash, again unable to perform. Leah knew a sensation of fulfillment she had never known.

The annulment came six months later. Most of that time Leah had spent with her mother in Baltimore. Hannah knew, Hannah consoled, Hannah had been right about men all along. In order to avoid a public scandal, or the airing of Leah's charges that Richard was impotent, the Schneiders gave up their claims for repayment of the contract money in view of the "damage" done to Leah's fragile psyche.

After the annulment papers were signed, Erma seized the wardrobe and four Gladstone bags. Leah returned to her mother's flat as impover-ished as when she had gone.

1917–1918

WAR!   WAR!   WAR!   WAR!

Leah checked the mailbox in the vestibule when she heard the shriek from upstairs, unmistakably the voice of her mother.

"*Gevalt! Vay iss mir! Got in himmel!*" Hannah cried in unabashed anguish. "God in heaven! Have mercy!"

Leah ran up the steps and flung open the door to see her mother on the overstuffed sofa, being ministered to by Fanny and Pearl with cold compresses to the forehead.

"Momma!" Leah cried. "What happened?"

"My heart! My heart!" Hannah wept, bouncing between Yiddish and English.

"Will somebody tell me what's going on!"

"That no good shmuck of a brother!" Fanny pointed to Lazar, who, with Uncle Hyman, cowered near the upright piano.

"He enlisted in the Navy!" Pearl cried.

"A thirty-year-old man with bad eyes and a weak back. What do they need him for, a cripple's brigade?" Hannah said, coming to a sitting position. "So, you're going so you should join your brother, Saul, in the ground?" Upon mentioning the deceased, Hannah went into another cycle of wailing.

"Shame!" Leah joined the chorus of banshees. "Shame, shame, shame."

"Momma," Lazar said, trying to wedge in a sentence edgewise. "I have a very special profession which is badly needed. It's not like I'm going to be a foot soldier."

"Need!" Leah shouted. "So maybe the great American Navy needs you more than your mother and sisters? *Nu*, be a great big mister hero and leave us here to starve."

"*Gevalt!*" Hannah wailed.

"Nobody under this roof is going to starve," Uncle Hyman interrupted as he pounded a proud hand on Lazar's shoulder.

"He's half blind," Hannah said.

"As my personal contribution to the war effort, I will continue to pay Lazar's salary to you, Hannahile. If I so much as miss a single paycheck, my name is not Hyman Diamond."

When the choir of rebuttals had simmered down, Uncle Hyman continued. "And what is more, you have my sincere word of honor that when this boy returns from the war, I will establish him in his own drugstore."

"And what if he doesn't return, or what if he comes back in a basket without arms and legs?"

"Or without eyes?"

"Or shell-shocked?"

"Enough, dammit!" Lazar snapped with an authority they were not used to. He walked over to Hannah and squeezed her shoulder firmly. "I'm going, Momma," he said softly; "that's all there is to it."

FOR THE FIRST time in its American experience, the Jewish population was sizable enough to respond to a national call to arms, and for the first time since biblical days the Jews had a country they loved fiercely. They were swept up by the war fever.

The initial hysteria of the Balaban women was soon transformed, like a miracle, into a feeling of thundering patriotism. A little pennant with a blue star was hung in the shop window, denoting a home with a son in the armed forces.

Lazar's photograph went up on the mantel in a place of honor, next to that of his brother, Saul. Lazar had, at last, won both liberation and lionization and was now the object of endless bragging, the new glory of his sisters and adopted mother.

Because Lazar had a profession much in demand, he was awarded the instant rank of Chief Pharmacist's Mate. He was immediately assigned to a hastily formed medical detachment of a few hundred naval physicians, surgeons, enlisted pharmacists' mates, and hospital apprentices, who were to establish a medical service for the Marine Corps, a small elite prewar force of fewer than ten thousand men.

A brigade consisting of the 5th and 6th Marine regiments was rushed to France in the vanguard of the American Expeditionary Force. The Marines were the soldiers of destiny, preordained to make up in valor what they lacked in numbers in some of the bloodiest and vital battles of the war.

The moment he boarded the crowded troopship *Henderson,* Lazar Balaban felt, for the first time in his life, a sense of freedom. He was free of his detested father, free of the red-necked bigotry that had killed his brother, and free of the Balaban women.

To most of his mates, the war was the answer to boyish dreams of high adventure and the stuff of spellbinding romance. Tough, apple-cheeked young men, untouched by the decades of warfare the Europeans endured, had come fresh off the farms and cities of a largely rural and unsophisticated country.

France! My God! France meant women . . . POON . . . doing it in the French way, whatever that meant. They listened to the nightly bull sessions of magically woven tales rendered by the old-time Marines who had been on the Shanghai detail and the Yangtze patrol.

For a young and naïve America, which had never engaged in a great international conflict, it was the end of innocence.

By mid-1917 the 6th Regiment had landed in St. Nazaire. The boys were so hyped up, they could not see the awful realities that lay beyond.

WHEN LEAH EMBARKED on her ill-fated marriage to Richard Schneider, Hannah used the contract money to take out a long-term lease on a building with a shop front on Fayette Street. Not only was the location more desirable for business, it afforded them living quarters such as they had never had. Hannah and Leah had private bedrooms for the first time in their lives, and look, such things existed . . . a separate living room with a genuine mohair sofa.

The Balaban women fell into lockstep with the war effort. Jobs in the garment industry, once scorned for their raw exploitation and working conditions, now became attractive and well paying. A former notorious sweatshop, Ginzburg Brothers, won a lucrative contract for making Army uniforms. The factory near the Camden Station of the B&O Railroad was only a skip and a holler away from their home. Leah and Fanny went to work as seamstresses at double peacetime pay.

Pearl, the youngest, found a fabulous job as a welder in the shipyards at Sparrows Point, so they were able to afford a full-time *shvartze* to keep the house. The Balaban coffers tinkled, another first.

There were numerous military installations about Baltimore, including a major overseas staging center at Camp Meade. Jewish soldiers and sailors on liberty found their way to the two synagogues on Lloyd Street and a nearby servicemen's canteen, and they were taken in and adopted by the community. The Balaban sisters got their share. With the war on and the large number of Jewish boys in uniform as a rationalization, the Balaban rage against the male species was suspended for the duration. There were nightly dances at the canteen and the Young Men's Hebrew Association, where the sisters could usually get the pick of the litter.

The Balaban house on Fayette Street was open to the boys and the table was filled with Jewish dishes so they wouldn't forget home. Although some foods were difficult to find, Hannah was an old-time *balabosta* and could always put something together from the vast Lexington Street Market, and her baking sent out an aroma of welcome.

Each Tuesday she closed the shop early and baked past midnight. Wednesday morning found her at the Central Post Office to mail a dozen or so packages overseas. Some fifty of her "boys" got at least one package a month. Their letters were read aloud, over and over, and their photographs lined an entire wall.

Fanny never got much better at the piano, but some improvement was bound to result from the nightly songfests. Bittersweet time. So they came through, Jewish boys from as far away as Texas and Alabama, and they went off to war with a lovely memory of Baltimore.

Since her exercise with Richard Schneider, Leah had grown bolder in setting the initial bait for men. Yet as each relationship unfolded, it began to take on a repetitious pattern. The deliberate lure, the pleasant romance—which Leah drank in as flattery of her beauty—a serious turn, and then, disaster: arguments, confusion, and a bulwark thrown up against further advances. In the end, Momma always turned out to be right about men.

During the war, the Balaban home was an enlisted man's domain. The Jewish officers belonged to the uptown German Jews. Rank begat rank. That was why Lieutenant Joseph Kramer of Joplin, Missouri, was a marked man when he stepped into the B'nai Israel Synagogue.

Never mind that Fanny saw him first. Leah, with her honed skills, snatched Joe from her sister with vampish boldness. Fanny never fully forgave her sister for years, but her initial pain was tempered when she became serious about a fellow of her own.

Leah reckoned that Alan Singer was more suited for her sister Fanny, anyhow. Al was a nice boy from Cleveland. Before he was drafted, he worked for his father, a small painting subcontractor. That was plenty good for Fanny, who wasn't exactly a knockout, but rather basic, dull, and giggly. Al was two cents plain, down on Fanny's level. Anyhow, they made each other laugh a lot. Leah's conscience was clear.

Joe Kramer: now, he was something else. Joe, with his gold bars, was not only an officer and a gentleman, but a member of the cavalry, as dashing a set of credentials as Leah had ever encountered. Here was a man of quality. His father and uncle were partners in the law firm of Kramer and Kramer. Joe was in his final year of law school at the University of Missouri. He was allowed by the Army to take his state bar exam early so that when he returned he would be able to hang out his shingle.

Joe was a go-getter and not a man who would be turned away easily. With such an attractive prospect, Leah came to realize that in order to win him, she would have to make some concessions.

It's a long way to Tipperary, it's a long way to go;
It's a long way to Tipperary, to the sweetest girl I know!
Goodbye, Picadilly, farewell, Leicester Square,
It's a long, long way to Tipperary, but my heart's right there!

The ferryboat *Emma Giles* steamed away from her dock at Tolchester Beach on the Eastern Shore and headed back across the bay with her fill of weary, happy passengers. It had been a lovely day excursion, starting from Pier 15 on Light Street, and the mood was mellow for the return trip.

A trio of aging ladies in quasi-uniform who called themselves the Doughgirls ended their foray of patriotic songs, marching in step and saluting.

The lights were lowered and the band played more sentimental stuff, and soldiers and sailors and their girls glided about the floor, forehead to forehead, cheek to cheek. As the space between their hips narrowed, couples broke away and made, hand in hand, for the deck outside, into the starlight for a little spooning.

Al Singer and Fanny Balaban danced with their eyes locked on each other, chomping their chewing gum softly in rhythm to the music.

"Al," Fanny said, "it's been a wonderful day, the most wonderful I've ever spent in my entire life."

"Yeah, me too," Al said. "Hey, let's go outside. I want to talk to you about something important."

On the deck above them, Lieutenant Joe Kramer balanced on the railing, following a shooting star. Joe could be moody, Leah had learned.

"You haven't spoken two words, Joe," she said.

"Uh . . . what?"

"Something's wrong?"

"No, nothing."

"Come on, out with it."

"Looks like we'll be pulling out soon."

"Oh!" Those dreaded words. "How soon?"

"Couple of weeks, maybe."

Leah came very close to him, leaned on him, and rubbed her cheek against his. It evolved into a long, deep kiss.

"I hate to see you leave," Leah said. "Things have been real different since I met you."

"I want to go," he said. "Most of us feel that way. I have to get my piece of this war. It's something that may be difficult for a woman to understand."

"I don't want it to be over between us."

"Neither do I," he said.

"I'm so glad."

"Leah, we've been seeing each other for a decent amount of time. There's something . . ." He halted.

"Go on, tell me."

"All right. Here it is. Straight. I've taken a room at the Belvedere Hotel for tonight. I'm not going to twist your arm to come with me. Just a simple yes or no?"

Leah's hand automatically clutched her heart. Her instinct was to feign modesty and then go into an impassioned denial mode. Joe Kramer was no Richard Schneider, or any of her other recent beaux.

"I love you, Leah."

There were no tactics of evasion she could employ now, and she knew it. There was either a chance of hooking Joe by consummating their affair, or the certainty of losing him by a rejection. No other choices. No games. His powerful, mournful eyes never left her.

Leah went tightly into his arms. "I'll come with you," she said.

As they kissed, Leah heard the unmistakably clumsy sound of Fanny flapping up the ladder from the deck below.

"Leah!" Fanny cried, grabbing her hand and leading her off as Al Singer honkered up to Joe, shyly.

"Leah, look!" Fanny cried, thrusting her ring finger out. The stone was so small, it was barely visible.

"Al just popped the question and I said yes. We're officially engaged. He wants to get married right away, before he goes overseas."

Leah embraced her sister, but her mind was whirling on something else.

"Then you can go to bed with him without shame," Leah muttered strangely.

"We've already been doing it, Leah."

Leah was struck with disbelief. "But why didn't you tell me? Weren't you ashamed? How long have you been doing it? Where?"

Fanny shrugged.

"Does Momma have any idea?"

"What's the difference? He's going to be my husband."

Leah looked down the railing to where Joe was shaking Al's hand. Leah realized she'd better not try any of her little tricks tonight if she harbored any hope that Joe Kramer would return to her. She had to go through with it. Moreover, she had to make love to him so fantastically that she and she alone would fill his thoughts in the months ahead.

THERE WAS A double wedding at B'nai Israel Synagogue underwritten by dear Uncle Hyman, the proud patriot, especially since his own son, Gilbert, had been rejected for service.

In less than a month Private Al Singer and Lieutenant Joe Kramer sailed from the port of Baltimore aboard troopships bound for France. They left behind a pair of brides in their first weeks of pregnancy.

Molly Kramer and Edith Singer were born only a few days apart at Sinai Hospital on Monument Street.

HANNAH BALABAN had mystic premonitions. High times could not go on indefinitely. How could such happiness be sustained?

Hannah was reasonably satisfied that Al Singer and Joe Kramer would not give her daughters a life of misery like that *putz* Moses Balaban had given her, and that was good news.

Hannah had two *eynikles*, a pair of beautiful, healthy grandchildren, both girls yet, and that was more good news. Finances had never been better and the war was now definitely being won by the Allies.

But nobody could go on living on such a cloud. Hard times were bound to return. She would be ready when they did.

True to her premonitions, bad news arrived by the bushel.

America's initial war fever had been diminished by the casualty lists. A stunned public came to realize that the war wasn't just one big happy adventure. When the first of Hannah's adopted soldiers was killed, she went into a depression that lasted the rest of the war, for there were others killed and many wounded. It was no joke, this war.

The second tragedy befell when beloved Uncle Hyman, their lifelong benefactor, passed away. He was in the prime of his life, a young man in his sixties, a godly man who gave to everyone: money . . . credit . . . love.

Hyman's only son, Gilbert, inherited the business. Would Gilbert be as generous and loving as his father? Maybe yes, probably no.

Fortunately, Hyman's last will and testament remembered them all, particularly his promise to set Lazar up in a drugstore of his own when he returned from France. If only some shyster lawyer didn't steal everything. The mourning for Hyman was one hundred percent genuine. His photograph went up on the mantel alongside Saul's and Lazar's.

Not so doleful was the news out of Havre de Grace. Moses, so he claimed, had lost everything to a couple of smooth-talking con men in a fraudulent get-rich-quick, phony-war-bonds scheme. When Moses learned what had happened to his money, he had a stroke, on the spot. He was forced to liquidate lock, stock, and barrel to cover his debts. Partly paralyzed and unable to work, he implored Hannah to take him in, after his brothers in Savannah had refused.

Scarcely able to turn away a stray cat, Hannah took pity. The rules she invoked were rigid. Moses could stay in a small alcove off her bedroom in a separate bed. He would have no power of decision over family matters and *no sex, whatsoever, positively*. Should he regain enough health to resume work, the whole matter would then be renegotiated.

Moses' stroke and the passage of time had aged him considerably. Moreover, his self-imposed loneliness as a miserly hermit had taken a toll. Moses was now on his best behavior every day, which made him almost palatable.

Perhaps, Hannah thought, coming so close to death might have given Moses a revelation about how despicable he had been. Whatever his reasons, he was no longer a force in their lives. He could read the Talmud until he went blind, so long as he didn't bother them.

Then Hannah's worst fears came to pass. Shortly after Moses was installed in his alcove, the dreaded telegram came from the War Department. Lazar had been wounded. He was hit, apparently by shrapnel, in the battle for Belleau Wood. For two weeks, Hannah could scarcely breathe until a letter came from a hospital in France. Lazar had not personally written it, because he had been hit in the arms and chest. He assured them all that he would fully recover, and as his letters came more regularly, and in his own writing, some of the pain and horror eased for Hannah.

After several months, during which Lazar appeared to be getting well, a shocker of a letter arrived. Lazar had married a Frenchwoman! A *shiksa* yet! And what was more, she was a widow with a small son. The trauma of this news was somewhat tempered when Lazar assured Hannah that his new wife, Simone, was not a serious Protestant and would be happy to take instructions on how to keep kosher and run a Jewish home.

"Look, it's not the end of the world. Lazar is nobody's dummy. I'll come to love Simone and her son, Pierre. God will provide me with wisdom."

Fanny and Leah left their babies at home when they went to work at the Ginzburg Brothers factory. It was an ultimate pleasure from heaven for Hannah. Little Edith and Leah's Molly were only a pair of matched dolls, that's all. Such *naches* from the little girls. Only a grandmother would know.

However, still another premonition disturbed Hannah greatly. Leah stayed out quite often and sometimes the entire night. Her "with a girlfriend" excuse somehow didn't quite add up. Hannah tried to perish the thought, but she could not help but feel that her daughter was screwing around on Joe Kramer. Hannah didn't ask. Leah didn't volunteer. But Leah sang to herself a lot these days and looked in the mirror even more than usual and spent far too much time in the bathroom primping up, just to be going out with a girlfriend. Joe Kramer had apparently given her a good time in bed, maybe too good for Leah's diluted sense of fidelity.

So, what else could happen? It did.

Pearl was now a young lady, but still Hannah's baby. She was a *shaynele,* a real pretty. Pearl strangely and suddenly dropped out of the nightly gathering of servicemen at the Balaban house. Gossip and rumor soon found its way back to Momma. Her baby daughter had been seen, not once, but several times in the company of a young sailor. The two apparently met at one of the stalls at the Lexington Street Market, of all places. Hannah was even furnished with the name of the family who owned the stall, the Abruzzi Brothers.

Hannah decided to conduct a quiet investigation on her own. Not that she was spying on Pearl, but a mother has certain rights to know. Pearl was a mere child and extremely delicate, as were all of her daughters. So, why not find out? She went shopping there twice a week, anyhow.

The Lexington Street Market was a century-old institution, where one could see a fantastic display from America's cornucopia. Hundreds of stalls in regimented rows overflowed with mountains of foods of all stripes . . . the produce of the rich earth of the Maryland truck farms . . . the harvest from the Chesapeake Bay . . . a conglomerate of ethnic tastes and aromas to stagger the senses. Hawkers hustled gawkers and eagle-eyed housewives pinched and bargained. Stall after stall displayed bakery goods adopted from a dozen different nations. Fish, vegetables, fruits, nuts, coffees, cheeses, meats, and sweets . . . a section with ham hocks, chitlins and catfish, catering to the colored folks. Weigh it, blend it, trim it, slice it, wrap it in yesterday's newspapers, here's a free sample . . . like it, lady?

Surrounding the market was a picket line of peddler carts filled with combs, mirrors, buttons, bows, and clothing and newspaper boys screaming war headlines and soapbox orators espousing forlorn causes.

Hannah stopped before the Abruzzi Brothers stall and drank in a deep breath and winced from the insulting smells of crabs, clams, oysters, shrimp, mussels, and other forbidden foods, alongside the iced bins of sixty varieties of fresh and smoked fish.

She studied the Italians in their fish-streaked rubber aprons and high boots, as they scaled, beheaded, gutted, and chucked from flat carts with oversized wheels into the bins and sang as they worked, as though personally anointed by Enrico Caruso.

The Jewish neighborhood was smack up against the Italian, whose hub was St. Leo's Catholic Church on the corner of Exeter and Stiles streets a block away.

Italians? Not too bad, Hannah thought, if you looked at the broad picture. A woman didn't have to feel afraid or particularly out of place walking through their neighborhood. They were certainly not like the Irish bums and hoodlums, who always gave the Jews a bad time.

The Irish never stopped drinking and fighting and they had swarms of kids they didn't really care for. On the other hand, the Italians liked to eat and drink and made babies they adored. Leah and Fanny sometimes exchanged nasty words with the Italian girls who worked at the factory, but by and large they lived quite well side by side, and it was even possible to make a good friend. Italians thought very much of the family as a sacred institution, like the Jews.

"Hey, lady, you like to sample some fresh shrimp?" Angelo Abruzzi, an ancient fisherman, said.

Hannah screwed up her face and turned away. "Over my dead body you'll catch me eating *traif.*"

"You Jewish lady? Forgetta the shellfish. I gotta bluefish, swordfish, shark, I gotta smelts and freshwater perch"—kissing fingers to lips to denote ambrosia—"I gotta white bass, snapper, and butterfish. I gotta smoked herring, cured herring, salted herring. . . ."

When the old codger wasn't hawking or singing opera, he was making eyes at the ladies. *Nu,* Hannah thought, a little flirting from an Italian was better than no flirt at all. Twice a week she stopped at the Abruzzi Brothers' stall, and in no time at all they were exchanging friendly banter.

Old Angelo and his brother Tony had seven sons between them. Six of them worked two family fishing boats in the bay, while he and his brother ran the stall. Angelo had retired when the war broke out, but when his sons started going off to the service, he returned to the market.

Hannah opened the locket she wore about her neck. Angelo wiped his hands and put on his glasses, aware of the proximity of the locket.

"My son, Lazar."

"Hey, lemme see. A Marine! Now, thatsa somethin'."

"He was wounded at Belleau Wood."

"I pray for him."

"He's recovered quite nicely. Married his nurse. A French girl."

"Oh, datsa great. Frenchwoman"—fingers to lips—"lika beautiful *vino.*"

Angelo returned the compliment, showing Hannah a photograph of a sailor boy. "This is my *bambino,* Dominick." Now a confidential whisper, as though the Kaiser's agents were listening from under one of the piles of fish. "He's a submariner. His boat is in dry dock. Even comes down and helps his poppa at the stall."

So! That was the culprit potskying *around with Pearl!*

"Thisa boy, he give his old man lotsa trouble. Fishing boat is good enough for my other sons, for Tony's sons, but not Dominick. He was a rookie policeman when the war come."

Abruzzi gloried in his knowledge of submarines and went on to explain that the United States had four submarines in service patrolling the European coast, namely, the L-1, L-2, L-3, and L-4. Earlier that year, the L-5 had been launched and commissioned at the naval shipyard in Newport News. Dominick Abruzzi was a member of the crew.

The L-5 started for Europe, but developed trouble two days at sea and sped home. The dry docks at Newport News, at the opposite end of the bay, were filled with ships. The L-5 was towed to the yard at Sparrows Point for repairs and modifications and the crew assigned to temporary duty in Baltimore.

That was where Dominick met Pearl, who was a lady welder assigned to work on the sub. Every night, Dominick would go to the Jewish servicemen's canteen to meet her under the name of Charlie Goldberg. Nature then began to take its course.

PEARL TOOK OFF her shoes to make her feet quiet, turned the key in the front door lock, and closed it ever so carefully. She went up the stairs with her feet pressed against either side to avoid creaking.

Hannah sat in a rocker in Pearl's room, knitting.

"Momma! You startled me. You're up late."

"I could make, perhaps, the same observation."

"Oh . . ."

"What are you carrying your shoes for, Pearl? They're too heavy on your feet?"

"I didn't want to wake up the babies."

"That's very considerate."

"Momma, what's wrong?"

"So, maybe you'll tell me."

"I don't know what you mean."

"You haven't been home a single night all week."

"I've been . . . at the canteen. You can kind of forget what time it is. So much fun and all."

"I'm your mother, Pearl. You shouldn't lie to your mother."

"Momma, what are you talking about?"

"One Mr. Dominick Abruzzi."

"Oh!"

"Momma already knows, *shaynele*. This is not a good situation you're getting yourself into. It would be better if you didn't see this boy again. I want you to promise."

"No, Momma, I won't . . . I can't."

When Hannah read her daughter's expression, she realized. "Have you been to . . . have you, God forbid . . . have you?"

"We're married!" Pearl wept, putting her hands over her face.

"Married? Married? Does his father know?"

"No, no one knows."

"But you're a child."

"I lied about my age."

"So, who would marry you? I demand to know."

"A priest. He did it secretly."

"A priest! A Catholic priest! *Vay iss mir! Oy*, let me think. Your cousin Gilbert knows a lawyer. It can be annulled."

"No, Momma. I'm going to have a baby."

"*Gevalt!*"

SUCH A MAJOR transgression was not to be easily forgiven. There was a tear-soaked banishing, as Pearl moved two blocks away to the huge three-story house belonging to the Abruzzi family on Albemarle Street. The place was filled from top to bottom with family. As though there weren't enough kids already, they spoiled Pearl as if she were the Virgin Mary carrying little Jesus.

Pearl fared well and got plump like her mother-in-law and sisters-in-law. Italians, she learned, could be extremely affectionate when they weren't fighting one another. Even the fights were largely playacting. Pearl never knew that people could devour so much wine and food and music. Caruso records and operas played day and night on the windup gramophone.

Moses, recovering from his stroke, learned what had happened and broke his silence. "That girl will not die a natural death!" he condemned.

Good, Hannah thought, serves Moses right. Look, the *momser* is happy! He's got something terrible to get his teeth into. The son of a bitch is taking to this tragedy as though it were a joy!

Hannah expected Pearl to come crawling back on her hands and knees, but such was not the case. After a few months, Hannah established an oblique, secondhand liaison. She would have neighbor friends just happen by the Abruzzi Brothers' stall and make innocent, offhand inquiries. Old Angelo sensed what was going on and he knew, in his heart, that Hannah was a fine, fine person and it would only be a matter of time until she made peace with the situation.

Hannah caved in when word got back to her that Pearl's water had broken three weeks prematurely. She plunged headlong into the strange world of Mercy Hospital, with all its crosses and somber nuns and candles and chapels and kneeling and God knows what else, to be at her daughter's side.

She met Dominick, her Italian son-in-law, for the first time, pacing the corridor with Angelo and a half-dozen Abruzzi women.

For such an infant as Anna Maria Abruzzi, only an animal could not find forgiveness. What a baby! From the absolute minute of birth she was a ravishing beauty, little Anna Maria with the huge deep dark eyes and a head already filled with little black curls. What normal grandmother could reject?

When push came to shove, one would have to admit that Dominick was not so much of a disaster as she first believed. A regular masher, just like his father. Dominick certainly seemed head over heels, crazy in love with Pearl. Likewise, a policeman in peacetime was nothing to be sneezed at.

After an overheated discussion between Dominick and his father, it was decided that, out of respect for Hannah, the baby need not be christened in St. Leo's. This endeared Dom to Hannah. What the hell, Dominick reasoned, his old man would get over it in a few years. They weren't Sicilians, after all, who kept a feud going forever.

1919

IT WAS OVER, over there! The boys came home. After the initial jubilation and victory parades, a more somber judgment was passed on the price of glory and victory. A wiser America withdrew into a shell of isolation and vowed it would never again become embroiled in a European affair. Let them fight their own wars from now on.

So Al Singer claimed his bride and daughter and repaired to Cleveland.

Joe Kramer had suffered a poison gassing and would never take another pain-free breath in his life. He, too, went west, to Joplin, Missouri, with Leah and Molly.

Hannah Balaban was left with a new French daughter-in-law, Simone, and her little son, Pierre, and Dom and Anna Maria Abruzzi. Hannah would sigh and shrug and say, "Well, *kinder*, this is America."

SUCH A FUSS the family was making over the returning soldiers. Gilbert Diamond harbored deep resentment about the veterans. Like maybe it was his fault he was physically unfit to serve. Maybe the family would be happy if he were dead in the ground under a Star of David, in some French cemetery.

Gilbert was frustrated, and who better to take it out on than a genuine certified war hero who had been with the United States Marines. Gilbert didn't like Lazar, even before the war when they both worked in his father's drugstore. Lazar was the super-salesman, always ready with the bullshit and the smiles to the old ladies. Johnny-on-the-spot, ready to help just to impress Gilbert's father.

Now Lazar comes home with a fancy braid around his left shoulder, a decoration awarded the Marine Brigade by the French Government for valor, and everyone treated him as though he were the messiah.

Lazar's wife, Simone, likewise was as glamorous as her husband. She arrived on a special ship filled with French war brides. Her picture and story were on the front page of the rotogravure section of the Sunday Baltimore *Sun*. By contrast, Gilbert's wife, Minnie, was a *shmatte*, a human dishrag.

Lazar had become everything Gilbert longed to be but wasn't and couldn't. Together with a shyster lawyer, Gilbert made it a living hell for his cousin to collect the four thousand dollars from Hyman's will. In trust and innocence, Lazar signed a half-dozen documents that guaranteed he'd be indebted to Gilbert for years.

"If your father, Hyman, God rest his soul, had lived to see this, he would turn over in his grave," Hannah declared.

"Business is business," Gilbert retorted.

"So, didn't I tell you?" Hannah moaned later to Lazar, wringing her hands in disgust. "Gilbert Diamond is a cockroach with the flat feet and bifocal eyes and the limp handshake. Not even the Czar's army would have taken him."

Lazar found a drugstore for sale in a good location, across from the trolley car barn, at the intersection of North Avenue and Pennsylvania. It was a transfer corner for the number 8 and 31 streetcars, and at five o'clock business was brisk in cigarettes and magazines. Along with active foot traffic, it had a nice six-stool, two-table soda fountain and a couple of *shvartzers* with bicycles for home delivery. It could have been a first-class money-maker, except that Gilbert cut himself in as the 51 percent partner before he would release any funds. Lazar was in for a struggle.

Gilbert's own inheritance from his father had been a bitter disappointment. Hyman had given away too much. Always with the relatives. No matter what the *mishpocha* carried out of his father's store, no one ever got a bill. Gilbert convinced himself that Lazar was lucky to get what he did: As for himself, he'd help the family only as a last resort.

No one took Moses into account, so Lazar became the titular head of the family. But if he had returned from France with Joan of Arc as his wife, she wouldn't have won Hannah's approval. Phew! What they'd heard about those Frenchwomen. Enough to make a cat stand on its tail. The Frenchwomen were all you-know-whats. Hannah prayed that their offspring didn't have congenital deficiencies.

It was traditional that the entire family, over twenty-five strong in cousins, aunts, uncles, and brothers and sisters, made a duty call to Hannah's house on Sunday.

Even Hannah's older sister, Sonia, and her no-goodnik husband, Jake, and their kids attended. Gilbert and Minnie and their pasty-faced children usually arrived late, so they could leave early and avoid a fight. To miss a week's homage at the matriarch's was unconscionable. When Lazar and Simone and her son, Pierre, failed to show up two weeks in a row, Hannah got the message. She was clever enough not to make a big *tsimmes* about it, for fear that Lazar might really leave the fold.

Simone's pregnancy, that agony shared by all women, was plenty enough reason for Hannah to worm herself into the good graces of her daughter-in-law. After a while the two women developed a genuine affection for each other, and also genuine respect.

As a war veteran, Dominick was given a choice of a number of "soft" beats. He took the first opening as a motorcycle cop for Druid Hill Park and the placid surrounding neighborhood. Moving out of Angelo's home was not accomplished without a major Italian family brawl. Dominick bought a small row house of his own, near his precinct station. As his reward, Pearl became pregnant again.

Hannah's two new *eynikles* were born a few weeks apart, one in Mercy Hospital and one in Sinai. Hannah muffled her consternation that Pearl had a boy. After all, little baby boys should not be condemned for the sins of their fathers.

OUT OF CLEVELAND, the Singers were not faring so well. Al was no go-getter. He hung out at the Jewish Veterans' Club, playing acey-deucey and cribbage day and night, between jobs. For Fanny, one winter in Siberian Cleveland was enough. Fanny nagged, the baby screamed, home had become a nightmare.

Al was no tower of strength. Faced with the loss of the only woman he ever loved, he gave in sheepishly. He gave up his neighborhood where he had lived since birth, his old gang, his beloved Cleveland Indians, and moved Fanny and the baby to Baltimore, to Hannah's home on Fayette Street.

"It's all for the best," Hannah assured her daughter. "What's the matter, Al, there's no houses to paint in Baltimore?"

The family was almost in place now, where they should be, Hannah thought. If only Joe Kramer would see the light. What was the great honor to live in Joplin, Missouri?

ON AN EVENING late in 1920, it was raining cats and dogs outside and turning to sleet and hail. Hannah was suspicious of such weather. It was usually a harbinger of bad news.

Moses, upstairs, had become almost completely useless. His big thrill in life came from helping to make up a *minyan*, a quorum, when needed, to sit *shiva* and pray for a dead soul. He thumped on the floor with his cane when he needed attention. This evening he pounded in tune with the falling hailstones.

Hannah, who was closing shop for the night, was unnerved. "Shut up, you *nudnik!*" She threw her hands open futilely and was starting up to him when she was detoured by a ring of the front door bell.

Leah stood there, drenched from the downpour, with little Molly clutching her momma's hand and shivering. A half-dozen suitcases sat on the pavement.

"My God! Leah! Molly!"

"Oh, Momma! Momma!"

Leah was hustled into the vestibule and sobbed as her mother dragged in the luggage.

Molly was taken upstairs and given a hot tub and fed and tucked in, before the two women settled in the kitchen. A glass tea and a hot water basin for Leah's feet.

"*Nu*, darling, what happened?"

"Momma, it's been horrible! Ghastly!"

Only then did Hannah notice her daughter's multicolored bruises around the left eye.

"Joe Kramer beat you up?"

"Oh, Momma," she wailed.

"I never trusted that boy. Not for one minute. He didn't lay a hand on little Molly, did he?"

"He tried, but I threw my body across her to protect her, and he doesn't care if he ever sees her again, his only child. He said a hundred times, if he said once, that he felt like a caged animal. A beautiful family I gave him. Momma, I tried. God in heaven knows that I tried. It's a terrible thing to say, but he should have died an honorable death in France. At least the memory wouldn't have to be so bitter. Don't look at my eye. Do you have any idea what a horror story Joplin, Missouri, is? Thank God he didn't find out about Richard Schneider. He might have killed me."

"Leah, Leah, you poor child. You're home now."

"Joe drank every night like a Cossack."

"Hub him in dreard."

"I did everything. I went on bended knees. I scrubbed. I baked. I gave in to some very weird desires." She whispered into her mother's ear.

"He made you do that! The pervert!"

"That's not half of it. The games he played, like making me dress up like a prostitute. It was disgusting. I worked my fingers to the bone. Don't look at my hands, they're raw. He'd go days without picking up dear little Molly. Not so much as a pat on the head he'd give her. I was a goddess on earth to that man."

The thump of Moses' cane on the floor interrupted. Hail pelted against the window. "I want somebody to take me to *shul!*" Moses shouted.

Hannah found Al sitting on the bed in his room, playing solitaire, dressed like a peasant in his underclothing. He played cards with himself, while his wife slaved at the Ginzburg Brothers factory.

"Al, take the *alter kocker* to synagogue."

Al flung the cards down. "Shit, a guy can't find no peace here."

"For three months you're sitting. Go find a house to paint."

"Shit."

"And the roof of B'nai Israel won't fall in if you join in the prayers."

"Shit."

Molly was awakened by the shouting and, seeing herself in a strange place, hollered at the top of her lungs for her mother, who had resumed weeping loudly.

Thump, thump, thump. "Will somebody take me to *shul!*"

LEAH FAILED to relate to her mother a significant part of the story. Joe Kramer returned from the war a sorely hurt man from mustard gas. He coughed and hacked day and night. His only relief came from drink and heavy medication, which often made him strange, and he grew bitter and surly.

Joe craved tenderness. For a fleeting moment in the postwar hysteria, Leah was consumed with an angelically noble desire to care for a wounded veteran. That urge was soon dissipated in the day-to-day grind. She saw a lifetime before her of caring for a semi-invalid.

Joe had a lot of attractive men friends, and Leah, in love with her concept of her own innocence, was a toucher and a brusher-up-against. This rankled the hell out of Joe.

Life boiled down to a cycle of arguments, drinking bouts, sullenness, and drugs. One day Joe found a packet of perfumed letters, bound with a satin ribbon, tucked away on a shelf in her closet. It contained love letters from over a dozen soldiers who wrote to her from France after she had become a married woman. Leah swore she knew the boys before she had met him. She just didn't have the heart to tell them, being in the trenches and all, that she was now married.

With bottomless sincerity, Leah asked Joe, "How could I write that I was married when they were facing death?"

"What the hell were you going to do, marry them all?"

"Oh, Joe, you just don't understand."

"How many of them did you fuck?"

"Joseph Kramer! How dare you! Don't you use those words when you speak to me."

That was when he punched her in the eye, threw her out, and then left Joplin for points unknown. It was back to the Ginzburg Brothers factory for Leah, with her sewing machine next to her sister Fanny's.

AFTER AN INITIAL postwar boom, America slammed the brakes on its overheated industrial machine. Billions in war contracts were abruptly canceled, resulting in massive layoffs and a deep national economic depression.

Everyone struggled, Lazar in his new store, Momma with her wed-

ding gown business, house painting. Even that *paskudnyak* Gilbert Diamond felt the pinch. Only Dominick, with his city job on the police
force, was untouched.

Hannah broke her head trying to keep the house on Fayette Street,
but it became a hopeless cause. She had no choice but to liquidate and
sell the business at a tremendous loss. She shopped around for smaller,
cheaper quarters.

Foreclosures were a common occurrence, and many of Baltimore's
little two-story row houses, with their uniform pearly-white marble
steps, were for sale at bargain prices. Alas, there was no Uncle Hyman
to come to their rescue.

Hannah found a house to lease, dirt cheap, on Monroe Street, out of
the downtown area. The neighborhood was only partly Jewish and
partly everything else. It was a crying shame to leave the sights, sounds,
and smells of Jewish Fayette Street, but there seemed to be little choice.

The house on Monroe Street consisted of a pair of flats. Downstairs,
the living room was converted into a dressmaking shop and the dining
room into a bedroom, which Hannah would share with Leah. Upstairs,
the three children, Molly and Fanny's two, would have the front room
and Al and Fanny the rear bedroom.

It meant there was no place whatsoever for Moses. When he learned
that Hannah had made an application to remove him to the Hebrew
Home for the Aged, a sudden miracle took place.

He walked down the steps by himself and stood humbly before Hannah and confessed. "I wasn't entirely wiped out. I'll buy the house on
Monroe Street, if you take me with you."

"You dog! You *goniff!*"

"I implore you humbly not to send me to the old age home."

"You can go shit in the ocean."

"Here, take the money."

"What's the difference? There's no room for you."

"All I ask is a cot in the shop. I swear to the Lord of Abraham and
Isaac, I won't make a minute's trouble. And what is more," Moses
continued, "some feeling is returning to my hands. Maybe I can even
take in a little tailoring work."

At first Hannah couldn't believe what she was hearing. But God
moves in strange ways. Well, what to do? Beggars can't be choosers. Off
they moved to Monroe Street, consuming every square inch of living
space. But there was a bright side. Hannah had all her children in
Baltimore and within easy walking distance.

PART FOUR

ARISE, YE PRISONERS OF STARVATION

TEL AVIV

DAVID BEN-GURION'S Tel Aviv office had been converted into a makeshift hospital room.

Exhaustion and tension, the black knights of battle, had taken a toll. Ben-Gurion was ravaged by inner fires. He appeared helpless, more like a needy cherub than a national leader.

The doctor took the thermometer from the Old Man's mouth and read it with concern. "You're still running a high fever," he said. "We don't want this spreading to your lungs."

Ben-Gurion chose not to hear the doctor. "Where is Dayan?" he grunted.

"On his way over," Natasha Soloman answered.

"What's going on?" B.G. asked.

"It's the American ambassador again," Natasha said. "He demands a meeting at once and he's getting nasty about it."

"You have to hold him off until I speak with Dayan."

The doctor rolled a portable stand to the bedside.

"What are you doing?" B.G. demanded.

"You're dehydrating again. I'm giving you another intravenous."

The Prime Minister's wife, Paula, entered with a fresh pot of tea, wearing her patented expression of combat.

"I don't want the needle," B.G. protested feebly. "Take it away."

"Do what the doctor tells you," Paula commanded sharply.

"Who let her in here?"

"Here, drink," she said, feeding the tea to him.

"What are you poking?" he said to the doctor.

"I'm having a bit of trouble finding a nice juicy vein . . . ah, here we go. Now then, are we comfortable?"

"No, I'm not comfortable. Why don't you go back to South Africa?"

"I might just do that if we get out of this mess alive. I'll be grabbing forty winks in the next room." He took Paula aside, beyond B.G.'s hearing. "Paula, he's very sick. He should be in the hospital."

"How can he leave?" she asked. "He's conducting a war."

"He's not going to be any good to us dead."

"Don't worry, he's too stubborn to die."

The doctor looked heavenward in a gesture of futility and staggered from the room to a cot in the secretary's office; he was asleep as his head hit the pillow.

Jackie Herzog, the Old Man's confidant, entered. "Natasha," he said, "a coded message is coming in from Paris. You'd better get over to Communications and translate it. It could be extremely urgent."

Natasha nodded, then tugged at Jackie's arm and motioned for him to come out into the corridor.

"Any word from Mitla Pass?" she asked hesitantly.

Her reddened eyes probed his. Jackie fidgeted with the *kipi* on the back of his head. "Apparently, some Egyptians crossed over during the night in rubber boats and are inside the Pass. We don't know how many. The Lion's Battalion is coming under both air and mortar attack."

She closed her eyes a second. They stung from weariness. "What else, Jackie?"

"Gideon Zadok was injured during the jump. We don't know how serious it is. He's refused to evacuate. Look, Natasha, the man is a former Marine. He knows what he's doing."

"No, he doesn't," she answered in a shaky voice. "Gideon is a little boy being driven by some kind of demon."

"He'll get back. He's got a book to write, remember?"

"Oh Jesus, what did we let him go out there for?"

"You'd better get over to Communications and get that message translated."

General Dayan, the flamboyant one-eyed Chief of Staff, turned the corner and moved crisply down the corridor toward them just as the Old Man shouted, "Where is Dayan!"

Dayan stopped for an instant and he and Natasha exchanged the wizened glances of former lovers. Dayan said nothing, but his strange, Cyclops-like expression told her the story. The situation at Mitla Pass was now in doubt. She turned quickly and made haste to the Communications center.

Paula Ben-Gurion helped prop her husband up, surrounding him with pillows, as his Chief of Staff arranged some pins on a large wall map, denoting the progress of the four sectors of battle. The Sinai was a huge tract of viciously hot desert, pocked with treacherous mountain defiles and little habitation except along the Gaza Coast.

Up to the last instant, Israel played the card that hinted they were going to attack Jordan, then wheeled about and hit the Egyptians in the Sinai, achieving a brilliant tactical surprise. The IDF was now engaging the Egyptians at a number of their primary defensive strong points.

The campaign had quickly reached its first critical phase. Control of the air had not been established. Israel's Air Force was a potpourri of aged piston planes from World War II, along with a few squadrons of modern French jets. Their pilots had but a few months' training in the jet craft and faced an overwhelming, state-of-the-art Egyptian air power, consisting of Russian MiGs and bombers. Mastery of the skies had to be attained, or Israel's ground forces could get caught naked out in the open desert.

The British and the French, who were scheduled to neutralize Egypt's air power, had not taken to the skies and both Russia and America were applying enormous pressure on Israel to cease fire.

"How far has Para 202 penetrated?" Ben-Gurion asked.

"They made a beautiful fake at Jordan, then crossed into the Sinai at Kuntilla. They are approaching the Egyptian defenses at Thamad right now."

"Thamad? They still have a hundred and fifty miles to go to link up with the Lions at Mitla Pass."

"I'm afraid that's right," Dayan answered.

"Moshe, I don't like it," Ben-Gurion said. "Jackie gave me a message a half hour ago that most of Zechariah's tanks and transport have been eaten up by the desert. What do they have left? Tell me the truth, Moshe."

"They have about half of their transports and about three tanks still in operation."

"About three tanks? What does that mean, 'about three tanks'?"

Dayan, speechless, knowing what was coming next, gestured defensively. A disaster was brewing. He hadn't told the Old Man that the Egyptians had crossed the Canal and reinforced the Pass.

Nausea swept over Ben-Gurion. He vomited and went into palpitations. A national catastrophe was shaping up, imperiling statehood itself.

"B.G.," Paula pleaded, "please, darling, calm down."

"Dayan," Ben-Gurion rasped. "Get the Lions out of Mitla Pass, now."

The air grew thick with an invisible terror.

"This is no time to panic," Dayan asserted. "Zechariah is just about on schedule. If he hasn't taken Thamad by tonight, we can talk about evacuation of the Lions then."

"No, get them out now."

"It's impossible by daylight. They would be sitting ducks for the Egyptian Air Force."

"Now!"

The Old Man's eyes fluttered closed and his breathing became pained.

"Get the doctor, Jackie," Paula cried.

The doctor was there in an instant and took B.G.'s blood pressure. It was going through the roof. He quickly fixed a syringe and applied it, and after a few moments the patient stabilized.

"Get the Lions out of Mitla Pass," B.G. rasped.

"I refuse. If we pull them out, the Egyptians will come out of the Pass in brigade strength, maybe more. They'll destroy our entire campaign."

"Now . . . now . . ."

"I'll have to give you my resignation," Dayan said unflinching.

B.G.'s two eyes stared at Dayan's one eye for a short eternity. "All right . . . don't talk resignation . . . but we will review it as soon as we have darkness."

Dayan nodded in agreement.

Natasha entered the room, looking stricken. Dayan snatched the message from her hand. The Old Man watched the juices run out of his Chief of Staff.

"It's from De Gaulle," Dayan said harshly. "He has come under unbearable pressure from the Soviet Union. The Russians threaten a missile attack against Paris if the French enter the Canal Zone. The message goes on to say that he and the British have decided to delay their air strike until at least tomorrow."

GIDEON

MITLA PASS

October 30, 1956

EVENING, D DAY PLUS ONE

"DEAD," the radio operator said.

Major Ben Asher grunted. He grunted the same way whether it was for pleasure or displeasure. Our main radio was FUBAR during the parachute drop—Fucked Up Beyond All Recognition. The backup set just caught a piece of stray mortar shrapnel. The Lion's Battalion was completely isolated. The severity of our situation sank in painfully. If we didn't get a major attack from the Egyptians, we could hold out through the night. Certainly our Southern Command would drop supplies as soon as it turned dark.

This wasn't the loneliness of a writer's office, small and confined. It was a vast loneliness. The desert had a hundred variations of stillness, a thousand haunted themes, God knows how many secrets. The sun wore itself out hissing all day at the rocky paths which lay agonized in the wadi beds.

Evening light brought on pastels. Blaring reds of the days toned down to muted purples. A sudden lizard flitted by, fearing discovery, and disappeared in a minute crevice. On the horizon, a gazelle leaped from nowhere to nowhere. The stagnant stifling air of the day began to drift about, stirred by tongues of coolness.

Silence had become contagious. Our brains had been dulled from the heat. Speech was unwelcome and movement floaty. This was going to be one long goddam night.

Canisters of flares were being set in beside the very guns, to keep lighting the entrance to the Pass throughout the night against a sneak Egyptian attack.

Look at these bloody paras. Real desert rats, most of them. They like it out here. Some probably prefer this destitution to having a woman. What insanity to succumb to a mistress like the Sinai.

What's that!

Hey, you're clear jumpy, Gideon. Get ahold of yourself. It was only some loose rock that has been peeling away from the mother boulder, perhaps for centuries. I watched it skid down a little draw.

Major Ben Asher huddled with his officers. He didn't seem to show an iota of anxiety. The officers synchronized their watches. I liked it when watches were synchronized. It reminded me of a movie script I wrote. There's always a stirring scene when the commander says, "This is it, men, big casino. Ready. Synchronize watches."

As darkness crept in, a pair of machine-gun squads moved up close to the Pass so its mouth could be covered by a cross fire, if needed. We knew the Egyptians had reinforced the Pass, but we didn't know how many of them there were.

Maybe the Egyptians had recovered from the initial blast of the invasion and had regrouped for a counterattack. Lord, if they broke through us here, they could cut Israel's forces in half. That's why we're here, boys, to prevent a breakout.

Shlomo returned from the officers' meeting. "Twenty-eight minutes to sunset," he announced. See, Shlomo's watch was synchronized. "I'm going to round up some gear," he said.

I stood and shook the old leg. It was fairly stable. At least it hadn't grown worse. I checked our lodgings for the night. We were quite well entrenched behind a boulder. I watched Shlomo draping bandoleers of ammo over his shoulders. The son of a bitch was itching for the Egyptians to come out.

Major Ben Asher was standing alone now, surveying his kingdom. He looked very comforting, like my colonel in the Marine Corps. He checked the wounded. Dr. Schwartz had them stabilized and doped up. If they survived the night, they should be evacuated in the morning.

I was honored. The major supped with me. We partook of the foul ration. The major pointed to my leg and grunted.

"It will be okay if I don't have to stand on my head again."

This drew his lame excuse for a smile.

"So, what do you think, writer?" he asked.

"I'd be a lot happier if I saw Zechariah and Para 202 crossing toward us. Anyhow, you asked the wrong guy. I went into the Corps as a lowly buck-assed private, and three years later I was discharged as a private first class."

"I must have read that goddam chapter of yours on the invasion of Tarawa twenty times," he grunted and plunged into the rations as though they were manna from heaven. "Are we in a better position than you were on the first night at Tarawa or not?"

"When you're up shit creek without a paddle, you're up shit creek without a paddle," I answered.

"I say it would take three Egyptian brigades to overrun our defenses."

"If you don't run out of ammunition and if the air drop tonight doesn't touch down thirty miles away."

"Well, we have the advantage of no choice. We do not have the luxury of a defeat. One thing for certain we have over the Marines. Our rations."

"You've got a taste for shit."

Ben Asher's mood became contemplative. "I never told you, writer, but I knew your uncle, Matti Zadok, intimately."

"No, you never mentioned him."

"I was only sixteen when I went into his Recon unit in the Palmach. I still carry his toe print on my ass. I wish he was here now. If we had to evacuate, he'd be the only man I know who could find his way out of here."

"My father hardly ever spoke about his brother," I said.

"Matti Zadok was always cloaked in mystery. I can tell you he was a great soldier. His major love was the desert. He's a breed of Jew who was half coyote. He could look out over this same scene and see things that would have escaped our eyes. He read the landscape as though it were his woman's body, sensing when there was water beneath the ground, ascertaining if a camel print was warm or two weeks old. No Bedouin could track him. Matti discovered dozens of minor antiquity sites, the kind that escape normal detection."

The major stood, a chunk to be respected, like Uncle Matti. He surveyed all that his eyes could reach, as night fell. Perhaps he was hoping beyond hope that Zechariah's column would suddenly appear on the horizon.

"Have you found what you were looking for here?" he asked me strangely.

"I'm not sure I know what I'm looking for."

The major left and Shlomo sauntered in, buckling under the ammo he was toting.

"Look," he said, handing me a new carbine with an infrared night scope. "I got it from one of the wounded boys awaiting evacuation."

"Neat piece."

"The password for tonight is Yad Shimshon."

I repeated it three times as Shlomo sighted in with his new toy.

Down went the sun! Deathly silence and coolness enveloped us instantly. I gulped down a pain pill. I was going to miss the morphine, but we were running low. There were two brave men in my family, Uncle Matti and Uncle Lazar. My father wasn't of their ilk. That's why he never mentioned Matti, because Matti had succeeded where he had failed in Palestine.

Why would my father remain silent about his brother, when he spent so much time bragging about me? Hell, I've never been anything to him but an alter ego. When I became a published author, he'd hold court on me, anytime, anyplace. He'd stand up at the cash register in the neighborhood deli and give an impromptu lecture about me to the lunch crowd. He'd walk around Rittenhouse Square with a pocket full of clippings and reviews and sit down beside total strangers on park benches and tell them the story of my life. He'd even go to the seminary and lecture about me to little sisters of the poor.

So, why the fuck doesn't he love me? Why hasn't he told me, just once, I was something very special as a writer? Why did he always pound a literary critique up my ass? Oh, Dad, you're a weirdo, a real weirdo.

I wrapped up in a blanket and used my helmet for a pillow, just like in the old days. Shlomo sat over me, staring at a sky that was beginning to twinkle. How lucky I had been to have him assigned to me. Luckiest break I ever got as a writer.

"Good night, buddy," I said.

"Good night, Gideon," he answered.

SHLOMO

I WATCHED GIDEON sleep fitfully as the desert entered night. It was my favorite time in my favorite place because the skies were almost always clear and the entire universe put itself on display for me, alone.

I have a theory that Moses and the tribes came through Mitla Pass during the exodus from Egypt. I wrote my master's thesis on the realities behind the biblical fantasies. Let me say, it didn't become a bestseller, but on the other hand, more than one biblical scholar broke his head trying to disclaim my paper.

Gideon grunted. His hip was bothering him. Poor fellow. He almost got away clean with the parachute jump. What I liked about him was that he was scared out of his mind, but he jumped anyhow. Has it only been nine months since this little *paskudnyak* Zadok arrived? It seems like three eternities. It was becoming hard to remember what life was like without him.

I WAS WORKING in the Foreign Office. The country itself was only seven years old, and things were upside down and inside out. We had a lot of brilliant men, ambassadors, and ranking officials, but crafting a Foreign Office according to the letter of international protocol was an impossibility during those times. Israel had too many other priorities—bringing in the remnants of European Jewry, building a defense force and a national air and shipping line, finding money to operate, bringing in the Jews from Arab countries, contending with enemies on every border. There was a lot of hit and miss, trial and error in the Foreign Office.

LOOK AT THE SHOW out there! First, the stars came out one by one, now hundreds every second . . . here I am, Shlomo! Look at me twinkle! Muffled voices can be heard from the command post. An order is given over the field phone and a flare bursts near the opening of the Pass. . . .

AT ANY RATE, I never knew my rank or title in the Foreign Office if, indeed, I even had one. It was "Shlomo do this, Shlomo do that." Shlomo Bar Adon became, as they say, a jack of all trades.

Monday morning I was taking a delegation of American senators around. It was quite important for us to gain credibility and sympathy from the American Congress.

Tuesday morning they left with a good impression and Tuesday night I was called to the office of Nimrod Newman, the chief of the American Section.

"Shlomo, you did a fantastic job with the Americans."

My mind immediately went to a promotion, a salary raise, a permanent position, accolades. My visions of glory were short-lived.

"Something interesting has come up," Nimrod said. "A request came in from the States a few months ago. We've been kicking it around. To make a long story short, I had a meeting yesterday at the P.M.'s office. Jackie Herzog was there with Teddy Kollek, Moshe Pearlman, and Beham. Dayan was also present."

Ah, here comes my promotion. Nothing less than ambassador to France would be suitable. "So what did you decide," I asked, "to parachute me into Damascus?"

Nimrod smiled. He smiled when he was happy, sad, hurt, unsure, in love, out of love. He smiled. What did Nimrod's smile mean?

"There's an American writer. You probably have heard of him— Gideon Zadok."

"Zadok? Yes, I've heard of him. Great first novel, then some kind of oblivion in films."

"Zadok wants to come to Israel to research a novel. He asks complete cooperation, short of top-secret material. We have agreed, among us, that such a book could do the country a lot of good at this time in our history, if he succeeds. We want you to make certain he succeeds, arrange his travel, get him appointments, set up his interviews, and we'll open the archives, up to a certain point."

"Nursemaid to a writer?"

"This would be the first American novel about Israel. It could be valuable in gaining favorable world opinion."

"I have a choice?"

"No," Nimrod answered with a smile. This particular smile I understood.

"How long do I have?" I asked.

Nimrod shrugged. "Probably several months."

"What is his security situation?"

"He looks like an excellent risk. We'll keep a close watch. You won't be involved unless he probes too much in sensitive areas."

"So, when does he arrive?"

"Next week. And one more thing. His uncle was Matthias Zadok. That alone demands some respect."

AN EGYPTIAN FLARE burst over our lines. So, we know you are in there and you know we are out here. I love to contemplate in the desert. The bastards are going to ruin my night. I felt my carbine for the hundredth time. It comforted me, especially the night scope.

ZADOK? It was, how do you say it, a love-hate affair from the beginning. Love? I loved the little *shmendrick's* mind. He didn't come to Israel to fart around. He wanted to know everything. He chewed up the country in great bites. His mind could retain a biblical battle, spear by spear, or the more recent battles, mortar by mortar. Gideon's days were dawn to midnight. He almost killed me with his schedule. On some interviews I translated for fourteen straight hours. He wanted to see everyone, go every place, even though the borders were extremely dangerous. He almost got us killed a couple of times near the Gaza Strip.

What else did I love? He was a good fellow. He couldn't resist a party and he was a happy drunk. I mean, the little *putz* could outdrink any Russian Jew in Israel.

Chutzpah was his middle name. When he got someone drunk, they'd spill their guts out to him. Even sober, people seemed to want to tell him their story. He got to the soul very fast. A few weeks and I began to feel his lust for life and tremendous energy. Maybe, just maybe, Nimrod and the others had made a good gamble. I started to believe in him.

The hate part? Oh boy, was he arrogant! It didn't matter who he wanted to get to, or what he wanted to know, he got it, often out of my hide. He drove me out of my mind. Push, push, push, two hundred, three hundred kilometers through the night to make a six o'clock meeting. Questions, questions, questions. History, anthropology, geology, agriculture, geography, military, archeology. Shlomo, what happened behind that rock? How the hell did I know what happened behind every rock?

And look, we were a small new country trying to make rules. He broke every one of them and left it for me to explain. I hated his tenacity and I come from a country of tenacious men.

He was often angry, a madman with a bad temper. Just when I hated him the most, he would turn around and weep for an hour after an interview with a concentration camp victim.

Love-hate. When I failed at something, he cursed me as though I were a peasant. When I got through on something difficult, he hugged and punched my shoulder like I had won an Olympic medal.

Bit by bit, I started believing in this little shlemiel. He didn't forget one fucking thing I taught him. So, maybe I was serving some kind of literary messiah. Besides, Nimrod refused to accept the three resignations I turned in during those first weeks.

SHIT! Gunfire from the forward observation post. I wrapped myself in my blanket and continued to watch the star show. I fished through my backpack and found a bottle of good old Israeli brandy. The rest of the world can laugh at us, but not at our brandy. Best cognac in the world. Ah good . . . the shooting had stopped. I made a short prayer that when the sun came up, I would see Zechariah's Para 202 crossing the desert floor toward us. If not, oh boy!

I could see Ben Asher pacing. Even in the semi-darkness his figure was unmistakable. Wait! Yes, airplanes. I could hear stirrings all over our lines. In a few moments we could distinguish the engines. Dakotas! An air drop! God, I hoped they sent a radio. I didn't like this isolation.

We popped off several flares to give the planes a fix, and silently several platoons moved out to recover the parachutes.

HE WAS ASLEEP like a baby now, the little *momser*. Jerusalem. That's when he started up with her. Gideon and Natasha Solomon, as crazy a pair of bedroom warriors as I have ever known, and I've been in some pretty good skirmishes, myself.

Jerusalem was a divided city with an ugly barbed-wire no-man's-land running through the Kidron Valley. There wasn't too much levity in the city. In fact, night life was downright grim. Of course, a party in someone's home would often turn out to be a good party.

A costume party at Joshua Hillel's flat showed promise. He was a very successful journalist, a stringer for a dozen American and European newspapers and magazines. His crowd consisted of actors, musicians, and newspaper people. A number of them had access to the foreign commissaries, so there was the promise of embassy-level food and real whiskey and vodka. Everyone would be in costume and some were very daring for Jerusalem.

Gideon and I came rather late and the evening was in full swing. Shoshanna Damari belted out Israeli songs and the more intimate revelry had found its way into the bedrooms, balconies, closets, and W.C.s.

Gideon had put together a cowboy costume, which was appropriate, and I was a handsome (so I have been told on occasion) Bedouin. Gideon immediately became a center of attention, as everyone in the country knew of his presence and not many real writers passed our way in those days.

What happened took place in the blink of an eye. Natasha Solomon, dressed as a belly dancer, was across the room, looking like she was ready to be eaten in layers.

I stood next to Gideon, who was immediately trapped by two women, and in that instant Natasha's and Gideon's eyes made contact across the room. I could almost swear the entire place had turned silent and they were the only two people left in it. If anyone had passed through the beam between their eyes, they would have been fried.

"Her name is Natasha Solomon," I said. "She works in the P.M.'s office. You want an introduction?"

"I'll introduce myself," Gideon answered and took off in her direction. I trailed behind out of morbid curiosity. Gideon pushed into the circle around Natasha, took her by the arm, and led her to a quiet corner.

"You're Natasha Solomon. I'm Gideon Zadok."

"Yes, I know," she said. "Can I have my arm back?"

As he let her arm go, he saw the tattooed number that denoted a concentration camp inmate. He stared at it for ever so long; then he looked into her eyes and tears fell down his cheeks.

"I'm sorry," he said, "I can't get used to it."

"That's all right, I'm in Israel now," Natasha answered. "Here now, no need to cry." And she put her arms about his neck so naturally, drew him close, and held him and let him finish his tears.

I, Shlomo Bar Adon, who rarely lies, could swear that I felt the walls of the Old City shake at that instant.

"Lunch, Hesse's at one o'clock tomorrow, all right?" Gideon asked.

"I'll be there," Natasha answered.

That was it. I don't know what I started by taking him to that party. At the very least, it looked like I had stirred up a couple of dormant volcanos.

THERE WAS A great deal of activity at the command post, so I went over. A new radio was in working order! Our operator was receiving the end of a long message from the Southern Command. He handed it to the major.

"Para 202 ran into heavy resistance at Thamad. Outside air support has failed to develop. That would mean the British and French. If the situation is not better by morning, we are going to attempt to evacuate."

"God in heaven, how are we going to get out of here?" a young officer asked.

"Don't worry, don't worry," the major said, "Zechariah will break through to us . . . don't worry."

JERUSALEM

THE HUGE STONE VERANDA in the rear of the King David Hotel offered a taunting view over the Kidron Valley to the Ottoman walls of the Old City. A gash of barbed wire ran through the valley, dividing the city and the country in half. One could almost reach out and touch the Jaffa Gate, it was so close. It had become an obsession with the Jews, for inside the Old City stood the most sacred place in all of Jewry, the Western Wall of Solomon's Temple.

Gideon was no exception. The sight of the Old City jolted his imagination to the threshold of pain. It was more than cruel for the Jordanians to deny access, he thought.

"Hello, cowboy," Natasha's voice said behind him.

"Hi," Gideon said coming to his feet. "You look great."

"Even out of costume?"

"Don't leave me an opening like that," he said.

"Hi there, it's me, Natasha."

"What?"

"You seem to be in a trance."

"Sorry. It's the Old City over there. It seems that every night I'm in Jerusalem, I dream about crossing over and going to the Western Wall. It can drive you crazy, I guess, if you live here."

"Yes, it does. We may yet live to see it."

Four days had flown by since the party. Four lovely evenings together. Fink's, a tiny five-table bistro, was the only place one could get a decent steak or Polish vodka and whisper romantic nothings. It had become their "in" place.

Gideon and Natasha hadn't done much about probing into each other's history or volunteering details of their pasts. They spoke in the abstract, gazed at each other in the abstract, and occasionally even touched in the abstract.

Both of them had their own intelligence networks. Natasha's story seemed commonplace on the surface: Hungarian, affluent professional family, lived undercover with false documents wearing a blond wig in Budapest for a greater part of the war, a survivor of Auschwitz. Her mother, father, two brothers were killed in the gas chambers, ran the British blockade of Palestine in a refugee ship after the war.

One could gather that Natasha was quite worldly and well traveled in Europe before the war. She had been married but said nothing about how it ended. Thus far in Israel, several names were attached to her romantically, but apparently not seriously.

But Gideon knew that none of the survivors were simple or commonplace. Their heads were labyrinths with pockets of secrets, tortured guilt, twisted and violent memories. Every concentration camp victim he had interviewed had raw nerves hidden in shallow places, waiting to be irritated. Natasha must have her share of them, but she covered them well.

Gideon spoke even less about himself. His mind, soul, and body were consumed by the book he was going to write. Israel had captured him more deeply than he imagined. He burned with desire to end the research and get at the book itself, but that was months off.

"The Knesset adjourned today. I'll be heading back to Tel Aviv tomorrow," Natasha said.

"Just in the nick of time," he said. "Shlomo and I are going on patrol with the paras in the Negev. We're going from Nitzana along the Negev-Sinai border down to Eilat. I'm really excited."

Natasha smiled the smile that every man wanted to see from the woman opposite him—sensuous, playful, knowing.

"What are you snickering at, lady?" he asked.

"I was the one who signed approval for you from the P.M.'s office. You're going out with the Lion's Battalion."

"Small country," Gideon said. "Well, are we Finked out? Any place else exciting to eat? How about here?"

"One of my girlfriends has a flat just a few blocks away and she's out of town. I'd like to fix you dinner. I found some fabulous baby lamb chops from the Arab side."

"How'd you get them? Come on, I'm curious."

"I have a friend with the United Nations peacekeeping force. Everything passes through the Mandelbaum Gate, except people. Shall we be off?"

"How about a drink first?" Gideon asked.

Natasha nodded knowingly. "What's on your mind, cowboy?"

"The story of my life in five minutes or less."

The sound of the muezzin calling the Muslims to prayer was heard from a minaret and drifted over the calm valley. A chilling moment in the divided city's life.

"Natasha, I've been a bad boy for a long time. Right now, my marriage is on tenterhooks. We've both made mistakes. Val's were small stuff beside my sins and transgressions. Mine were whoppers."

"Whoppers? What's that?"

"Big ones. I rationalized my screwing around because I blamed her for nailing me to Hollywood. But, you know, in the end we've all got to own up for our own actions. So, the marriage is on hold, more or less on trial."

"Do you still love her?"

Gideon wavered just long enough to give Natasha an answer without words. "You know how it goes," he finally said. "We've been bedmates for over a dozen years, good lovers . . . even great sometimes. We're comfortable around each other when we're not fighting. We've got two beautiful children and I guess you'd say, they're my life. Who knows about love? We do care for each other. That may have to be enough."

"That's sad," Natasha said.

"When you invited me up to your room last night, I did something I never believed possible, especially to a woman like you. I said no. I said no because I was determined to stay clean here in Israel. Val and I left on very good terms and I wanted, very much, to be trusted again as a husband. God-damned lies pile up on each other. Tell one lie and you need twenty more lies to back it up. It's shit living that way."

Natasha's eyes grew mournful and moist. "That's very commendable," she said.

"I don't know, Natasha. If it were a quickie or a one-week stand, maybe I'd give in, but I've got a gut feeling that once we get our hands on each other, we aren't going to want to let go. Am I right?"

"Maybe," she answered.

Gideon sighed heavily, then took his drink down to the bottom of the glass. "There's even the possibility I might ask the family to come to

Israel if this research runs too long. If my wife comes here, I want to be able to look her straight in the eyes."

Natasha laughed a bit bitterly. "Well, you're not a Hungarian, that's for certain." She took his hands and demanded his eyes. "You're a damned fool if you don't grab at whatever promises compassion and what we have in the making."

"Natasha, don't lean on me. I'm not the strongest guy in the world when it comes to this."

"What we have brewing is beautiful, wild, madness. We've been looking for each other for a long time, cowboy."

"I know that and I'm scared to death of you."

"You only want a woman you can walk away from. I know that because I'm cut out of the same dirty cloth."

"Sorry, Natasha."

"Funny, I've never been rejected before," she said. "I don't know how to behave." She took a pad and pen from her purse and scribbled out a street and telephone number. "Here's where I'll be tonight if you have a change of heart."

Lord, Gideon thought, lead me not into temptation. He tore the paper to bits and put it in the ashtray.

Natasha spouted something in Hungarian.

"I don't speak the language, but I get the drift," he said.

"Up your mother's you know what," she said.

"See, it's wrong already," Gideon said. "People should be happy in love. We're grim and we haven't even made it to the bedroom." She got up abruptly. Gideon grabbed her arm tightly. "You don't want love, Natasha, you want combat."

NATASHA

COMBAT! HOW DARE HE! Gideon the cowboy writer, big shot. Interviews us as though we are cattle . . . Which concentration camp? . . . What was your relationship with your parents? . . . What dreams do you have?

Dreams! I have only one dream . . . only one. Where is it? Venice? Auschwitz? The Cornwall Coast? It is the same, always covered in billowing fog. I see him emerging from the white mist. "Father!" I call. His eyes are so cruel and filled with lust and anger. He smiles, thin-lipped. His Van Dyke beard coming to a sharp point.

I shiver. It is so cold.

"So you have won again," Father says.

"It wasn't my fault they found the note. I didn't want to send you to the ovens. Father! Don't go away this time! Father!"

Just as I am about to touch him, the fog envelops him and he is gone. I run after him . . . nowhere . . . nowhere . . . "Father!"

We were once the Solomons of Budapest, a great affluent family. Thirty, forty, fifty at a gathering. Doctors, teachers, merchants. So highly respected. Monarchs of Jewish society.

I loathed him . . . Professor Doctor Hubert Solomon. He was so cold, so unloving. The pain he caused my brothers as he sliced them down, never letting them rise to his level, and the pain he caused my mother when he went to bed with her.

It was me, Natasha, you wanted, wasn't it, Father? He touches me, pats my head . . . I cringe. His eyes follow me all the time. Yes, I want to love you, Father, so I can plunge a knife into your back.

The Nazis came and took us all . . . uncles, aunts, cousins, brothers. Father and I escaped. I lived over half the war in a blond wig and sharing false "Aryan" documents with three other Jewish girls.

They found us and took us to Auschwitz. Luck had to run out. Or were we betrayed? Who will ever know? When we got to Auschwitz, we found out who carried messages and we learned the entire family had been killed . . . everyone . . . everyone . . .

Just Father and I were left. We found a secret way to get messages to one another from the clothing factory where I worked to the school where he taught the children of the SS officers. *It was one of my messages that got him killed. The guards intercepted it and thought it was a coded message to the underground. It was only a birthday greeting. They never discovered me as the sender, but they sent him to the gas chamber and crematoria.*

Father would have survived if I had not sent the message! But hadn't we said all along that only one Solomon would survive?

Oh, Father, I did love you, really.

I hated you!

I loved you.

And you . . . and you . . . and you. Ah, you look just like Father. . . . Come in, come in.

I love you till the strength is oozed from your stupid body. Till you can no longer move, function. Oh, Natasha has gotten you so tired you can hardly stand up. Well, get the hell out of here! You're dead! Oh, I'm so sorry. I hate to see you beg and whimper. Get on your knees like a dog!

Natasha, you naughty girl, you've got to stop doing this.

. . . I would stop, but the dream keeps returning. He is in the fog luring me. So I will go to another party and another and another until I see him again . . . the fog . . . the smoke . . . the smoke from the ovens of Auschwitz!

The costume party in Jerusalem? Wonderful!

There he is! The American. He swaggers toward me. I want him! "Hello, cowboy."

The son of a bitch is a clever one. I will do it more slowly to him. The bastard. Doesn't he ever get weary? He tells me things that make Natasha cry. His fingers always play over my tattoo number. It brings him pain, but he refuses to weaken like the others. Bastard!

I hate him.

I love him.

I hate him.

I love him.

What do you know about refugee camps and swamping blockade runners and barbed wire and guard dogs and the crematorium? I sent my father there! You understand what that means! The fog! The fog! . . . bloody fog again . . . even in Jerusalem . . . what do you know, cowboy . . . everything is hunky-dory in America . . . oh, the wife and daughters are coming to Israel, how lovely . . . but you will not leave Natasha. No one leaves Natasha until she is ready. . . .

A week later Gideon returned from a routine Negev patrol with a company from the Lion's Battalion to his base at the Accadia Hotel. He was so grungy, one could almost smell him across the lobby.

He glanced at his mail, then stared at the telephone. He stared and stared and stared . . . picked it up, set it down. An hour passed and he still stared. It rang, startling him.

"Hello," he said.

"All right, you son of a bitch, I called first. Are you now satisfied?" Natasha said and slammed her receiver down.

"Oh Jesus," Gideon moaned.

The phone rang again. Gideon lifted the receiver, a bit gun shy. "It is Natasha," she said in a sudden soft voice. "I'm sorry. I knew you would be back today and I hoped you might want to see me."

Gideon closed his eyes and clenched his teeth . . . then broke. "Yes, I want to see you, God damn you. You haven't left my mind all week. Where are you?"

"In the lobby. I'll be right up."

MITLA PASS

October 31, 1956
0400 HOURS, D DAY PLUS TWO

GIDEON ROLLED OVER in his sleep and lay on his bruised hip long enough for it to irritate him into wakefulness. He blinked his eyes open and saw Shlomo sitting with his back against the boulder, one eye open, one eye shut, like a coyote.

"What time is it, Shlomo?"

"Four in the morning. They made a good air drop, right on target. We've got a radio working. A message was sent to you from the P.M.'s office. The American evacuees were taken to Athens and will be flown to Rome tomorrow. I'm sure Val will wait for you in Rome."

Gideon sat up, heaved a sigh of relief, and massaged his leg. "What's happening?" he asked.

"Para 202 broke through at Thamad. They were approaching the Egyptian fortifications at Nakhl. It isn't clear if they made a night attack or will try it in the morning. If Zechariah clears Nakhl, we'll probably see him late tomorrow. If he gets stopped, Southern Command is going to try to evacuate us."

"Jesus. How are we getting out of here?"

"Don't worry, they'll take Nakhl. You don't know Zechariah. He is a bulldozer."

"Hey," Gideon said, "wow, look at those stars. How many do you think there are?"

"A billion billion? A trillion trillion? You will never see it again like out here in the desert."

"You're a desert rat. Once, a long time ago when I was a kid in Norfolk, I saw it like this. Someone took me flying out over the ocean. Man, it is cold."

Shlomo fished through his pack and came up with a half bottle of brandy. Gideon took a swig, coughed, and grimaced.

"This stuff is weed killer, buzzards' puke."

"You have to understand the subtlety of Israeli brandy."

"Val used it as nail-polish remover."

"Speaking of Val, are you going to join her in Rome?"

"Honest to God, I don't know, Shlomo. I'll face up to that one if we get out of this mess. Maybe I'll just disappear and turn up someday in a Tibetan monastery."

"Tell the truth. You love Natasha?"

"I've tried to walk away from her a half-dozen times. I can't."

"But do you love her?"

"Every time we make love, we go out to another part of the universe. It happens every time. It has to be some kind of love, or lunacy, I guess. I know there are things I love about Val."

"You're greedy, that's your problem," Shlomo said, taking a long drink and banging the cork back on the bottle.

"Let me ask you something, Shlomo. Your wife ever cheat on you?"

"Naomi? That's a fair question. I don't know the answer and I don't plan to find out. We started as kids together in the Palmach. When we were in training or forced marches, we slept together in the fields. Americans have a crazy thing about all women must be pure. It's not the way life works. I've been on diplomatic missions to Burma, to Uganda, to America. Two, three months without her. She'd stay at the kibbutz with two kids. We are people, just people. We're not saints. If Naomi has needed a man, she's been extremely careful. I come home, I don't ask her, she doesn't ask me. I cannot get more love from anyone than I have from her. Americans are always worried about it. Why should it be bothering you in the middle of the Sinai?"

"I'm up to my eyeballs in guilt."

"Natasha?"

"Natasha and others before her."

"You should be guilty. You've been a real shmuck."

"You don't know the half of it," Gideon said. "Suppose you found out by accident that Naomi had been screwing around. What would you do?"

"You know how it goes. When you're young and sitting around the campfire and life is just beginning and this question comes up, everyone says they would kill, they would break bones, they would walk away. Today? If she still loved me, I'd probably forgive her. It would kill her inside if I didn't forgive her. You don't kill the woman you love because she makes a normal, human mistake. Hell, anybody can get hot pants. The trouble with you Americans is you're always playing Jesus, Joseph, and Mary."

"I didn't forgive Val," Gideon said, as though he were speaking to himself, "and it's bugging the hell out of me. I wish I could shout out to her so she'd hear me in Rome . . . Val, I forgive you."

"What's with Val? She worships you. She does not love anybody else. I don't believe it."

"It happened a long time ago, years ago."

"Then forget it. She'll be waiting for you at the Leonardo da Vinci Airport and she'll kiss your feet with love."

"I can't forget it. Maybe I'll never forget it."

"Then stick it away in a little closet in your head and close the door and lock it and throw away the key. Every day people have to make the decision to live with infidelity."

"Maybe it would be dead and buried if I hadn't run into Natasha." And then Gideon's voice quivered. "I need it as an excuse for what I've been doing. I started up with the women as soon as I became a published author. Up till now, I blamed Val for holding me back as a writer . . . the old lady doesn't understand me at home, sweetheart, so let's you and me get it on for the weekend. It was my justification for a lot of crap I pulled. All Val's fault. I didn't realize it then, but I was giving away pieces of my soul."

"Hey, don't talk about it. Jumping from airplanes, morphine, the desert. Everything makes you crazy out here."

"I never talked to anyone about it, because I was Mr. Macho Man. I wouldn't admit my wife could or would do that to the great Gideon Zadok."

"You know, we may be dead tomorrow at this time. What do you need to punish yourself for?"

"That's right. Maybe we'll be up in the stars looking down. I have to square it before the trip starts."

Shlomo shook his head that he understood.

"It happened a few years ago," Gideon continued.

"You're still married, aren't you?"

"Yeah, but I handled it very badly. When I learned what Val had done, I went ape shit."

Sherman Oaks, 1954

GIDEON HAD COME home from the studio early, aching all over, running a fever, and it was growing worse. He groaned and crawled his way into bed. After getting him settled in, Val left for the afternoon to pick up Roxy and Penny and deliver them to Girl Scouts and a piano lesson, respectively.

Within the hour, there was a frantic call from Gideon's secretary, Belle Prentice.

"They're having a hemorrhage over here, Gideon," Belle said. "They rehearsed the garden scene today and it didn't play. They're shooting it tomorrow and there's no cover set. The colonel wants to go back to your original idea."

"Belle, you've got to be kidding. I'm sicker than a dog. I'm going to start upchucking any minute."

"They want to send me over with the studio doctor."

"Isn't there some kind of state labor law against this sort of thing?"

"Honey, be a big Marine. It's only three or four pages."

"All right. Look, I'll sketch it out and phone it in to you, so they can set up the lights and sound. I'll have the dialogue in, sometime tonight. You going to be home?"

"I'll stand by here at the studio."

"Later." Gideon moaned and rolled out of bed and dug the screenplay out of his attaché case. His legs were wobbly. God damn it, no foolscap pad! His office was in an outside building, so he began to fish around in Val's desk, which occupied an alcove in the room.

"Ragpickers' ball!" he mumbled as he waded through the nests of papers and God knows what in the desk drawers. Come on, Val, he thought, give me a break. Where's a note pad?

What's this! Gideon pulled out a key with a large black tag reading "King's Court Motel—Santa Monica Blvd & La Cienega St. Room 357."

He blinked in disbelief. He had used that motel on several occasions. Oh my God, he thought, his heart racing, Val has found the key! No, wait a minute. Gideon always asked for a certain corner room on the second floor. He'd never been on the third floor. What the hell was this all about?

Johnny Brookes had told him about the motel when he needed a hot sheet joint for a matinee. In fact, Johnny even registered him in on one occasion and brought the key over to him.

Johnny Brookes! Hold the phone!

Johnny and Cindy Brookes were part of "their" crowd, close buddies. John was an ex-Marine and was now a minor but promising director. He and Val and the Brookeses had been together a few dozen times, anyhow. Lots of nice, clean, grab-ass late barbecues and skinny dips at the Zadok pool and an equal number of trips to Johnny and Cindy's place on the beach.

The Brookeses didn't have any children. Cindy preferred poodles. John was a good sort, but he had become very unhappy and the marriage was floundering. He and Gideon bowled on the same team, played tennis as doubles partners by day and occasionally bummed around together in the evenings, particularly after a late working day. John didn't monkey around too much, but he needed a quickie more often as the marriage soured and he had a yard-long list of available ladies.

Gideon began thinking back. Six months ago, Johnny was doing a film at Goldwyn and Gideon ran over for lunch from Pacific Studios. That's when the King's Court Motel first came up.

VAL AND JOHNNY IN THAT CRUMMY MOTEL! Val naked in front of him! Johnny going down on her. Sixty-nining in front of those lousy headboard mirrors! Had he fed her pot or some of his goofballs? Did she wear the black lace garter belts? What about the filthy music and the oil baths and the water beds!

Gideon reeled into the bathroom and threw up. He tore back into the bedroom and took the pistol down from its high shelf and staggered about like a water buffalo who had taken an arrow in the chest.

God damn! There's honor among thieves. A man doesn't go screwing around with his buddy's wife! They balling the shit out of each other at that sleaze joint—and then she comes home and makes love to me. Next day, a little doubles at the club and good old partner John. Holy Jesus!

Two and a half hours ticked by tortuously until Gideon heard the front door being opened and the girls ran in jabbering.

"Hon, I'm home," Val called.

In a moment she entered the bedroom to find Gideon sitting on her chaise longue by the fireplace, with a lap robe over him and his head wavering from rage, weariness, and fever.

"You shouldn't be out of bed," she said.

"Close the door," he rasped, "and lock it."

Val smiled. Oftentimes, the sicker Gideon was, the more passionate he became. He looked terrible. She'd try to talk him out of it. She stood over him and reached to feel his forehead. He took the motel key from his robe pocket and flipped it down at her feet.

Val stared at it a moment, then sagged into the easy chair opposite him. "Thank God it's over with," she croaked, "it's been a nightmare."

"You and our old pal Johnny been making a little bang-bang. Funny, John came over to my studio for lunch yesterday. He never mentioned a word about it. We had a lot of laughs about a couple of hookers he'd been seeing. Now pick up the phone and call him. Invite him over tonight, without Cindy. Tell him I'm out of town and you're hurting. Don't take no for an answer."

"Hadn't we better talk about this first?"

"No, ma'am," Gideon answered as his hand came from under the blanket and he leveled a pistol at her. "Do as I say. Maybe you guys will put on a little dog and pony show for me . . . if I don't blow his head off first."

Val tried to dial but was unable. The receiver fell from her trembling hand.

"Leave it for now," Gideon commanded, "and start talking."

"Can I get a glass of water?"

Val staggered into the bathroom and fought for composure. Half the water spilled down her front and she gagged as she drank. She returned and sat, hands folded, rocking back and forth in misery, eyes cast down.

"What do you want to know?"

"Everything. Every God-damned last thing!"

She tried to look at him, but it was not possible. "Maybe you want to know where my head was at that time, maybe not."

"Just start talking."

"You were writing *The Tenderloin* and you were very unhappy. You kept going up to San Francisco alone, as often as you could. You didn't want me with you to clutter up your prowling."

"Our daughters were in school!" Gideon snapped.

"Mom always came up to take care of them before that. You didn't want me."

"It was too filthy a job for you, Snow White. You didn't want to come, so don't give me that shit."

"All right, but you let me know you were taking off for parts unknown without us, just as soon as you could . . . Israel . . . China . . . always trying to run away. I felt, so . . . so unwanted. And then there was that visit to Dr. Murray. No more children, he said. It meant we couldn't try for a son. I was depressed as hell and you were gone.

Then I came to realize that my going back to art school was just a sham. I had to face the fact I didn't have the talent. So, I was alone and low and terrified of losing you. Oh, baby, let me take your temp. You look terrible."

"Keep talking."

"You went up to San Francisco over the Fourth of July and we were angry. You missed Penny's birthday. . . ."

"So it's my fault and Penny's."

"It was my fault! Mine! There were lies I had to tell myself in order to do it. I had to justify it! I even pretended that if you knew about Johnny, it would turn you on."

"Oh God!"

"You and I . . . we . . . we had been talking about swinging. I'm not making it as an excuse. If I've learned one thing out of this, it's that we all have to take the responsibility for our deeds. But I needed excuses because there was some kind of bile starting to come out of me and I couldn't stop it. So, I turned on the one man I loved to justify failing him."

"What happened?"

"Johnny popped over one afternoon looking for you. He was about to start shooting that Western at Fox and he wanted you to clean up a scene for him. You had just left for the airport and I was really down. He told me things were very bad between him and Cindy. He . . . he said they hadn't made love in almost three months . . . and that started it going. . . . I was . . . more aggressive than he was . . . and we did it!"

"Where?"

Val shook her head.

"Where!"

She pointed to the bed.

"In our bed?"

"Yes . . . we slept together in our bed."

"You mean fucked, don't you?"

"Yes!" Val screamed. "I fucked him!"

"Did he go for rubbing his face around where the black stockings end and your soft white thighs begin? Did he bury his face in your muff!"

"Come on, Gideon, stop torturing yourself."

"We've seen that son of a bitch bare-assed. He's got a *shvantz* on him like a horse. How'd you like giving head to that great big salami? Did you soap him down in the shower and give him a super-deluxe job?"

"I did it. We did it like people do it. I swear to God, I don't remember half of it."

"Bullshit. He had you up on speed."

"Yes . . ."

"And you kept fucking him in our bed?"

"No, just that once."

"How many times, where?"

"Out at their beach house a few times. And . . . three . . . four times at the motel."

"You came, didn't you? Screams and flailing and sweating and moaning. You had one orgasm after another! You enjoyed every minute of it, didn't you? Especially when he had you put on a show. You put on a show with your fingers up your pussy and he came all over you!"

"No . . . I don't remember, I tell you. Neither of us knew why we kept coming back. He's . . . he's a fair lover. But, Gideon, he wasn't you. Nobody is you."

"Sure, that's right, baby. Let's establish the fact that he was a lousy lover. That makes me feel real good. Oh, he was just terrible, a real bum in the sack."

"I wasn't doing this to hurt you. I was messed up, baby, just messed up. At the end of a few months, it was over with. We both became just . . . disgusted with ourselves."

"But he came back to our dinner table. We all went skinny-dipping together, didn't we? God damn, what a laugh you two must have had behind my back."

"We thought it best to go on like nothing had happened. And nothing did happen after we quit. Only the God-damned lie. It has been like a cancer in my soul and it wouldn't stop growing."

"Take a look in the mirror!"

"I can't."

"You'll see a slut, a whore, a tramp, a pig, scum. The Admiral's daughter and all her Protestant bullshit. The only thing you're sorry for is that you got caught."

"Sometimes I swore you wanted me to be a whore. We've played at it a hundred times. It's no excuse. I got mixed up between fantasy and reality. Look, honey, it's no excuse. I could've always said no to the games you and I played . . . but I loved playing them with you. Honey, honey, I just want to live long enough for you to trust me again. I love you, man. . . ."

"How about Penny and Roxy? You love them too?"

"Please don't. I beg you. Please don't."

"What are you going to tell them when it comes time to let them know they've got to learn to keep their legs crossed? You going to tell them what a sweetheart Momma was to their daddy? You junky whore, going down for a toot of speed, just like the two-bit pigs in the shooting galleries. Give me a sniff and I'll give you a fuck."

"Kill me!"

"Why don't you be quiet. Our daughters will hear you."

Val became hysterical, and after a time she took her hands down from her face. It was wet with tears, and her eyes screamed silently in pain. Val clenched her trembling fists and pulled herself together once again. "I'll tell them their mother is a human being and human beings make mistakes. I'll tell them to try not to make mistakes as a woman, because there is no free lunch in that game. I'll tell them, if they make mistakes, there's no escaping having to pay the price. I'll tell them their own consciences will drive them crazy. I hate myself, Gideon, almost as much as I love you."

Gideon's face became wet with perspiration, and his eyes fluttered and his head rolled. "Get out of here. Pack your shit and go visit your mother. I'll take care of the girls."

"I'm not leaving them," Val said. "If you want me out, we'll take a place nearby, so they can finish their school term."

Gideon picked the pistol up from his lap, stared at it, then tossed it on the coffee table. He dialed the studio.

"Good afternoon, Pacific Studios."

"Gideon Zadok's office. Hello, Belle, Gideon. What the hell's the name of the hospital near the studio?"

"You mean St. Joseph's? Say, you sound terrible."

"Get me a private room and have the studio doctor come see me later. Get a typewriter and whatever we'll need to write over there. Then, come pick me up."

"What the devil is going on?"

"Will you do what the fuck I say!"

"Let me speak to Val."

"Just do what I say, Belle." He hung up and he wept.

"Oh God, baby," Val cried, "forgive me. Gideon, you've got to forgive me."

"In a pig's ass I'll forgive you."

MITLA PASS

October 31, 1956

0800 HOURS, D DAY PLUS TWO

THE FIRST KISS of daylight began to melt away the darkness and the stars blinked themselves off. There was the soldiers' anger at morning, stretches, groans, bitching all along the Lion's foxhole. The paras took their morning piss, brushed their teeth, and dug into their rations. The night had gone fairly well. An Egyptian patrol had come out of the Pass after midnight to probe, but was easily beaten back. Word from Para 202 was that the attack on Nakhl had already taken place, or was about to begin. It wasn't clear. The next few hours would tell the story.

A distant sound of bombing was heard coming from the other side of the Pass and the Canal. Someone might have been hitting the Egyptian airfields.

"So, you never forgave her?" Shlomo asked Gideon.

"No, how could I? I was playing around all over the place and now I had an excuse. If I had forgiven her, she would have had to forgive me. I wanted to keep on doing what I was doing . . . balling starlets . . . going out on pot at my agent's house in Malibu . . . gang bangs . . . fun and games. I never forgave her, but I know from how much she hurt me, how much I have hurt her. I never knew about that kind of pain until then. I'd give anything . . . anything if I could tell her now."

"And Natasha?"

"I suppose we deserve each other. I was smug. There wasn't a woman in the world I couldn't walk away from. I had my fortress home. I had a guilty wife, well fixed inside the moat, and the castle walls. I was safe . . . until I got messed up with Natasha." Gideon squinted out to the endless sea of rocks and sand. "Come on, Para 202, where are you, you bastards? Come on, Zechariah, stop farting around."

"That's the worst thing two people can do to each other," Shlomo said. "If you live together, have children, share the same bed, if there is a morsel of love left, you have no right to withhold forgiveness. You have no right to hold it over her head."

"Tell me about it," Gideon snapped sarcastically.

"There's an evil streak in all of us," Shlomo went on, "which we must control. When it takes over, we become the devil's advocates on earth."

"Yeah . . . I know and Val knows."

"Do you trust Val?"

"Yes, but not all the way. Not like it once was."

"Do you trust any woman?"

A sudden smile lit Gideon's eyes. They were no longer sad. "There are two women in my life . . . yeah . . . I trusted them all the way."

"Your mother and . . ."

"No, not my mother. One, Miss Abigail Winters, a teacher. She thought I would become a writer one day. The other woman? Molly, my sister. I wouldn't have made it without her. I love Molly. When I knock this book, I'm going to bring her to Israel and show her around . . ."

They were suddenly interrupted by a half-dozen jets screaming over the Pass. Shlomo spotted the unmistakable twin tails of enemy Vampires.

"Egyptians! Hit the deck!"

MOLLY

1922

MY MOTHER, Leah, worked at the Ginzburg Brothers clothing factory in Baltimore, and so did my Aunt Fanny. All of us lived in Bubba Hannah's house on Monroe Street. Zayde Moses lived there too, but nobody counted him.

I was four years old in the spring of 1922 when Momma and Aunt Fanny went out on strike, and don't remember much of it, but in our family the strike was discussed for years and years, so I was able to fill in all the details.

Conditions at the factory were very bad and the strike was long and bitter. Just when it seemed that the strike was going to be smashed, two union organizers came down from New York from the Jewish Workers Federation. One of them, Nathan Zadok, was to become my pretend daddy.

I've heard the story a hundred times of how the union organizers tricked the Baltimore police into making a mounted charge against the women pickets at the Ginzburg Brothers gate. They were clubbed and twelve of them, including my mother, Leah, were taken off to jail and received six-month sentences from a crooked judge.

This created an incident to exploit, because the women became known as the Ginzburg Brothers Twelve and eventually the union won the strike. Although my mother spent only ten days in jail, she seemed to like being a martyr.

WELCOME HOME, LEAH! a big sign read over the front door. A

hundred people must have jammed into the house. The whole family was there, Uncle Jake and Uncle Lazar and all my cousins and Aunt Pearl, even though her husband, Uncle Dominick, was a member of the police force.

Later that night, when they had all gone home, Bubba heated a pan of hot water, added Epsom salts, and placed it on the floor so Momma could soak her feet.

Momma had given me a thousand kisses that day, so I'll never forget it. She was braiding my hair when Bubba said to speak Yiddish so the child won't understand. Even at the age of four, I could understand Yiddish pretty well, but pretended not to. That way, I could learn more family secrets like just how much Bubba hated Zayde Moses.

". . . There was this huge woman jailer, who takes you into a little side room and orders you to take off all your clothing in front of her, down to the last stitch. I promise you, she hadn't had a bath in three weeks," my mother said. "You could see in her hair, little white lice eggs." I found out later that any woman my mother didn't like had lice eggs in her hair.

"Don't worry, darling," Bubba said, "every uphill has a downhill."

"Oh, she enjoyed her job, if you know what I mean. She implied to me that in exchange for favors to her, I would be given special treatment. She couldn't take her eyes off me. It gave me a chill all over."

"I always have said that the road to hell is just as bad as arriving there."

"We learned that the strip-search room had a two-way mirror, so the policemen could watch. They were looking upon me without a stitch on. You can't believe my humiliation. One of the girls, the Italian, Teresa, was having her period. It didn't make one iota of difference."

"Here, darling, eat, I have to put some flesh back on your bones."

"I nibbled a bit here, a bit there, until we called the hunger strike. But there were mice droppings on everything, and the cockroaches were the size of dogs. It was almost a relief to go on a hunger strike."

"I tried to get food to you," Bubba said. "I begged on bended knees. That police sergeant was a regular hoodlum. Maybe they thought I'd baked a gun inside the cake already."

"As a principled human being," my momma said, "I don't hold it against Dominick Abruzzi that he works with animals, but Pearl, God help her, would be well rid of him."

"Let me tell you, darling, that for five days after your arrest the yellow journalist rags hardly printed a word about it. They are as dirty as that judge who sentenced you. Only when it became a national scandal did they put it on the front page. A mother could die."

"Thank God I was in prison with them," Momma said. "The others weren't as strong as I was. Frankly, I became their inspiration. Only when I thought of Molly here, of never seeing my precious child again, did I falter."

I was hugged and kissed and patted. It was nice.

"On the third night of the hunger strike, I began seeing visions," my momma went on. "I swear, on Molly's name, as I sit here, I heard—get a grip—the voices of Saul and Uncle Hyman. I felt myself growing weaker and weaker."

Momma ate and scanned the coverage in the newspapers. She mumbled that her photograph in that Hearst rag did not do her justice.

"I found something in the dark horror of my prison cell, a cause, a cause I knew I would die for if necessary."

"Don't throw yourself into causes so fast," Bubba answered. "You're just coming into the bloom of life, Leah. You put this behind you. Life is life. Always remember that."

"Momma, I've met Nathan Zadok. It was he who brought the lawyer who got us freed."

Bubba did not react with joy. "Leah, you had a bad, bad experience. Tomorrow life starts all over."

"Yes, you're so right. A new start and maybe, just maybe, Nathan . . ."

"Nathan Zadok is a fast-talking Charlie. I've known these radicals all my life. It's not that I'm saying marry a Rothschild, but a church mouse is wealthy beside a Nathan Zadok."

"Wealth? What is wealth? This little man, can you believe, speaks fifteen different languages. He knows Tolstoy, Shakespeare. He reads Jack London in Russian. The Communists are going to do something about the class struggle, the poverty, the lynchings in the South. They want to make a better world for children like Molly."

I once again came in for a round of hugs and kisses.

"Don't go falling hook, line, and sinker for no fast-talking Charlie," Bubba repeated.

"I hear you, Momma, but my heart doesn't hear you. Do you know, Nathan saw me on the picket line and fell in love with the back of my head."

"So, that proves he's a stupid as far as I'm concerned. Leah, I'm hoping that your next marriage, God willing, will be your final one. These boys coming in from the old country are damaged merchandise.

Wild radical ideas foam from their mouths. They don't understand half of what they're talking about. I have never, never seen one of those shmucks laugh."

"I have so very much to learn from Nathan."

"What you'll learn is the inside of a tenement, with a leaky roof and no heat. Let them save themselves before they save the world."

"Shakespeare . . . Tolstoy . . . Jack London . . . and he will teach me what Marx and Lenin will accomplish for the proletariat."

"Leah, you've always been a fragile little flower. You've just gone through a horrible experience. Give yourself a chance to breathe."

"The Jewish Workers Federation is making enormous plans for me and the others of the Ginzburg Brothers Twelve."

"They're nothing but a bunch of Communist sheep in wolves' clothing, using the misery of a slave shop to exploit you. Once, please, for God's sake, be sensible. Nathan Zadok is a little *pisher* with a big mouth, who will never have two nickels to rub together. And where was your Mr. Hero today?"

"He was on important Party business."

Guess who rang the doorbell? Nathan Zadok came in with copies of the *Freiheit*, the Yiddish-language Communist newspaper, with a front page filled with pictures of the release of the Ginzburg Brothers Twelve.

Bubba picked up the hot-water pan and emptied it and suddenly began to mop up the kitchen, which didn't need mopping, while Momma fed Nathan. He ate like he had just gotten off a hunger strike himself.

In no time at all, Bubba and Nathan Zadok were arguing about America.

"So let me tell you about America," he said bitterly. "I arrive without a penny to my name. My Uncle Samuel, who owns four department stores in New England, didn't have for me the time of day. He said, 'I give you America, Nathan, now go get it.' "

"That's the way we all start here, with nothing," Bubba slashed back. "You want that you should be a millionaire on arrival?"

Nathan recounted how his family had dumped him in New York with a few dollars in his pockets. "They hated me because I knew about the failure of Zionism and Palestine, firsthand."

"Don't you speak against Zionism under my roof," Bubba threatened.

He went on about a room he had in Harlem with a mean landlord. "Every morning I got up at four-thirty. That's when the *Forward*, a reactionary newspaper, no better than Hearst, was put out on the streets. I read the job ads and, with the help of some Jewish-speaking people, found the right subways to get to the garment district. We were greenhorns, what did we know? Half the ads for jobs were for scabs to break strikes. The other half, for a day's work in a shape-up, you had to bribe two dollars of your wages to the foreman. So we ended up most days cheating the H & H Automat for a cup tea, a slice bread.

"And the rest of the day? There was no heat in the apartment, so we gathered at the public library on Fifth Avenue to read the Yiddish periodicals and stay warm. The end of every day I put part of the *Forward* in the soles of my shoes, to cover the holes."

During Nathan Zadok's first winter, he went on, he got jobs as a floor sweeper, a shoveler on city snow removal crews, a custodian of the mounted police stable, also as a shoveler of horse manure.

"By springtime I got a permanent job with Barney Bloom, the *goniff* coat maker. Most of the garments were subcontracted to family sweatshops in the Bronx. I delivered unsewn parts and picked up finished coats. I had to fight my way into the subway, with two boxes that weighed forty pounds each, and walk six, eight blocks and up five stories with my *shmattes*. For eleven hours a day, six days a week, I was paid the glorious sum of ten dollars. This is your America, Mrs. Balaban? I'll tell you about America . . . with its lynchings and Jim Crow and KKK. With chain gangs, racketeers, police brutality, union busting, sweatshops, a yellow press, slums, sharecroppers, political prisoners."

"Oh, Nathan," Momma cried, "it's so awful!"

"What did you expect, gold on the streets?" Bubba argued. "We are all like salmon swimming upstream. Some make it, some don't."

The rest of Nathan's story we already knew. Nathan became a Communist to fight all the evils in America. The Jewish branch of the Party published a small Yiddish-language newspaper, called *Freiheit,* and he was sent to Baltimore to form a secret Communist cell and get subscriptions for the *Freiheit.* Also, to infiltrate and gain control of the Garment Workers' Union.

MY MOTHER and Nathan Zadok and four women from the Ginzburg Brothers Twelve went on a victory tour. At first they wanted to leave me at home, but someone in New York decided I could be useful.

Every day we went to a different city by train or bus. We were put up in the homes of comrades. At night there would be a meeting at the local Workmen's Circle hall, and I became a very important part of the evening.

"Fellow workers! Comrades!" Nathan Zadok would yell. "We serve notice that we will no longer accept the exploitation from the bourgeoisie like cattle to the slaughter! The Jewish trade union movement of America is on the march!"

He would get everybody stomping their feet and screaming and collections were made and people signed up for the *Freiheit*. Sometimes it was scary, because plainclothes police and stool pigeons tried to get the names and addresses and photographs of the people in the audience.

The Freiheit Choral Society would stretch across the stage and the big bosoms of the women heaved and the bald heads of the men shone.

> *Schwab! Schwab! Charlie Schwab!*
> *Life's unhappy lest you rob,*
> *From the bakers in your mills,*
> *And the miners*
> *In your hills.*

I never really knew who Charlie Schwab was, except that he exploited the workers.

They would introduce Momma and the other four ladies of the Ginzburg Brothers Twelve and the building would creak because the noise was so thunderous. Mother would come up to the speaker's rostrum and all the lights would be dimmed. Momma would then recite a poem she wrote in jail:

> *"Shackle me not to any machine,*
> *I am flesh, I am real,*
> *I want to see my child play in daylight,*
> *In the sun.*
> *Therefore I labor, I toil, I sweat,*
> *And we will march,*
> *From this sewer of debasement*
> *To a golden throne,*
> *Where only the masses are allowed,*
> *Immortal!"*

I really didn't understand it then and don't understand it too much now, but people would be crying and clapping and whistling and Momma would cross her arms over her bosom and bow.

Then came the pledges.

"I have a pledge from the Furriers' Union, Local 24, for fifteen dollars!"

Cheers.

The biggest night was in Detroit. We collected over three hundred dollars.

Now was my turn. Even though I was only four and not old enough to be a Young Pioneer, I was dressed in uniform with a blue skirt, white blouse, and red kerchief and I would march out with fifteen or twenty Pioneers behind me and we would sing:

> *"Fly higher,*
>   *And higher,*
> *And hiiiiigher,*
>   *Our emblem is*
> *The Soviet star,*
>   *With every propeller*
> *Roaring RED FRONT,*
>   *Defending the U.S.S.R.!"*

When the cheering stopped, we would sing our encore:

> *"One, two, three*
>   *Pioneers are we,*
> *Fighting for*
>   *The working class,*
> *Against the bourgeoisie,*
>   *HEY!"*

And we'd hold up our fists in the Communist salute. Momma and the Ginzburg Brothers ladies would come to the front of the stage and she would hold me up to the audience. The Freiheit Choral Society returned to the stage and everyone in the audience arose.

> *"Arise, ye prisoners of starvation,*
>   *Arise, ye wretched of the earth,*
>   *For justice thunders condemnation—*
>   *A better world's in birth.*
>
>   *No more tradition chains shall bind us,*
>   *The earth shall have a new foundation,*

We have been one
WE SHALL BE ALL

'TIS THE FINAL CONFLICT
LET EACH STAND IN HIS PLACE
THE INTERNATIONAL SOVIET
SHALL BE THE HUMAN RACE

THE INTERNATIONAL SOVIET
SHALL BE THE HUMAN RACE"

Sometimes we sang it in Yiddish. And once, in Boston, we sang it in Italian. And then we would go on to Cincinnati, or Chicago, or Pittsburgh. It was wonderful.

The last stop on the tour was Hartford. Momma and Nathan Zadok were married in a rabbi's home, because it was Sunday and they couldn't find a judge or justice of the peace. The manager of the tour, Comrade Dworkin, was there for the ceremony. I remember him vividly because he had an ugly, round face and two of his fingers were always brown from nicotine stains and he pinched my cheek with that hand all the time and it smelled bad. Nobody liked Comrade Dworkin, but they couldn't say so.

I found out later that Comrade Dworkin was a spy for the Central Committee and Nathan had gotten into a lot of trouble. Nathan was called to New York on charges made by Comrade Dworkin, for various crimes against the Party. The worst of these was getting married without permission and getting married by a rabbi in a religious ceremony.

Normally, he would have been thrown out of the Party, but they gave him a year's probation, because Momma still had some value as a member of the Ginzburg Brothers Twelve.

I was told to call Nathan Zadok "Daddy," even though he wasn't my real father. My real father was named Joseph Kramer and Momma told me he had been killed in the war.

1924

I HAD BEEN promised a baby brother or sister for my sixth birthday. I hoped it would be a brother. On my birthday, I looked everywhere, even in the scary cellar, which was filled with rats and where Zayde made Concord grape wine. I couldn't find my baby brother anywhere. When Momma and Bubba discovered me, I was shriveled up in a corner, crying.

"So, what's the matter with my Molly darling?" Bubba asked.

"I was promised a baby brother," I wept.

"Don't cry, Molly," Momma said. "The stork got very busy and he's running a few days late. Believe me, you'll get your present." I did believe her because, in those days, kids my age didn't know how babies were born. I thought it had something to do with the word "pregnant" and Momma's belly, because a few weeks later my brother was born and Momma's belly was gone.

I was allowed to hold him, and from the moment I saw him, I loved him because he was the only thing in the world that really belonged to me.

Bubba took him from me, held him up, and said, "This child is a genius."

IN THE FIRST seven years Nathan was married to my momma, we moved to seven different cities. The first four were Party assignments and the other moves came when Momma got restless, approximately every ten months.

We always lived on the third or fourth floor and had to walk up, because in the few places that had elevators, they were always out of order. I also remember packing suitcases and going to catch a train. As soon as Gideon saw the suitcases come out of the closet, he would scream. He told me later he had dreams all his life of running for the train.

The neighborhoods in all the cities looked pretty much alike, East Coast dinge, with row houses that were derelict on the day they were finished. The worst building was inevitably the one that Nathan leased for the Jewish Workers Federation. It held a few offices, and a couple of the rooms were used as Yiddish classrooms. The big meeting hall could be converted into a Yiddish theater. This was where the Freiheit Choral Society rehearsed and performed. Their emphasis now was songs about the South, usually about a lynching.

Nathan came to a new city with a nice letter from the federation, stating he was a local editor for the *Freiheit* and his salary was forty dollars a week. Actually, he was paid twenty dollars, but could buy repossessed furniture on the installment plan. Later it would be repossessed from us.

Gideon and I almost always slept together on a Murphy bed in the living room, except for those nights the cell held a secret meeting, usually to discuss a plan to infiltrate and seize the leadership of a union, or break up a public meeting of the rival Socialists.

We were dressed in hand-me-downs. The relatives were generous, but the clothes were either too big or too small. In some cities a Party member would be the butcher, grocer, or baker. As their contribution to the movement, Nathan was never sent a bill.

In other cities, our credit at the grocer and butcher was soon canceled. Momma would give Gideon and me a note and we would stare at the grocer like we were real hungry.

When things were really desperate, Momma would go to the Italian, or German, or Chinese neighborhood and plant a banana peel near the doorstep of a shop and then do a monumental pratfall, screaming as she went to the pavement, "My God, I hope I don't have a miscarriage!" At that instant a lawyer happened by and it cost the grocer at least ten dollars to drop a lawsuit. Momma and the lawyer split it, five dollars apiece.

Once Gideon had a real bad toothache. Momma didn't have any money and there was no Communist dentist in Akron. She told me to wait for Gideon and stay with him in the reception room until she came to pick us up. Six hours went by and Momma didn't come back. Finally the dentist caught on and sent us home with a note pinned to Gideon, threatening to turn us kids over to the juvenile authorities.

Nathan would come to a city that had, like, six hundred Jewish Workers Federation members and half of them would be secret Communists. He would recruit and sell new subscriptions to the *Freiheit*. But as fast as he could recruit them, other older members were always brought up on some kind of charges and expelled. When we would leave about a year later, there were still six hundred members.

One small benefit of being a *Freiheit* manager was that Nathan got free press passes to the symphony, opera, concerts, and sporting events. He always gave the sports passes to Italian comrades on his premise that they were hoodlum games. He never went to the concerts, except if there was a Russian artist. He was afraid the Jewish artists might not be Party-approved. Momma took Gideon and me to everything, even when he was in diapers. I remember walking up as many steps as there were to our apartment to reach the second balcony and the fright of looking down the steep pitch to the stage, but the music and acting were wonderful and my brother and I became enthralled by them. Momma was always a lead singer in the Freiheit Choral Society and was certain she would have made the Metropolitan Opera chorus if she hadn't given her life to the movement.

By the time Gideon was in second grade, he could sing the tunes of all the arias in ten operas and he had also memorized all the Beethoven symphonies and would spend hours before Uncle Lazar's or Uncle Dominick's windup Victrola, pretending he was leading the symphony orchestras.

Momma also believed Gideon was a genius in music, and she sent him to Bert Weinstein for piano lessons. Bert was blind but a gifted musician. Lessons didn't come for nothing. They cost twenty-five cents, and Gideon had to walk thirty blocks to Bert's apartment and thirty blocks back home. Bert needed the money, but he finally had to tell Mother that her son's genius lay in another field.

"Well, just how badly does he play?" Mother asked angrily.

"When that boy sits down and plays 'Für Elise,' I wish it was my ears that had gone instead of my eyes."

But that didn't keep Gideon from loving music all his life and he was really super singing duets with Uncle Dom.

Old man Abruzzi heard them once and remarked, "That boy's voice is going to kill somebody—we'd better start him on a fishing boat."

I read aloud very well, because I aspired to be a great actress, and every night I read to Gideon. Books like *Jews Without Money* by Michael Gold, or we would act out all the parts of Clifford Odets's *Awake and Sing!* and *Waiting for Lefty*. When he learned to read, Gideon couldn't get enough, and that's when we began thinking, maybe he will become a writer.

As I said, I was going to be an actress, and usually the Jewish Workers Federation had a Yiddish acting group in every city. I got so good that Maurice Schwartz, the great Yiddish Shakespearean actor, came to see me perform to possibly recommend me for a scholarship to study in Brooklyn.

It turned out to be a disaster. The play was a sort of Yiddish Communist children's version of the American Revolution. In the last act, George Washington gives his farewell speech to his troops and tells them they must always be on guard against colonialism, imperialism, deviationism, and cosmopolitanism. Then George Washington tells everyone to free their slaves. It was a stirring moment.

The only trouble with my acting was that I got stage fright sometimes. After the farewell speech, there was a finale in which I rode a wooden horse, rigged up to gallop on a treadmill. I was Paul Revere, and as the horse "galloped" I cried in Yiddish, "The fascist redcoats are coming!" Gideon was a drummer boy and also on the treadmill, running with all his might to stay even.

Well, the stage manager never did get the treadmill to work right. On the night that Maurice Schwartz was sitting in the first row, the electrical circuit got overloaded and blew all the fuses. The treadmill stopped abruptly, but Gideon and I kept on going and shot off the stage like cannonballs. We landed on Mr. Schwartz and all of us went to the floor.

My career was over before it began.

But every day and every week, Gideon kept opening secret doors through reading, and I knew he would be a real writer someday, because he was always thinking about stories.

AMONG THE FIRST WORDS Gideon remembered must have been Momma saying, "This is not a well child." Momma kept six huge scrapbooks filled with articles on symptoms, diagnosis, and treatment of everything from the common cold to rare tropical skin diseases.

Because Momma was often out of the house on some kind of Party business, I was left to take Gideon to the clinics. We spent long, morbid hours in the cavernous, peeling waiting rooms of the university hospitals and charity clinics. Gideon would be squeezed in between an old man in a wheelchair and a kid with braces, while I filled out the endless forms required for proof of inability to pay. He didn't mind, though, because the long hours gave him a chance to read more and more novels.

Sometimes I went with him and Momma, like during the summer. I remember her litanies to those snotty-nosed interns who were barely shaving. "I held this child in my arms the entire night, pleading with him to keep breathing. All he has to do is look at a cottonwood tree and he's gasping for air. He went on a hayride against my wishes and came back with a rash, from head to foot, the color of a bowl of strawberries. His Uncle Hyman, may his soul rest in peace, had the most horrible case of hives Johns Hopkins had ever seen."

Momma located a clinic of specialists in asthma, hay fever, and sinus problems in Richmond, Virginia, and was convinced Gideon should be examined there. She *shnorred* Uncle Lazar for enough money to keep Gideon in Richmond for two weeks of tests. His back was covered with little quarter-inch scratches, an inch apart, into which they rubbed powdered ragweed, or wheat, or a variety of dusts. If the scratch became inflamed, another allergy had been unearthed.

Still more tests were applied to his arms and legs by means of injections under the skin of other allergic materials. If an injection blew up and discolored, another culprit had been found. He had dozens of scratches on his little back. It made me cry to see it.

My brother was allergic to milk, wheat, red meat, fish, shellfish, eggs, butter, most cereals, most fruits, most vegetables, ice cream, chocolate, most kinds of dust found in most of the air, flowers, all weeds, reeds, most trees, cats, dogs, newspapers, all cooking oils, and peanuts.

He could safely eat turnips, stewed rhubarb, and certain varieties of onions. Every week he got allergy shots and silver protein Argyrol packs way up his nose, to clean out his sinuses. He spent a lot of school days in bed.

You would think, with his ability to read and stuff, he would be a good student, but he wasn't. The main reason was that neither Gideon nor I completed a full term in one school, without changing neighborhoods or cities, until we moved to Norfolk, Virginia.

Most Sundays found Gideon and me in the lecture hall of the local Jewish Workers Federation, or a hall in which Communists were allowed to speak. We listened to a rotating show of out-of-town lecturers and sometimes the big guns of the Party like William Z. Foster and Earl Browder and the beloved Ella Reeve "Mother" Bloor, who was always just back from the Soviet Union with another glowing report.

Sundays for us were torture, sitting on hard-back folding chairs and trying to understand Marx and Lenin's manifestos.

We would alleviate the hours by staring at the cracks in the ceiling, or a repetitious design on the wallpaper. Gideon learned to sleep with his eyes open, an accomplishment I was never able to master. This is not to say that being a Young Pioneer was all drudgery. Sometimes the entire family would travel to New York for a giant rally in Madison Square Garden. When twenty thousand voices sang "The Internationale," it was a very stirring moment. The comrades did everything together: lectures, picnics, social events, picket line duty. The best was May Day, when the workers of the world marched in unity.

Being in the movement, we had to be careful of which comrades were our close friends, because after we'd known them well for a year or two, some would simply be called up on charges and expelled. We couldn't acknowledge members who had been thrown out, even if we passed them on the street. So we were both afraid of making close friends.

The same Comrade Dworkin who had managed the Ginzburg Brothers Twelve victory tour had become a much feared member of the Central Committee. But Dworkin came under suspicion when the Arab riots broke out in 1929 and, as an editor of *Freiheit*, he supported the Jewish settlers. Orders came from Moscow to reverse this position and support the Arabs. A lot of Jews quit the Party on that issue.

Dworkin was eventually expelled when something inside of him cracked at the death of his father and he committed the cardinal sin of going to synagogue to sit *shiva*. None of us were really sorry to see him leave, but Nathan was called up for being a "Dworkinite" and received a humiliating demotion to Norfolk, a post considered one notch below a sewage treatment plant.

The Party allotted him a meager twelve dollars a week, which meant he had to take a second job. One of the comrades, Harold Sugerman, was in the wallpaper business and, on Party orders, took Nathan in as an apprentice.

"I tell you," Nathan moaned, "that, worse than killing chickens, worse than the coal business, worse than splitting rocks in Palestine, is the paperhanging trade."

Norfolk had a few new homes requiring quality work. Sugerman subcontracted for the worst type of slumlords who slapped on a coat of paint and new paper to conceal the rot. Sometimes, after forty or fifty years and a dozen coats of wallpaper, the wall could hold no more and everything had to be scraped off by hand. The job always fell to Nathan.

If a place was furnished, everything had to be moved and covered. Then came the shlep, the stevedore's work. He lugged ladders, sawhorses, planks, and pasting tables up two or three stories. In the beginning, he was unable to match rolls on the walls and ruined a half-dozen jobs. Sometimes the walls were too crooked. At other times the paste wouldn't hold and the whole roll fell down on top of his head.

"It's up the ladder, down the ladder, three hundred times a day, then shlep everything down three flights and move all the furniture back. I'm getting varicose veins."

There was little work in the winter, so Nathan taught Yiddish for fifty cents a student a week and Leah picked up a few dollars as the director of the Freiheit Choral Society.

In springtime, Nathan left to go to one of the "gold rush" cities such as Pittsburgh, where the out-of-town paperhangers worked seven days a week for two or three months straight to fill the larder for the coming winter.

Our second year in Norfolk, when Nathan left on his route of the gold rush cities, Momma suddenly lost interest in lugging Gideon from

clinic to clinic. In addition to school, I kept the flat clean, did most of
the cooking, and took care of Gideon.

Both of us started to feel the eyes of the comrades on our backs when
we would enter a home or meeting hall. It seemed that Momma was
being very friendly to a lot of the men comrades. I know that the
Freiheit Choral Society was suddenly overloaded with male singers for
the first time.

When Nathan slipped home for an occasional weekend, he and
Momma always argued.

"I tell you, one more year of this paperhanging business and I'm
going crazy."

Momma always had a new and mysterious malady. "My gallbladder is
wrecked from too many hours and days in the Ginzburg Brothers slave
shop."

Then Nathan would always turn on Gideon. "My son is a disgrace to
me. Look at this report card. What's this business of engaging in reactionary pleasure-seeking activities? Baseball, football. It is a shame for a
proletariat child. And who let him bring Mark Twain into the house!"

Sometimes the only way to have a truce was for me to get a head-
ache, or Gideon to have an attack of asthma.

But Momma knew how to laugh a lot and even joked about herself.
She did keep our clothing neat and patched and shopped for the best
day-old food that could be found, and we never missed any concert, or
opera, or play that came to Norfolk.

She learned to read beautifully and lifted us into the world of Ernest
Hemingway and Eugene O'Neill. If nothing else, Gideon owes her his
love of literature and I owe her my love of acting and music.

NORFOLK-BALTIMORE

1935

MISS ABIGAIL WINTERS was no ordinary sixth-grade teacher. The children at J. E. B. Stuart Grammar School held their breath at the beginning of the term, praying they would be assigned to her class. Miss Abigail was not much of a looker. She was a gangly type, almost awkward in her movements, and she didn't go to too much trouble to pretty herself up. Most men were intimidated by her, because she was a very rare person, a woman flier, an aviatrix, and this commanded fear and respect.

Her father, Clarence, had been a war ace and she and her brother, Jeremy, were, as it were, raised in an open cockpit. Miss Abigail did a lot of other extra-special things like playing the guitar and composing songs. She knew dozens of songs in many languages. She was the drama coach of the school, as well.

She took her students on field trips to the sand dunes at Spencer's Point—the air shows, the walks through the swamps and marshes near the creeks, and the creeks themselves—so they could explore the animal and plant life that would evade the untrained eye.

It was no secret that the Norfolk school board had their eye on her to make her an assistant principal as soon as there was an opening.

There was something further that was unique to Miss Abigail. One or two of her students ran off with most of the honors every year. During the first days of a school term, she scrutinized her pupils quietly until she found the children she was looking for, and she'd work with them hard for honors, but only if they wanted to.

Gideon had been sick with a severe asthma attack when the school opened. He came into the class several days late and slipped into a seat in the last row—a dubious distinction—because his last name began with the letter Z.

"I think I see a new boy," she said. "Would you please stand up and give your name to the class."

Gideon arose. "Gideon Zadok."

"So you're the missing culprit. In my classroom we reverse the alphabetical order so that the Z's are in front. We don't get many Z's, so I saved your seat, right up in the first row, please."

"Wow!"

There was an immediate eye contact established between Gideon and his teacher, which told them both that this was not going to be an ordinary relationship. It broke into words two weeks after he entered her class. Miss Abigail ended a lovely songfest with a medley of Stephen Foster tunes which had been requested by a number of the students.

I hear those gentle voices calling,
"Old Black Joe."

As she took the sash from about her neck and set the guitar on her desk, she and Gideon exchanged another of their instantaneous glances. She detected sudden rage in his eyes. It lasted but a fraction of a second and was gone. Miss Abigail bided her time and, in the course of the day, asked Gideon to remain after school to help her clean the blackboards and erasers. Gideon sensed that it was going to be no casual encounter, and he closed up.

After the blackboards were erased, he got a pan of water to wash them as she corrected papers. "I was curious about something, Gideon," she said. She saw the boy's body stiffen and his lips tighten. "I'm not going to bite you, relax." She smiled in a certain way that made the recipient also smile. "What do you have against Stephen Foster?" she asked.

"I . . . I . . . nothing."

"They are very lovely songs, aren't they? I've never been around a campfire when he wasn't sung. Well?"

"I guess they're beautiful, if you say so."

"Then why weren't you singing?"

Gideon broke into a fit of sneezing. "Excuse me. It's the chalk dust."

"Oh, I'm sorry. I shouldn't have asked you to do the blackboards."

"It'll go away in a minute . . . ka—chooo."

"Does Stephen Foster make you sneeze?"

"No, ma'am."

"Then why don't you like him?"

"I don't sing Christmas carols either, Miss Abigail. I'm Jewish and I don't believe in Jesus. I pretend to mouth the words, but I really don't sing. I . . . I just don't like what Stephen Foster is saying."

"How is that?"

"Well, because he makes it sound like the negroes enjoyed being slaves and he treats them like they were ignorant little children, or dogs licking the feet of their white masters. You know, 'Massah's in the cold, cold ground and all the darkies am aweeping.' You know."

"What?"

"They didn't want to be slaves. Nobody wants to be a slave."

"Do you know any colored people?"

He did. His dad had meetings with them sometimes, and many times he had gone to hear a Communist speaker in black churches. "No, ma'am," Gideon fibbed, "I don't know any negroes."

Miss Abigail chewed on it all for a moment. "I agree with you, Gideon," she said at last, "but I'm in a difficult position. Every school in America, or certainly every school in the South, sings Stephen Foster. Here it's required. The school is named after a Confederate general. Can you understand that I agree with you, but I still want to be your sixth-grade teacher and have to do some things I don't always like."

Gideon blinked at her and frowned. No adult had ever said anything so grown-up and honest to him before. Molly was always honest with him, but she wasn't a totally grown-up adult yet.

"Can you understand it, Gideon?"

"I think I can, Miss Abigail."

"It's a secret we have to share, because I could get into a lot of trouble," she said.

"You can trust me," he said.

"I know I can," she said. "That's why I told you the truth."

GIDEON DID NOT know how deep their secret was until a strange incident revealed everything.

A comrade picked him and his father up one evening and they drove south for a meeting at the Zion-Afro Baptist Church just over the North Carolina state line. James Ford, the leading black Communist in the country, was to speak. It was a special event and had to be held in a negro church because it was the only place where they allowed unsegregated audiences. James Ford always ran on the Communist ticket for Vice President. He didn't get many votes, because negroes couldn't vote in the South, but he ran anyway.

They arrived at the church, which was packed with black farmers and whites from as far away as Raleigh and Newport News. It was a hot, stifling night as Gideon and his father crammed into the rear of the church. The word was passed that James Ford would be a little late, and the pastor led everyone in a hymn-singing session. Gideon had a fit of sneezing and went outside to catch a breath of air and take a pill.

The church was set back in a stand of oaks near a crossroad of the state and county highways, with sharecroppers' farms all around. As Gideon stepped out into the night air, the singing followed him. It became uproarious as a number of people began seeing Jesus and screamed and several fainted.

There was a light on in the pastor's house in the rear of the church, and he made for it to find the water pump, so he could swallow his pill.

He stopped dead in his tracks as a car coming down the highway pulled off and drove toward a shed alongside the pastor's cottage. Gideon watched as a soldier and another huge man emerged from the car. He felt something was not right and ducked behind a tree to observe. The driver, the huge man, was a comrade whom he had seen at several meetings and who had been to his own home on occasion. He was another of those mysterious Party functionaries no one spoke about.

The soldier took off his clothing, down to his underwear, and the comrade handed him a package which he opened, containing civilian clothes. As the soldier dressed, Gideon saw some headlights blink on and off from inside the shed, and a second car drove out.

The soldier, now in changed clothing, jumped in the back and lay on the floor and was covered by some kind of canvas tarp.

There was a moment's conversation between the huge comrade and the driver of the second car. It was then that Gideon was able to make out Miss Abigail behind the wheel. Not believing his eyes, he slipped in closer for a look. It was indeed Abigail Winters, and she whisked away and sped down the highway with the soldier.

GIDEON HELD HIS tongue for two weeks. Not a word of it, not even to Molly, but he felt he would burst. How to go about telling Miss Abigail he knew about her? Or should he?

Sometimes kids left their desks messy or misplaced something and she would have them stay after school.

Gideon decided to leave a story he had written on the floor near his desk. Sure enough, the cleaning lady put it on the teacher's desk and Miss Abigail asked Gideon to remain after class.

"I believe this is your composition book," she said to him after the room had been cleared.

"Yes, ma'am, thank you. I thought I'd lost it." She gave him a sly look and he cracked a smile. "I guess I did leave it so you'd find it," he confessed. "I'm really sorry."

"Well, you did want me to read it, didn't you?"

"I guess so. I mean, yes I did."

"Well now, next time you just come up and hand me a story and say, I'd like you to read this."

"Can I?"

"Of course you can. Your stories are very, very popular with the class. I think the kids look forward to rainy days. Your storytelling has replaced my singing act."

Gideon straightened up, threw his shoulders back. She made him feel proud. "When I tell a story to the class," he said, "I make up kids' stuff, you know, prince and princess stuff for the girls and baseball stories for the boys."

"They are very entertaining."

"They're okay, Miss Abigail. Not my real good stories. Kind of the reason I left that story for you to read was that I didn't want you to think I was a trivial writer."

"My goodness, son, you're not even twelve years old."

"Sure, but I'm behind schedule. I've just started my serious writing."

"Why do you want to be a writer so badly?"

Gideon's face reddened. "It's a secret," he said.

"We already share one secret."

"I don't even share this secret with my sister."

"All right, have it your way."

Gideon looked at the floor and shoved his hands in his pockets, then remembered Miss Abigail didn't like the boys putting their hands there and pulled them out quickly. "Miss Abigail, I want to be a writer because writers know when a person is lonely. I mean, when Molly read me some books, those writers reached out and said, Look, Gideon, we know about your loneliness and we know that you feel downtrodden. And they said . . . I'll stand up for you. You're not alone anymore."

"You know that?"

"Yes, ma'am."

"Don't you think a writer should develop a balanced view of life? Writers have to know how to laugh, to drink, to be ridiculous and just a little crazy. That takes time."

"I know writers have to be crazy. But more than that, they have to get mad and stay mad. If things don't make a writer mad, he'll end up writing 'Flopsy, Mopsy, and Cottontail.' "

"What makes you angry, Gideon?"

"You know."

"You mean the situation with the negroes?"

"I cry about it some nights. It's much worse than Jewish people are treated and we get treated pretty badly, sometimes. I can't understand what keeps them from rebelling."

"When people have been reduced to slaves, it takes a long time to mount the rage needed to rebel. They accept their misfortune passively. It's a lot easier than fitting oneself for a noose. Perhaps their children will rebel."

"Well, that's something I'm going to do as a writer, make people angry. I'm going to stir them up."

She stared at the boy for ever so long. He was so small, so meaningless in the grand scheme of things. A billion or so other young men had frothed in anger before him and they were never heard from again. Yet there was something about this child. He was already accepting the pain of other people. Of course, the cheapest commodity in the world was unfulfilled genius. He craved recognition as a unique human being. What kind of bloody curse was he putting on himself? Or can the poor little fellow even help himself? In her ten years as a teacher, she had searched for, longed to find that kind of wild spark in one of her pupils. Good Lord, he was it. She knew. There was something about the way he looked into her eyes . . . no, there was something haunting about this boy.

"Tell me, Gideon. Do you want to have, or do you want to be?"

"I'm going to be," he answered without hesitation.

She hefted the composition book. "This is a very good story," she said. "I don't think Hemingway wrote it much better."

Gideon turned his eyes away in shame. "You, uh, read *A Farewell to Arms*, then?"

"Yep, partner, I read it."

"Yeah, I should have known. Well, maybe I did use a few of his ideas."

"There's nothing wrong with that. We all start out following our hero and then, somewhere along the line, we start to put our own stamp and style on things. There was an awful lot of Mozart in Beethoven, until Beethoven found his own way to say it."

"I'm glad you told me. I always felt I was cheating."

"When you're telling your stories to the class, I have detected a lot of Jack London, as well as Eugene O'Neill."

"To be honest and absolutely truthful, Miss Abigail, I've fooled a lot of other teachers."

"I'll bet you did. Why did you set this story in Mexico?"

"My sister Molly and I just finished reading *Tortilla Flat* together. John Steinbeck is going to be my favorite writer."

"I don't believe I know him."

"He's new. He'll be the greatest of them all. *Tortilla Flat* is about the Mexicans . . . the Chicanos in Monterey. Boy, does he stand up for those people."

"We mentioned Eugene O'Neill. Have you actually read him?"

"Yes, ma'am, everything he's written so far."

Holy Christ, she thought, holy Christ! She handed him the composition book.

"Got any more of these filled up?" she asked.

"Yes, ma'am, seventy-two of them, to be exact. I should have known you'd figure out where I got my plots and characters."

"You're too much!" She laughed. "All right, how about you whipping up a little play for me. Nothing too serious. It's for the kids. A fun play. And I'll steal a few tunes from my favorite composers—not Stephen Foster—and you can do the lyrics with me and I think the drama club might just like to put it on."

Gideon's mouth was agape. "Oh boy!" he shouted and ran up to her and threw his arms about her neck and kissed her on the cheek. Then, realizing his transgression, he nearly fainted with fright. "Oh, I'm sorry."

"Forget it, partner."

He turned and started to go, then walked back to her bravely. "Miss Abigail, I went to the meeting to hear James Ford at the Zion-Afro Church in North Carolina. I . . . I . . . I saw you there. I saw everything that happened."

It was her turn to show fright.

"The secret is safe with me. My father is a Party organizer."

"The young man you saw was a soldier working in the Army, recruiting other soldiers into the Party. He was so good that it was arranged for him to go to Moscow to study. We waited until a Russian ship was in port for him to desert."

"I swear to you, Miss Abigail, that I'll never tell another person. Not even Molly."

"I know, Gideon."

THE BALANCE OF the school year was the happiest Gideon had ever known. He was not absent because of illness for a single day. He wanted time to stand still, because when the semester ended, he would leave J. E. B. Stuart and go on to junior high school.

To Leah's horror and Nathan's disgust, Gideon made a sandlot baseball team, the feisty little player who made up in gall and guts what he lacked in size and talent. Joining his list of writer heroes came baseball heroes, Jimmie Foxx and Lefty Grove.

There was a lot of forbidding and scolding at home when Gideon came in scuffed-up, but he and Molly noticed that if they made a stand against their parents together, both Leah and Nathan gave in quietly.

Molly had come to an age when she was interested in boys and boys in her, and she established her right to have dates.

Leah was spending less and less time with Gideon. It came down to going to the odd concert with him or taking him for a doctor's visit. She was immersed in Party activities and whatever else she did later at night, after the choral society rehearsals, when Nathan was out of town.

Nathan had even less to do with his family. Except when he took them to Party functions, Nathan Zadok engaged in no activities with his son and stepdaughter. He never set foot on a playground, in a restaurant, at a movie, the theater, a sporting event, the beach, a department store, school. Nor did he listen to a radio program, or read a book, or newspaper except the *Freiheit*, or help with homework, or take a walk around the block, or go to an amusement park, or a museum, or fish, or net crabs, or see a parade, except for May Day.

"SO, WHAT'S THE big surprise?" Nathan asked.

"Your son . . . fanfare . . . Gideon Zadok, aged twelve . . . has won the Alice B. Merriweather prize for the best short story by a sixth-grade student in the entire Nawfalk, Virginia, district! Ta da! This story will go on to the state finals. I have here a check for ten dollars as the winning prize." Molly finished by holding the check and story aloft.

"I'll take care of that," Leah said, snatching the money deftly.

"Aw, nothing, folks, really nothing," Gideon said, "just another ordinary day in the life of Gideon Zadok, red-blooded American boy and future writer of renown."

"I think that's just marvelous," Leah said. "Here, let Momma give you a kiss."

"Now, folks, if you will relax," Molly continued, "I will read you the winning story by your son and my baby brother."

"I have an important meeting for the Free Tom Mooney Committee," Nathan said, in reference to the jailed labor leader and martyr. "But go on anyhow, I'll be a few minutes late."

"Tom Mooney will still be in jail tomorrow," Molly said indignantly.

"Er, how long a story is it?" Leah asked. "The choral society, you know."

"It meets on Thursday," Nathan said. "Today is Wednesday."

"Some of the members need special coaching," Leah said.

Nathan gave a "humph."

Leah wanted her husband to realize that she was not a happily married woman and might be doing something about it. She had been leaving a few of her mash notes around, like mouse droppings, to be discovered. Nathan did not nibble at the bait. He'd grown used to the hot meals and pressed shirts, and didn't want to risk losing those conveniences in warfare over Leah's petit-bourgeois romances. Moreover, a divorce would send the Central Committee into an uproar. And my God, once out on his own again, he would have to take a pay cut and resort to rooming in the homes of comrades.

Gideon had become clearly disturbed.

"Well . . . how long is it?" Leah asked.

"It's only five pages, Mother," Molly snapped, "and it will take less than fifteen minutes."

Leah leaned over and pinched her son's cheek, "for Momma's baby."

"*Nu*, go ahead already," Nathan said testily.

Molly was unnerved and read the story too quickly. Nonetheless, it was a simple and beautiful little fantasy of a boy who daydreams about being a great athlete. The hero plays out a complex football game in his mind, naming all the players after his schoolmates and friends. The hero reserves for himself the role of star running back, who always scores three or four times in the final quarter to save the game. It is not until the last paragraph that the reader realizes that the game is a fantasy and the boy is crippled.

Molly ended the reading, as she ended reading all of Gideon's stories, with tears streaming down her cheeks. It didn't matter if it was humor, a murder mystery, a tragedy, or a Western, Molly was always brought to tears. "It's so beautiful."

"Well, it's off to the choral society," Leah said, patting her son's head. "This is no surprise to me. From the minute you were born, your bubba said you were a genius."

"Wait!" Nathan said, storming to his feet in a manner that they had seen at a hundred meetings. "I think that this calls for a literary critique by the Soviet Committee on the Arts. To begin with—" He shrugged and gave a gesture of futility. "This story cannot be passed by the committee on the grounds that it lacks social significance."

"The Norfolk School Board didn't make social significance a requirement for a sixth-grade writing contest," Molly said angrily.

"In that case, just what does such a story do for the plight of the masses?" Nathan continued and then informed the poor illiterates around him of his credentials in literature, in untold numbers of languages.

"If I were in the Soviet Union today, I would be the editor of *Pravda*. Baseball? How can you make from such a hoodlum game a story of lasting value?"

"It's not about baseball, it's about football, Dad," Gideon said.

"Baseball? Football? What's the difference? It's played in America not for idealism of sports, as in the Soviet Union, but for money. Now, if the boy had been a coal miner, crippled in a mine because of the treacherous working conditions, then you would have a story."

"But, Dad, that's what you would have written," Gideon said. "This is what I wanted to write."

"Exactly. You had better start thinking in terms of the proletariat, the class struggle." Nathan picked up a copy of the day's *Freiheit*. "You should start thinking in these terms and someday you will be writing for the *Freiheit*. They, and they alone, will tell you what you can write and what you can't write. Such decisions can only come from your leaders, and believe me, they know how to enhance a young man's career. However! You had better start taking seriously your Yiddish. If you don't learn Yiddish, *Freiheit* wouldn't publish, not a single word."

"Why should I write in Yiddish? I'm an American. English is my language."

Nathan's finger leaped skyward and waved furiously. The good wrath was in him now. "Don't ever, ever let me hear such bunk baloney again. What do you want to write? For Hearst? For the yellow press?"

"Well, I must go, toodle-oo, darlings," Leah said, folding the check and plunking it into her purse. "It's a very nice story, no matter what the grim reaper says. When was the last time you went to an opera, a play, Mr. Know-it-all? These children would be culturally starved without their mother. Good night. Oh, Molly, fix Gideon something from the icebox. There's American cheese and baloney. But no peanut butter. He's allergic."

Nathan did not skip a beat as his wife left. "Someday you will realize that with Yiddish, which is an international language, you can express real emotions, not like this hotsy-totsy English. Yiddish, mind you, is becoming the most important international language in the world."

"For immigrants," Gideon mumbled inaudibly.

"It's a crying pity that a boy going on twelve years can't yet read the *Freiheit*. Look, J. J. Frumer, the poet laureate of the Yiddish language. Now, he is an important writer!"

When Mother and Father had departed for their respective meetings, Molly comforted her brother.

"I don't understand why Dad can't understand," Gideon said. "I think most kids of my age play out make-believe baseball and football games. It's fun because you can do anything in fantasy. I honestly feel that a lot of grown men play sports games out in their heads, in which they are always a superhero. That's the only way they can accomplish what they can't do in real life. Fantasy is very important for a writer."

"I understand the story very clearly, honey," Molly said. "You just keep on thinking inside other people's heads. That will help make you a writer."

"I am already a writer," he answered, taking the story from her. "Only I'm not renowned yet."

Danny Shapiro, who was fast becoming Molly's steady beau, knocked and entered with the grin on his face that he always wore when he set eyes on her. Danny saw their bitter mood. Molly winked quickly. "Danny promised me he'd buy you a chocolate banana split if you won a prize in the contest. Didn't you, Danny?"

Danny, who was not very fast with a buck, gulped, then nodded in agreement. "Yeah, and I'm a guy who pays off his debts." What the hell, he thought, twenty cents would win another round in the battle for Molly's heart. He forked over two bits to Gideon, hiding his pain.

"Thanks anyhow," Gideon said; "I'm allergic to chocolate, bananas, nuts, cherries, and whipped cream."

THE DREADED DAY had arrived. The school term was over. Gideon helped Miss Abigail pack up her personal books and clean her desk. She went to the bookshelf behind her desk and took down a half-dozen volumes.

"These should take care of some of your summer reading," she said. Gideon beamed. "What else do you plan to do?"

"I've got a gang of guys I'm starting to hang out with. We're going to do a lot of stuff. I also plan to write a three-act musical play about the fall of Ethiopia to the fascists."

"I'll be keen to see it," she said. "Before we call it quits, I've a little surprise for you. I'd like to take you flying with me."

"Jeeze."

"Get a note giving permission from one of your parents."

His spirits plummeted. His father would never give permission. As for Momma, she did not like Miss Winters. The two had met during the school year. Leah was aware of how deeply influenced her son had become by his teacher.

"She has a terrible body odor," Leah remarked, sniffing the air after their first meeting. "I know that woman has lice in her hair." Leah had even discussed with a doctor the possibility that Gideon was allergic to Miss Abigail and ought to change classes.

It was much the same with Molly's friends. The suggestion of a dangerous and highly contagious social disease (that one does not mention by name) generally followed Molly's second date with the same boy.

"It's really neat of you to offer me a plane ride, but I'd never get permission."

Miss Abigail became downright morose. "Do you have any idea how much I'm going to miss you, Gideon?"

"Me too," he said shakily.

"Then, to hell with it," she said, "let's go flying. There's something I have to share with you before we split up."

"Okay, ma'am."

IT HAD JUST turned twilight when the Granby Street trolley stopped at the cemetery near Dead Man's Corner and Gideon jumped off. He took in a deep breath to reinforce his courage and trotted over to the airstrip. It was a small three-hangar affair with a dirt runway, mostly used for barnstorming shows and air races. On the other side of the field the Navy had a facility.

Miss Abigail greeted him wearing a leather hat with goggles, a fleece-lined leather jacket, and knee-high boots. "Come meet my dad and brother." The older fellow, Clarence, was her father, the famous war ace. He was attired in mechanic's overalls. Another man, in his late twenties, was her brother, Jeremy, the famous stunt pilot on the southern barnstorming circuit. As he was introduced, Gideon wore an immediate expression of hero worship.

Clarence tousled Gideon's hair. "So you're the culprit who's stolen my daughter from me," he said.

"Not really, Mr. Winters."

Clarence turned to his son. "Jeremy, is that goddam cockpit heater working?"

"It tested out fine, Dad."

"Well, what the hell was it?"

"Just a wiring connection in the blower."

"Goldurn thing. Kid, there's some clothing your size in locker number twenty. Andy's kid's stuff should fit you."

As Gideon dressed, Abigail and her father and brother went over the flight plans.

"New moon. Should be like silk up there tonight," Clarence said.

The two men put their backs into opening the hangar door and were greeted by the outstretched arms of the most magnificent flying machine one could envision. They unlocked the wheels and each got behind a wing and pushed her onto the tarmac. The craft was a monowing Consolidated P-30, a two-seater pursuit fighter.

The Army had tested a number of prototypes and made a number of modifications, until it abandoned the craft. The test planes were sold off to former fliers like Clarence Winters. New, the plane had cost the taxpayers the staggering sum of over fifty thousand dollars.

Clarence, Jeremy, and Miss Abigail got the plane for a pittance and tinkered endlessly with it. They named her *Jenny* after Miss Abigail's mom. *Jenny* was one of the hottest barnstormers on the southern circuit. She had everything, a turbocharger that could push her to the lightning speed of 275 miles an hour, at over twenty thousand feet.

They turned the tail gunner's seat around and set it under a sleek sliding canopy and added a variable-pitched three-bladed propeller.

"Well, what do you think of her, son?" Clarence asked.

"Nifty," he replied with a voice that suddenly shot up to falsetto.

"Then let's go flying, pardner."

Clarence stood on the wing and leaned into the rear cockpit, which had all but swallowed Gideon up, and he explained the gadgetry, use of the oxygen mask, and how to speak over the radio.

Gideon did a white-knuckled clutch as the plane zipped down the runway. He caught a fleeting glance of Jeremy and Clarence waving to them. Off the ground they went! After a stunning loop around Norfolk and the grand flotilla of warships at anchor, he could see the amusement park at Ocean View and make out the cars shooting around the roller coaster and even see the flagpole sitter! They flew parallel to the beach for a while, then banked out over the ocean, straightened out, and climbed. Higher . . . higher . . . to infinity and a blanket of enveloping darkness.

"Gideon, can you hear me?"

"Yes, ma'am."

"Everything okay with you?"

"It's wonderful, Miss Abigail, wonderful!"

"Are you scared?"

"No, ma'am."

"All right. Put on your oxygen mask. We're going to climb. Got that?"

"Got it."

She opened the throttle. "Hang on, pardner, we're shooting for the moon." Higher and faster Miss Abigail pushed the craft until the coastline and Norfolk were but tiny toys. Two great arms of darkness wrapped about them. Gideon could see the back of Miss Abigail's head and her hair flowing out under her leather cap. How he worshipped her doing all this just for him.

"Gideon?"

"Yes, ma'am."

"I'm going to change the pitch of the propeller so that the engine makes the least amount of noise. When I do that, it may sound as if the engine is sputtering, but it's quite normal. Do you understand?"

"I've got it."

"We're almost there, son."

"Where?"

"Heaven."

Miss Abigail found the darkest part of the sky and settled *Jenny* into a huge circular pattern and slowed her down to a glide.

"Now! Open your canopy!"

Hands trembling, Gideon unlocked and slid the glass cover forward.

"Look up, son! Look up!"

Gideon, Miss Abigail, and *Jenny* seemed to be one and the same, flirting like a dolphin among a trillion lights, blinking, taunting, beckoning, and then a trillion more. Here and there bolides and shooting stars and comets rocketed by to what almost seemed touching distance, some for a blink of a second, some with showy flashes that made him gasp.

Round and round *Jenny* played, a darling little elf poking around in an infinity of splendor. But all they could really have was a peek, a tease. Take me higher! Can't we stay forever, Gideon thought. He felt as though he could step out of the plane and hurl himself outward and catch the tail of a flamer and hang on.

But nothing is forever, especially a gas tank. Well, maybe he could freeze this time into memory and live it again and again, nothing is forever.

He slid the canopy shut and sat stunned as Miss Abigail revved up the little bird and they rejoined the earth . . . and Communist rallies . . . and redneck Jew-baiters . . . and wheezing for breath when Momma crushed him in her arms . . . and Dad ripping up the Sunday Hearst paper that Molly had brought home.

When they landed, the field was ghostly. Clarence and Jeremy were gone and Miss Abigail eased the plane into the hangar. Gideon went to the lockers and changed and met her in the rickety office, where she had fixed some hot chocolate, which sent shock waves of wonderful warmth through him, even though he was allergic to it.

"Do you know why I took you up there?" she said.

"I think so."

"Why?"

"It embarrasses me," he said.

"No, go on and tell me."

"You took me up there because you think I'm one of those comets. Because . . . because . . ."

"What, Gideon?"

"You want me to know what it's like to live up there."

"You're pretty smart for a writer," she said. "You're going to have to be very tough to get through. And you're going to have to take a lot of pain."

"I know," he said, "but I can't help myself."

She filled his cup from the pot on the hot plate. "I'm going to Spain with my brother to fight for the Loyalists."

They did not speak for a time.

"I'm not going to Spain as a Communist. I've quit the Party. I'm going as an American. You see, the people of Spain have voted for a democracy and the Fascists are trying to destroy that. There is a strong Communist Party in Spain, in the government, but that doesn't mean Spain will go Communist. It means there is a chance for a democracy with the Communists as one of many parties. The French and the British are afraid that the Communists will take over if democracy wins. So they are acting neutral. That means they've let the floodgates open for Hitler and Mussolini to help the Fascists."

"I understand all that," Gideon said.

"If Franco and the Fascists win in Spain, it will lead to another world war. A war in which you will probably have to fight. We have to stop them now. It must remain another of our secrets, Gideon, but I have to go. I'll write to you as soon as I can."

The boy shook his head.

"Let me drive you home," she said.

"No, ma'am, I'd like to walk for a while. I'll always remember my sixth grade, Miss Abigail. And when I write something worth publishing, I'm going to dedicate it to you."

"Gideon . . . Gideon . . ."

"I love you, Miss Abigail," the boy cried and ran from the shed.

MOLLY WAS MOSTLY seeing one boyfriend, Danny Shapiro. Danny worked in his father's grocery store. It was a small neighborhood store with groaning, sagging wooden floors and bins of beans and a coffee grinder that could send you into ecstasy with its aroma and gunnysacks filled with flour and sugar and a long pole with grips to snatch the cans on the top shelves and a glass case filled with penny candies.

Irv Shapiro, Danny's father, couldn't say no to a neighbor out of work, or on the shorts. He made a living, but barely. He always said if he collected all his IOU's he could buy out the entire A&P grocery chain.

Although Molly was Gideon's security, particularly with Miss Abigail gone, the boy knew his sister was entitled to her own life. Not only did Danny not pose as a threat, Gideon took to him as an older brother. He could always shake Danny down for a nickel or even a dime, to send him off to the ice cream parlor, so Danny could neck with Molly on the front porch swing.

Moreover, Danny had use of the family car, an Essex, and let Gideon tag along on a picnic, or to the beach, or the movies. Sometimes Gideon and Danny would go off to a ball game by themselves, which made Molly sore, but she wasn't much interested in sports and kind of liked the closeness between her brother and her beau.

Molly got a summer job as a salesgirl at Kress's five-and-dime store and bought a radio with her earnings. It livened life up considerably. On Sunday nights there was "The Jack Benny Program" and it seemed as if half of America was listening. There were other great programs, like

"The Fred Allen Show" and "Major Bowes and His Original Amateur Hour" and "The Shadow" and "The Texaco Star Theater."

Gideon sorted out and studied the really fine and original writing, particularly the radio dramas of Arch Oboler and Norman Corwin and Orson Welles and the adaptations of the great plays on the "U.S. Steel Hour." There was "Metropolitan Opera Broadcasts" and Toscanini leading the NBC Symphony.

Nathan had shunned buying a radio because the programs were either "bourgeois trivia" or "reactionary propaganda."

"That Gabriel Heatter is a fascist with his dirty news."

When Molly brought home the Atwater-Kent table model set, Nathan realized he wasn't going to get rid of it. It sat in the kitchen, which also served as the living room. If Nathan was caught listening, he'd quickly shrug in disgust and leave the room, or place himself between the radio and the family, open his copy of *Freiheit*, and read to himself aloud and make so much noise rustling the paper no one could hear. Nothing seemed to interest him but the Party. The hard-and-fast rules of life had been laid down by the Central Committee, so there was nothing further for him to explore.

Even Leah, with all her comings and goings, was reduced to tears by the soap operas, Bess Johnson in "Hilltop House" and "Orphans of Divorce," which reflected the daily agonies of ordinary people she could identify with.

Life between Leah and Nathan had become rotten. Their arguments quickly turned into shrieking matches filled with terrible verbal violence. Nathan's veins would protrude on his forehead almost to bursting, and Leah, of late, was given to beating herself in the face with her own fists. On other occasions, she would throw open the front window and scream out her misery to the entire neighborhood and constantly threaten suicide. The police knew the address well.

"I'm going to throw myself out of the window!" she'd yell. Nathan would then open the window and stand aside. Leah would invariably faint and lie "unconscious" until it was time to revive and drag herself off to a meeting, bravely.

Gideon had become an accepted member of the neighborhood gang, even though his mother and father were considered crazy. He told too many good stories to them and had become nifty with the glove as a first baseman. He was one of the guys even though he was a Jew boy.

There was a garage in the rear of the flat, but all it held was an excess of old furniture and piles of junk. It had a small loft and he could bury himself there and read and write stories by the hour. Only Molly and a few close pals knew of the secret office. His greatest joy was corresponding with Miss Abigail.

Getafe Air Base
Madrid
August 3, 1936
My Dearest Friend Gideon,
Jeremy and I have made it to Spain, at long last. To get here we had to endure a difficult route through the Pyrenees Mountains from France. I'll write more about it later. Fliers are desperately needed and we were immediately assigned to the Malraux International Squadron. My plane is a Boeing P-12, an old bird, but she does what I ask. We are up against the Italians and Germans of the Nazi Condor Legion, who are running the latest Fiats and Messerschmitts. The Condors were okay as long as they didn't have any real opposition, but in our first three patrols we've given them flying lessons. Jeremy has shot down his first enemy. . . .

Norfolk
October 11, 1936
Dear Miss Abigail,
. . . A crisis is brewing in my house. I am about to reach my thirteenth birthday, when Jewish kids (boys) get confirmed in a ceremony called a bar mitzvah. My grandmother and grandfather are really after me to be confirmed and want me to make a trip to Baltimore next summer and get instructions. But my father says he'd never forgive me, and besides, he'd get into trouble with the Party. . . .

Getafe Air Base
Madrid
November 15, 1936
My Dearest Friend Gideon,
. . . You must realize that even though I'm no longer a member of the Communist Party, I believe, very powerfully, about what we are doing here in Spain. When I became a Communist, I honestly thought I could help change some of the injustices in America. But later I watched the Communists devour each other brutally. And while they preached they had created the ultimate democracy in Russia, they showed themselves to be the most un-

democratic organization on the planet. They certainly are not the answer for America.

I have come to love Roosevelt and I realize now that a true democracy doesn't have a patented answer for every ill in its society. We cannot and do not fear our neighbors, our country, and ourselves as the Communists do, in order to exist.

I am in Spain to fight against Hitler and Italian fascism. I wish to God Americans understood that better.

If you are truly to become a writer, then you must have freedom. The Communist writers I've followed have either left the party in protest or have become mimeograph machines and bitter automatic liars. Writers cannot flourish in an atmosphere of tyranny. Free yourself, Gideon . . . free yourself!

Norfolk
January 25, 1937
Dear Miss Abigail,
. . . My family is really shaken up by the purges in the Soviet Union. Thousands of Jewish intellectuals, doctors, artists, and politicians have been put on trial and either banished or killed. A lot of Jewish members of the Party here have quit in protest. My father doesn't allow the subject to be spoken of in the house, but my mother and Molly are having second thoughts.

After four years of being told to hate Roosevelt, the Party is now telling us to support him. They do that on a lot of issues, say one thing one day and the opposite the next. . . .

Getafe Air Base
March 15, 1937
My Dearest Friend Gideon,
. . . We have recently fought two huge battles at Jarama and at Guadalajara and it is difficult to tell who won. As you know, Madrid has been under siege from almost the first day of the war and it is still under siege, only now Fascist artillery can reach the city and it is a pity to see the magnificent buildings, centuries old, being demolished. It is more pitiful to see the starvation because of the blockade. I wish to God the democracies would end their terrible boycott. They are helping squeeze a fellow democracy to death.

Our five international brigades have over thirty-five thousand

volunteers now, from everywhere in the world, and are holding
the republic together while they build up a Spanish home army.

You can be proud of our Abraham Lincoln Battalion. They
have fought well on every front although they've suffered terrible
losses. . . .

Norfolk
June 12, 1937
Dear Miss Abigail,

. . . I have just read the new book by John Steinbeck. It is called
In Dubious Battle and reminds me of your fight in Spain. He is
truly going to be the greatest writer of our times. . . .

. . . You certainly remember the boys at the Turney Boys
Home Orphanage. You remember how much fighting they did at
J. E. B. Stuart? Well, my team played them in baseball and we
beat them. I hit a single and a double and stole two bases. Afterward we visited them at the home. I learned that they fight so
much out of fear. They're really scared as I am of things. I wrote a
play for them, which was loosely based on *The Front Page,* and it
was a riot and went over very well. I'm just like one of them
now. . . .

Getafe Air Base
Madrid
July 7, 1937
My Dearest Friend Gideon,

. . . It is with terrible sadness that I must tell you my beloved
brother, Jeremy, was shot down. . . .

. . . Every night since his death I have dreamed not only of
him, but of the boys I have shot down, strafed on the ground and
bombed. I realize they are Nazis and Fascists but I cannot get out
of my mind the sorrow in their homes now, because I realize the
sorrow in my home. What might these young men have become?
Have I killed a writer, an artist? How many beautiful boys lie
under the Spanish soil. . . .

Oh, Gideon, my dear Gideon, I want to come home, but I
continue to be enraged by what they have done to this beautiful
land. . . . If only I knew that you wouldn't have to fight a war,
it could all be worth it.

Norfolk
August 10, 1937
Dear Miss Abigail,
. . . I see your mom and dad every chance I get. They are hold-
ing up very well, but they wish you'd come home. So do I. You've
done enough, really enough. . . .

Getafe Air Base
Madrid
October 20, 1937
Gideon! I HAVE MET ERNEST HEMINGWAY! You know, I'm
sort of a curiosity, being a woman flier, and I went into Madrid
for him to do a story about me and we've fast become drinking
pals.

He has a room in the Florida Hotel, as do most of the journal-
ists. The whole Republican territory has been half starved. No one
has seen fresh meat for months. Well, Hemingway was on the fifth
floor of the hotel (the two top stories have been blown away by
artillery). He ushered me in, and there, hanging near the window,
was a side of beef.

He covers the war with special maps, binoculars, pistols, com-
pass, hobnail boots, and canteens filled with Scotch. The front
lines are only a twenty-minute taxi drive from Madrid, so he
showed me what the war looked like from the ground. . . .
"Papa" started off as a neutral, but has gone heavily to the Loyalists. For such a great writer, he's really strange in his fears about
becoming politically involved. . . .

Remember how we discussed his personality? He does have a
terrible masculinity problem. He has a lady friend on call and his
escapades are notorious. He tried to collect my scalp but I told
him I was desperately in love with a young man of thirteen and
intended to be faithful to him.

The problem with "Papa," as I see it, is that as soon as another
person is in his presence, he has to put on a show of his bravado.
He has created an image that sometimes makes him, as a person,
larger than his writings. Everyone around him caters to him, even
up to speaking "Hemingwayese." I think that deep down inside,
he is a very insecure man and had to create a public version of
himself to deliberately mask his many fears.

One day "Papa" is going to have to take a long look in the
mirror and realize he is not nearly as huge as he has inflated

himself. When he realizes he can't live up to the image he created, he's going to be in serious trouble.

But he is a thing of beauty to watch at his work. He lets no one or nothing stand in his way when he's after his story. He sloughs off bureaucrats and red tape and is powerfully arrogant and he is *always* right (in his own mind). I tell you these things because you might have to do the same in order to become a great novelist.

When I told him about the story you had written using the plot of *A Farewell to Arms* and setting it in Mexico, he roared with delight and penned to you the enclosed note. . . .

Dear Gideon Zadok,

Abigail Winters tells me you are going to become a great writer. Well, you're off to a good start, stealing my plot. Someday I'll tell you how many plots I have "borrowed." Remember, boy, only steal from the best.

A novel takes the courage of a marathon runner, and as long as you have to run, you might as well be a winning marathon runner. Serendipity and blind faith in yourself won't hurt a thing. All the bastards in the world will snicker and sneer because they haven't the talent to zip up their flies by themselves. To hell with them, particularly the critics. Stand in there, son, no matter how badly you are battered and hurt. I hope to hear of your success someday.

Your friend,
Papa Hemingway

Gideon entered the kitchen, tossed his books on the oilcloth-covered table, and sampled the icebox. It was mostly empty, as usual. A few lingering packages of sandwich meat looked unappetizing. There was the standard note from Leah pinned to the bulletin board. It read that Momma had to go out on business and wouldn't be home that night. Molly could fix him a deviled egg sandwich. There was also an apple. Momma loved him very much.

Leah was getting bolder in her outside forays. Gideon shrugged and was turning to his homework when he looked up and saw Molly in the doorway. She looked absolutely awful.

"Hi," Gideon said. "What's the matter? You sick?"

"Have you seen a newspaper or listened to the radio today?"

"No."

"Get a grip on yourself, Gideon."

"Hey, what's the matter, anyhow?"

Molly set the afternoon *Ledger Dispatch* on the table, put her hands in her face, and wept. Gideon stared at the headline.

NORFOLK AVIATRIX KILLED IN SPAIN
Abigail Winters, daughter of WW I Ace, shot down in dogfight

Abigail Winters's death was the most crushing and tragic experience of young Gideon's life. For days he was in a stupor, barely eating, barely sleeping. He spent hours on end in the garage loft that held his "office." Then came a final thunderclap, the news that his mother was going to take him from Norfolk. He all but refused to leave the loft, spending the days and half the nights curled up in a ball, staring blankly at nothing.

Molly came to him often, virtually force-feeding him, demanding he open up with a word or two.

"Are you angry with me?" she'd ask.

"No."

"Momma probably made the decision to go to Baltimore a long time ago. She was just waiting for an opportunity for Dad to be out of town. I've done everything I could, but I can't change her mind."

Suddenly Gideon burst out, "I don't want to leave Norfolk! I've got all my pals here. They just made me captain of the baseball team. I hit over three hundred. Some guy wanted to pick a fight with me and four of the kids from the Turney Home jumped him. I'm writing another play for them. Abigail's dad has taken me flying and wants to teach me how. He treats me like I was his own son, and he really needs me."

"Gideon darling, it's not going to be that bad. You've got a dozen swell cousins around your age and you know how Uncle Lazar and Uncle Dominick love you."

"I don't want to live in that house on Monroe Street. It's got rats all over and the schoolyards are all made of concrete."

Tears came to Molly.

"Don't cry, Molly."

"I'm so sorry I won't be with you to take care of you," Molly wept, "but Bubba loves you so. . . ."

"Sure . . . sure. . . ."

"Honey, I'm nineteen years old. I should have graduated high school a year and a half ago. Every time we moved I got put back a class. I made some of them up, but if I go to Baltimore, they'll put me back another term. I'm staying here in Norfolk so I can graduate with my class. As soon as I'm out of school, I'll be able to get a decent job and send for you or come to you."

He jammed his hands into his pockets and clenched his teeth.

"Okay, baby? Tell me it's okay."

"Sure, I understand. I really do. It would be just plain selfish of me."

Molly put her hands on her brother's shoulders and looked at him with a half smile. "Hi, blue eyes."

Gideon stiffened and fought for courage. "God always makes writers suffer. God's always testing to see if we can take it. *He* wants tough writers."

"There's something else I have to tell you, Gideon. Look at me. Danny and I have been secretly married for three months. Not even Momma knows. We both love you very, very much. Danny wants you with us as much as I do."

"I love Danny," Gideon said. "I'm glad you have each other."

"Oh, Gideon! Put your arms around me and squeeze me as hard as you can."

THE NEGRO STEWARD rapped on the cabin door. Leah slipped into her dressing gown and opened it.

"Your tea and toast, ma'am," he said, "we'll be arriving in Baltimore in about an hour."

Gideon climbed down from the upper bunk, splashed his face in the tiny sink, and brushed his teeth. Momma edged in, pushing him aside. She applied her makeup, a chalky powder to make her appear sallow and dark eye shadow to make her look consumptive. Gideon had seen her put on that special pasty face when she was going to have an argument with Dad, or when she applied for welfare, or a free clinic for him, or to otherwise indicate she was suffering.

"I'm going over for breakfast," he said.

"Be careful what you order," she said, "remember, no eggs or bacon and be sure you drink buttermilk."

Gideon went out on the deck to catch the early morning zest in the air, as the overnight steamer from Norfolk to Baltimore chattered up the bay. The boy was still suffering badly from the death of Miss Abigail. He leaned on the railing and thought about the novel he was going to try, which would let the world know what a great woman Abigail Winters was.

Leah had laid the groundwork for her departure carefully, over a period of several months. She had ascertained that the Norfolk water was filthy, all but poisonous, the climate unfit for human habitation, and the very air filled with dangerous pollutants. All of this was far too detrimental to Gideon's health.

Molly and Gideon had figured out the true reason for Momma's conniving. She had had enough of her marriage to Dad. A rash of secretive phone calls from a dentist in New York indicated that the caller was interested in something more than Leah's teeth.

Leah had been very good at securing work, not for herself, but for Nathan. She had gotten numerous jobs for him to moonlight on numerous weekends. The children realized that she did it not only to fill the perpetually bare cupboards, but to get him out of the house so she could attend to her equally numerous amorous rendezvous.

Just before school vacation, Leah informed her husband that she had obtained work for him, through relatives, in Pittsburgh for the entire gold rush season. As soon as he headed north, Leah began packing and gave as her reason the unhealthy climate, water, and conditions in Norfolk.

At first she refused to allow Molly to remain, but when Molly threatened to spill the beans to Nathan, she relented.

Many times Gideon had traveled on the Old Bay Line to Baltimore. It was mostly fun. He and Uncle Dominick took in a lot of ball games at Oriole Park. It was big-time stuff, a triple-A team, just under the major leagues. There were concerts and opera at the Lyric Hall and sometimes some real good touring plays at the Ford Theater. His cousins were neat and he particularly liked Uncle Lazar, who had been a Marine, and Lazar's big-busted French wife, Aunt Simone.

As they eased into the Baltimore basin, Leah's hand danced nervously on her son's shoulder. The *President Warfield* turned toward her berth and was deftly maneuvered dockside and the gangplank rolled into position.

"There she is!" Leah called. "Momma! Momma! Here I am."

Bubba Hannah saw them and waved vigorously as they disembarked. "Momma! Momma!"

Hugs! Tears!

"Gideon! Look at how that boy has grown."

"He's a sick child. Norfolk was killing him. Thank God we're here."

"Come, come, Leah. Lazar brought his car. It's parked on the other side of the pier."

THE LITTLE RED brick row house with the white marble steps on Monroe Street seemed smaller to Gideon and more jammed than he remembered. What space would there be for him? How could he write with other people sleeping in the room?

Zayde Moses barely looked up from his sewing in the front-room shop as they spilled in jabbering. Ho hum, Moses thought, Leah is home again.

Bubba was older and slower, but did not forget Leah's footbath routine. Gideon curled up in a broken, legless, spring-protruding, overstuffed couch, placed randomly in a corner of the kitchen. Moses slipped out of his shop to eavesdrop from the back porch while setting his rattraps, a dozen of them, some heavy enough to stop a cow.

As Leah's feet soaked, Hannah went about her Sabbath baking, rolling and curling dough and twisting it deftly into knots, to be baked into challah bread. She gave Gideon a bowl to lick the last of the cookie batter from.

"Momma, I slaved, I scrimped. That little *momser* Nathan squeezed every penny. If it hadn't been for me going from door to door to find him work, we would have starved."

"I told you from the beginning, he was a no-goodnik. So, maybe you'll listen to Momma, now."

"I had to steal milk from the neighbor's doorstep for that child."

"A no-good Charlie, that's what. Those Communists make nothing but trouble. Good riddance," Bubba said, with a mock spit to the floor. "So, where's Molly?"

"A mother's heart could break," Leah said. "She insisted on staying in Norfolk with the excuse, now hear this, so that she could graduate with her class. Like Western High School in Baltimore was a garbage dump. The truth is that Molly may be up to some monkeyshines with this Danny Shapiro boy. It's no secret what he's after."

"Kenst shtarben aveck."

"He's from a family of Mongolians, or something. They're one step above the *shvartzers*. I begged her, 'Molly, don't throw your life away on this boy. What kind of a future will he give you?' I might as well have been talking to the wall. Children these days don't listen to a single word you tell them. Just pray she doesn't come to Baltimore with a little present in her belly."

"The head of a shmuck has no conscience," Hannah agreed.

"So, where will we put up Gideon?"

"Upstairs in the front room with Al and Fanny's children."

JESUS, Gideon thought.

A hair-trigger rattrap sprung and Moses cursed, outside. The front door bell rang.

"Moses!" Hannah called. "There's a customer. Probably Mr. Sachs for a fitting."

Moses shuffled into the kitchen, the fringe from his prayer shawl showing beneath his greasy vest. He pointed a bony finger at Gideon. "You didn't have your bar mitzvah. You go to *shul* and learn so you can be called to the Torah."

"I'm not going to Hebrew school," Gideon said defiantly.

"You're a *goy!*"

"Shaddup and see who's at the front door," Hannah commanded.

"This boy is not going to die a natural death," his grandfather bellowed and shuffled out of the room.

"Hub em in dread," Hannah said after her husband left. "He doesn't earn enough money to feed a canary. Three dollars' earnings for him is a big week. And Fanny's husband, Al Singer, is no prize. We've been living on the five dollars Lazar gives and maybe a few dollars from that wop Abruzzi."

"And Gilbert Diamond with his millions?" Leah asked.

"From him we get *bupkes.*"

"Jake Rubenstein also doesn't contribute?"

"When has Jake Rubenstein had two nickels to rub together? *Nu,* let me go next door and phone Pearl and have the wop bring over a rollaway bed. Leah, you'll sleep in the middle room with me."

Leah pointed to the front door in inquiry about Moses.

"The *alter kocker?* He has a cot in the shop. It's too good for him. He doesn't put fifty cents on the table for the kitchen."

"Well, never you mind," Leah said, "I won't be here for very long. Momma, sit down, I have something to tell you. Sit, sit. Speak Yiddish."

Gideon understood perfectly, as had Molly before him.

"Momma, I'm only here till after Sabbath. I have been invited to go up to New York City, can you imagine?"

Hannah looked at her daughter knowingly, wiped her hands, and sat and sighed.

"I met . . . I think this is Mr. Dream Man, a dentist."

"So soon, already?"

"Actually, I met him last summer, quite by accident. I was at Virginia Beach and he was down on vacation with his family from New York."

"With his mother and father?"

"Not exactly. With his family, his wife and children."

"But, Leah, you're a married woman and this is a married man."

"He is a very, very unhappy person. He and his wife haven't slept together for almost a year."

"You believe that crap? You've got to watch out for dentists, especially when they give you the gas. Your Great-aunt Sylvia, God rest her soul, woke up suddenly to find you-know-what you-know-where."

"Momma, I know the difference between love and infatuation. This is a gentleman dentist. In Brooklyn. With a three-story brownstone house in the Bensonhurst district. He has a car, a 1937 Terraplane, and he gets a new one every other year. Believe me, Momma, I didn't do one single thing to arouse him. But when he saw me coming from the dressing room in my bathing suit, that was the finish of him. I didn't so much as give him a 'how do you do?' "

"Of course you didn't. What happened?"

"Not a thing, Momma, but the man was smitten, he couldn't help himself. I did nothing to provoke it. So, comes the love letters, the flowers. So you know . . . I went for a weekend in New York. It was strictly social. My God, I had to invent such stories for Nathan, that little weasel."

"I don't like this, Leah. You are going to break up a home with children."

"Momma, how can you say that! This poor man has been in utter misery for years. A little sympathy, a little understanding, is the least I could give him. He's longing for culture. So, what's wrong with a little culture?"

"I . . . I . . . can't . . . I can't . . ." Gideon cried suddenly.

"What's the matter with the boy?" Hannah asked, alarmed as Gideon clutched his neck and gasped.

"I can't breathe!"

"Oh my God!" Hannah screamed.

"It's all right, Momma," Leah said. She slipped as she stepped out of the water pan and made for her purse. "I have an adrenaline spray in my bag."

NATHAN NEEDED a weekend at home, desperately. His eyes widened in horror as he entered the flat. Devoid of furniture, which had been repossessed, the flat looked like an old whore whose makeup kit had been stolen.

He was extremely tired. The job in Pittsburgh had been a back-breaker, the usual slavery for a cunning, lying slumlord. When he tried to collect, *gevalt!* He wouldn't have wished it on that other paperhanger, Hitler! A month's profit went up in smoke.

The anger welled up. His forehead vein grew violet. He threw open the window and screamed, "I'm going to make a scandal!" The neighbors, accustomed to Leah's suicide threats, took it all in their stride.

A note pinned to the bulletin board indicated that Molly was still in Norfolk, at the home of a comrade, and there was a letter for him.

My Dear Nathan,

. . . How I have lasted until now, beyond all human endurance, only speaks for my loyalty and faithfulness as a human being. But the strongest human being sooner or later has to break. . . .

Norfolk was slowly draining the life from our dear son, Gideon. For his sake . . . it is with terrible sorrow that I have reached a final conclusion that you are an unfit father and provider and probably are the cause of much of the boy's illnesses. I have filed for a divorce . . . if you threaten to make a scandal I shall have to take severe measures to stop you. . . .

Certain government authorities may be very interested in your activities, if you know what I mean. They do not fool around with undesirable aliens and I am certain you don't want to go back to Poland. . . . I tried, God knows I tried, but you have crushed the love out of a delicate flower, me.

Sincerely,

Leah

Leah had played it perfectly. The Party was Nathan's life, but Jewish members were leaving in droves. Some, like Nathan, dreaded the thought of life away from the comrades and stayed and kept their mouths shut. Through all the Stalin purges of great old venerated Bolsheviks and intellectuals and professionals and artists, he was quiet. They had been liquidated after extorted "confessions."

In America, the Party had become a shell of itself. It could no longer afford to expel loyal foot soldiers, like Nathan Zadok. He was transferred to a higher post in Philadelphia, to pick up the scattered remains of the Jewish Section. His immediate job was to gain control of the Jewish paperhangers' union local. He was also ordered by the Party to go through the divorce quietly and to pay three dollars and fifty cents per week child support to Gideon.

My Dear Son,

First of all let's get some things straight. I have not come to Baltimore in the past month because I have been ill. I am papering at night, sometimes until the morning, to meet my obligations. Have I ever failed to send a money order for $3.50 a week, even if I don't have what to eat? Have I? And what about the extra dollar I include, even sometimes when I have to borrow it? So, if I don't come to Baltimore it is because I'm sick. The doctor says my condition won't be better for some time yet, so I shouldn't travel. That should put that bunk to rest. I would be there in a minute if I were physically and financially able to travel.

Under no circumstances can a boy from a progressive home endure the humiliation of a ceremony such as a bar mitzvah. You will not be forgiven if you submit.

Now, to more serious business. I don't know what to do with you. Just think of it, you are already not a little boy and here I am worried because you don't write to me. Every day I look for a letter. You don't want to satisfy me even with a few words to tell me how you feel. I ask you, sonny! Is that nice?????

If you don't want to write to me, why don't you tell me?

Well, be a good boy, sit down, and write to me a nice letter. You know I love you. Bad news. I have no future work and no money. You don't know me anymore. When I start to work again and have some money, then you'll recognize me again. So, you are against the poor and for the rich? Oh, I cannot believe that. Unless you write to me regular, I may think that you are against the poor. So let us see. Be good, write, and keep well.

Your Daddy loves you.

Nathan

LAZAR

1939–1941

I AM GIDEON'S UNCLE, Lazar Balaban, the pharmacist. I became an important part of his life from 1939 through 1941, a very difficult period.

When Gideon arrived in Baltimore from Norfolk, my own situation had greatly improved. After the great depression and years of virtual bondage, I was finally able to buy out Gilbert Diamond. Once on my own, I did very well.

My darling wife, Simone, proved to be a true gift from God. She was thrifty. She had ideas. She made things happen.

During those days a man could pick up a good pharmacy for a song. We sold our old location and moved "uptown," so to speak, into a first-class establishment in a pleasant residential neighborhood with trees and lawns, with doctors and teachers as customers. It was a mixed neighborhood, a lot of Jewish families, Italians, Irish. Most people were making a nice living. It was peaceful. My store was at the intersection of Garrison Boulevard and Liberty Heights Avenue, a prime crossroads location.

After being raised by my stepmother Hannah, whom I considered my real mother, and after living with my three half sisters, what did we go and do? Simone and I had three daughters, Priscilla, Tracey, and Laurie. My lovely wife made our daughters into a rose, a diamond, and a pearl. We had a lively, beautiful home on Belle Avenue, a few blocks' walk from my store.

When I married Simone in France during the war, she was a widow with a small son, Pierre. I adopted the boy and he grew into a fine young man. He was away at college, MIT no less, studying engineering.

I was always happy to see Gideon. He came over often to work in the store and bum a dinner from Simone, who was God's gift to the culinary art. Gideon was a gifted boy. Everyone in my house loved him and I offered to take him into our home. Leah refused, stating that Gideon would be better off living in Monroe Street with her and Bubba Hannah. Well, the truth of the matter was that Leah did not like Simone, and in her warped thinking, Simone posed as some kind of threat to steal her son. What could I do?

We had a lot of very bright kids among my nieces and nephews and my own children. They would set the world on fire, some of them. We were going to be an American family this country would be proud of. But it was Gideon who had always borne a burden, even a curse. He was expected to be the miracle child.

When he returned to Baltimore he was a troubled lad. It didn't take long for him to become a leader. Not in school, where he struggled to make passing grades, but out on the streets. When little guys get tough, watch out. Gideon started smoking cigarettes, ran with a gang, and generally flirted with trouble.

There was a street called Herbert Street, which ran off Monroe. It was not much more than an alleyway lined with tiny, tiny row houses mostly inhabited by poor Irish and poorer Portuguese fishermen. It was a mean street with mean kids and there were nightly brawls between neighbors and inside the homes.

Gideon Zadok was able to control his gang and lead them with his sharp little mind. They heisted stuff out of neighborhood stores, prowled for other gangs to fight, stole bicycles and sold them for spare parts, and otherwise spoiled for trouble.

The kid was on his own. His father, Nathan, was in Philly. Molly was in Norfolk and Leah was gone from the house most of the time. Bubba Hannah did most of the raising. She loved Gideon powerfully, but she had grown old. When we had a matriarch as strong as Hannah, we thought she'd never age, but each Sunday now, we saw it happen.

Bubba would darn his socks, keep his clothing clean, and feed him, but that was it. She could not cope with a wild teenager who had fast turned into a street fighter.

Dominick Abruzzi had worked his way up to detective sergeant and we had become close, over the years.

"I'm worried about Gideon," he said.

"Me too, Dom."

"Up to now I've been able to talk the juvenile officers into keeping the kid's name off the blotter. He's got no record, but Uncle Dom can only do so much."

"I think we've got to bring his father in on it. Maybe he can take the kid in Philly a little more, give him something to look forward to."

Dom and I agreed to give it our best try, even though we didn't like Nathan Zadok or his Communist shit. We phoned him.

"I'm in the neighbor's apartment, I can't talk, and he needs the phone," Nathan said.

"The boy is getting into trouble," I answered.

"It would be very hard to have him in Philadelphia. We barely have room to breathe in now. Look, I'll write you a letter."

Dom had his ear against mine so he could hear. He snatched the phone from my hand. "Listen, Zadok, your son is one step away from going to the detention home. How are the comrades on the Central Committee going to take that one?"

"All right, all right, calm down, Abruzzi. You Mussolini Fascist," he hissed under his breath.

"Now, you get him to Philly as often as you can and spend some time with him."

"I'll get things arranged, no matter what the cost, the extra train fares, the extra cooking, laundry, clothing. You do know that I send him support money, without fail," Nathan whined.

When we signed off, both Dom and I shook our heads. "He's not going to help. Jesus . . . Jesus . . ."

We took it upon ourselves to wean him away from his gang as carefully as we could. As a detective sergeant, Dom had free entry to all the sporting and cultural events. If it had anything to do with baseball or music, Dom took care of him.

I encouraged Gideon to come and see us anytime he wanted. With Pierre away at college and three nonathletic daughters, it was fun to have somebody to shoot baskets with. We both liked to run and we'd spend many an early evening trotting around the neighborhood. We would pass Garrison Junior High School and Forest Park High, modern schools set in lawns and trees and serenity. It wasn't difficult to see how much Gideon wanted to attend these schools.

So I went into a little conspiracy with him. He'd use my Belle Avenue address as his own and get a transfer out of his inner-city school. It worked, and the boy became very attached to Garrison. After-school activities, particularly the drama club, did a lot to keep him off the streets.

In the evening, we'd sit on the porch swing and rock, and as we got closer and closer, he told me about what it was like to go to Philly.

I'd be pretty much asleep when the conductor called out, "Chester, Chester, next stop Chester." The train pulled into an open-air elevated platform station. There were red brick factories all around from the turn of the century and, on a corner down the block, the flashing neon lights of the Colorado Café. Funny name for a diner. Outside the window I saw the big sign painted across a building: WHAT CHESTER MAKES MAKES CHESTER. *Philly was the next stop. Christ, I hoped I'd never see that sign again. Sometimes my dad met me, but most of the time I'd take a streetcar.*

Dad moved quite often, but every place looked alike. They all seemed to be second- or third-story apartments and they were spooky because they were usually in the rear of the building and the halls were never lit. There was a lot of dark mahogany paneling and a uniform mustiness and gloom. When I entered, the first thing that got to me was the smell of mothballs from the front hall closet where Dad's only good suit hung.

Dad had married a Party member with two sons older than me. They weren't bad guys. We'd all sneak off to the ball games together, and when I was able to see major leaguers, Dizzy Dean and those guys, it was almost worth the trip. Dad was always on his stepsons with his temper and I stood up for them against him. All pleasures were forbidden, even the funny papers.

Dad's wife, Lena, was a kvetch, a complainer and nagger. Every sentence she spoke started out negatively, to put you on the defensive. "What's the matter, you don't like Philadelphia?" The big joy of her life was stuffing food down everyone's throat. "Eat, eat, eat, eat" . . . like she was getting sexual satisfaction out of cramming your belly; or, if you didn't eat until you burst, she'd take it as an insult: "Jewish cooking is not good enough for you?"

Little varied between me and Dad. Almost every conversation turned out to be a lecture. "Do better in school," "Don't hang out with hoodlums," "Read important works by Party members," "Pay honor to the Soviet Union."

The Second World War had started and France had fallen and England stood alone. At first the Communists had been ordered to berate and denounce the war as an imperialistic war. Then Stalin made a pact with Hitler. I heard that members quit the Party in droves over this, but Dad justified the pact. Then, later, Russia was attacked and overnight the bad war became a good war, according to the Communists.

I had reached puberty and the whole new world of masturbation was a wonderment, really fantastic. I read a lot of books and could even talk to Aunt Simone, who was a lot different than Bubba and Momma. She taught me not to feel guilt and shame and that stuff. Also, not to seek answers to my curiosity with her daughters. I'd never touch my cousins. I loved them.

One night in Philly I was in the bathtub and I started jerking off. Dad came home from a Party meeting in a fury. I could hear by the way he slammed the door. He always kept a key to the bathroom door so my stepbrothers and I couldn't lock ourselves in. He broke in and caught me and beat the hell out of me. I was slipping and sliding all over the tub, unable to stand, and he just kept pounding me with both fists. I could have whipped him, but a guy doesn't hit his father, no matter what.

"Filthy, rotten, dirty little pig!" he screamed.

I swore I was going to get even, and I did. As summer came to an end, Dad's temper got worse and worse. One night, out of the blue, I came home to see the kitchen filled with a half-dozen comrades. One of them was on the Central Committee.

"Sonny boy, I have a big surprise for you," Dad told me. "The Central Committee has decided, due to my faithful years as a Party member, to waive your age requirements and swear you into the Young Communist League, now . . . before you go back to Baltimore."

. . . So there I was holding up my fist in the Communist salute and repeating an oath after the comrade from the Central Committee. . . . I don't know what happened, exactly, maybe Miss Abigail's voice came from the beyond but . . . I couldn't help it . . . I started reciting the Pledge of Allegiance: "I PLEDGE ALLEGIANCE TO THE FLAG OF THE UNITED STATES OF AMERICA AND TO THE REPUBLIC FOR WHICH IT STANDS, ONE NATION, INDIVISIBLE, WITH LIB-ERTY AND JUSTICE FOR ALL."

The comrades like to shit their pants.

My dad screamed and slapped me in the face in front of everybody. I went to the door. "I'm an American! I'm an American!" I shouted.

"Come back here," my dad demanded.

"Go fuck yourself," I said and ran for it. I ran all the way to the train yard and jumped a freight part of the way back to Baltimore and hitched the rest of the way.

Well, the next week Dad was expelled from the Party and wrote me that he'd never forgive me. Two weeks later he was all over me to start writing

*him letters again. He never admitted it, but I had done him the biggest
favor of his life.*

My brother-in-law, Al Singer, had always had a struggle. Al had
painted many houses so well that he finally got an opening to buy out a
retiring contractor.

"Lazar, I need your help," he petitioned.

Al was no go-getter, but he was honest. I loaned him the money he
needed to buy the business. I had to wait a little too long, we had a lot
of fights, but he paid me back every dime. Al and Fanny and their
children finally moved out of the second-floor flat on Monroe Street to a
place of their own.

With space now available in Bubba's house, Molly and her husband,
Danny, moved from Norfolk, mainly so she could take care of Gideon.
What that boy needed more than anything else was something of his
own. I gave him a little dog as a present. Gideon worshipped that
animal. Dinky he called it. A mutt, but, like Gideon, he was a street
fighter. He rode in Gideon's bicycle basket and slept on Gideon's chest.
The tricks that dog would do for that boy.

For a brief moment, with Molly now in Baltimore, life looked a little
better for Gideon. Then disaster struck, bang, bang, bang.

Leah returned from one of her affairs and just moved right into the
boy's bedroom, so he had to sleep on a couch in the kitchen. Gideon
went on a weekend field trip with his schoolmates, and while he was
gone, Leah had the animal shelter people pick up Dinky and put him to
sleep.

Leah didn't tell Gideon about it and he was certain the dog was
stolen, because Dinky would never have run away from him. For a
month the boy searched high and low, walking through all the adjoining
neighborhoods and shouting for his puppy. It was pathetic.

One night he heard his mother speaking in Yiddish to Bubba and
confiding that she had sent the dog to the pound.

"He was filled with fleas. Gideon was terribly allergic. I only did what
I thought best. I didn't know he would carry on like this."

I don't know if he ever fully forgave his mother for that, but it was as
though a part of him had died, and what came back in its place was
anger.

A few weeks after Gideon learned Dinky had been put to sleep,
Danny Shapiro was hit by a truck and hospitalized for an indefinite
period, with a fractured skull and several broken bones. Molly was a
poorly paid secretary and her salary couldn't cover the medical bills,

much less support herself, her husband, her mother, and her brother. Dom and I dug into our pockets again.

But, thank God for small favors, there was one less mouth to feed because Leah was soon gone again. This time it was to Washington, where she married a little shoe clerk who worked in Sears, Roebuck and did nice things with women's feet and got to steal a quick glimpse up the leg sometimes, when offered. It actually appeared that she would settle down with this guy for a while.

Then came the third blow, the terrible blow, the death of Bubba Hannah, God rest her soul. She went in her sleep, thank God, from a heart attack. The impact on the family was shattering, the most terrible event of our lives. Gideon, already weakened from blow after blow, seemed to be the one hurt the most.

Bubba always loved him a little extra-special. For years she had taken pennies and nickels from the food money and put it away, so when she died each of her grandchildren received . . . eighteen dollars. For Gideon, she left fifty dollars. "That boy is a genius," she always said. "Someday he will make us proud."

Dom and I had to clean up Hannah's affairs and had no choice but to sell the Monroe Street house to pay off a large accumulation of debts. Who should take in Zayde Moses but Al and Fanny.

Gideon passed his sixteenth birthday, but his heart was not in high school. He always managed to be pleasant as a member of my family and sometimes he'd put on a hilarious skit with one of my daughters. But mostly the boy was very sad and depressed. To read his stories had once been a joy, but now the pages were filled with an overwhelming sense of despair. Sometimes I got a terrible feeling that he was searching for death. Simone and Molly also picked up on this.

Gideon was in Forest Park High School, a co-educational institution. There were lots of pretty girls—this was the time of life when tight little blooms opened into flowers. There was a nice Jewish center for the kids in the neighborhood and dances every weekend after the Sabbath. It seemed that every girl Gideon met, who liked him, became the object of a fantasy.

He was desperately, desperately seeking someone of his own. Someone who could love him more than an uncle or a sister. And he pretended that every new little romance was a matter of life and death. He was a charmer and got all of the girls he wanted, but many became frightened of him. He was far too serious, far too soon.

DANNY SHAPIRO was finally released from the hospital, but he had to find work where he could sit at a bench. The accident had left him with one very weak leg and he had terrible headaches from the fractured skull. I took him in as an apprentice pharmacist and let him and Molly fix up a little room in the rear of the drugstore to live.

It wasn't exactly paradise, but I had three children in college and was sending support money for Zayde Moses, as well as taking care of Gideon, Molly, and Danny. I was stretched and it would be a year or two of real hard work for Danny to get certified. So, we made do. Nobody starved.

It went like this for a year. Danny improved steadily and worked like a horse. Gideon . . . he raged inside and failed in school and had the drudgery of summer school. Can you imagine that boy flunking English. No reason for it, except he just didn't care.

A letter came from Leah in Washington. We always dreaded that envelope. She wrote that she was coming to get Gideon and take him to live with her and her Sears shoe salesman.

"LAZAR! LAZAR!" Simone screamed.

I tore down to the basement, where Gideon had his "office." He was face down on the floor, unconscious, an empty pill bottle in his hand. I pried it loose and read the label. Oh God, God, God! Phenobarbital . . . one-grain tablets. It appeared to be a new bottle he had taken from the store . . . oh God . . . one hundred pills were in him. I put my head to his chest. He was breathing, but his breath was becoming labored.

"I want an emergency police ambulance!" I shouted. "Tell them to bring a doctor and a tube. They'll have to flush him on the way to the hospital."

Simone responded instantly, without panic. My daughter Priscilla came in and I screamed to her, "Get the ipecac out of my medicine cabinet and put on coffee! Go!"

She returned with the ipecac and I grabbed him by the hair while Priscilla held his mouth open and I poured the medicine into him, pulling him to his feet. "Give me a bucket!" We held his head while he vomited.

"Let me die . . ." he mumbled with slobber and puke running down his chin.

"Come on, buddy, keep walking. Here! Take some more of this ipecac. Come on, buddy, keep walking! Quick with that coffee!"

The siren of an ambulance was heard.

"Let me . . . ! Let me die!"

THE LORD SMILED on us that day. If we hadn't found him that moment, he would have done himself in. We all broke down and wept when the doctor told us later that he would pull through without permanent damage.

"I'm sorry for all the trouble I caused. I'm sorry," Gideon said.

We were deeply, deeply troubled and knew the lad had to stay under our wing. Neither Molly nor Danny could apply for legal guardianship because of their financial situation.

With a little inside help from Dominick, Gideon's case was placed in the hands of a sympathetic judge, Paul Sklar. Dom and I had to confide in Paul that the boy's father had tried to force him into the Young Communist League and Leah had legally deserted him. Gideon was called into the judge's office to confirm this.

The case against Leah was open and shut. Tears fell down Gideon's cheek as he confirmed her many absences.

"And your father tried to coerce you into becoming a Communist?" the judge asked. "Is that true?"

Gideon's mouth clamped shut.

"It's all right, son. It won't go any further than this office."

He refused to speak.

"You want to stay with your Uncle Lazar, don't you?"

"Yes, sir."

"Well?"

"Nobody's going to make me rat on my dad," Gideon answered.

"Wait outside," the judge ordered. He turned to Dom and me and we nodded that it was true. The judge shook his head and signed the decree for me to be his guardian, but God alone knows what damage had been done to Gideon in those two minutes.

December 7, 1941

WAR!   WAR!   WAR!   WAR!   WAR!

JAPANESE ATTACK PEARL HARBOR! FDR ASKS CON-
GRESS FOR A STATE OF WAR. SNEAK ATTACK CAUSES
MASSIVE DAMAGE. CASUALTIES HIGH. BATTLESHIP *AR-
IZONA* SUNK.

I turned off the radio, but could not stop looking at the newspaper.
Awful! Awful! Simone's eyes were rimmed with red as she patted my
back and stroked my hair. The woman had been so badly damaged by
war, and now, so soon again. I reached back and touched her hand.

"Pierre called from Boston," she said. "He's talking about enlisting."

"I'll get back to him right away. Pierre has always listened," I said.
"They don't want college boys. It's just not his time to go. I assure you,
darling, he will finish his postgraduate work."

"God, the madness. I'll cut Pierre's finger off before I let him go."

No use talking to her when she got like that. I poked through the
icebox. The hell with it. I needed a drink.

"Here, I'll fix it for you," she said.

Molly entered the kitchen with Danny limping behind her. She
looked the color of a corpse.

"Gideon has enlisted in the Marines," she blurted.

I banged on the table. "That's crazy! He's just turned seventeen!"

"He's up in his room packing," Molly said shakily. "He says that if
you don't sign his papers, he's going to run away and enlist somewhere
where he can pass for twenty-one."

"He's got to prove his age and he only started shaving last year."

"He's got an altered birth certificate and they aren't checking ages
too closely."

Oh boy, oh boy, Gideon was going to be one tough customer.

"You want me?" Molly and Danny said together.

"Let me see what I can do," I answered. I went up to the room he
used when Pierre was away, knocked, and entered. He was filling up a
suitcase on the bed.

"Going someplace?"

"Did Molly tell you?"

"She mentioned some *chozzerai* about you trying to enlist in the Marines."

"I have enlisted. There's a consent form on the desk. If you sign it, I can leave from Baltimore tomorrow. Otherwise, I'll just keep going from city to city until one of the recruiting stations takes me."

"An ultimatum? You are talking to your Uncle Lazar, young man. You don't give me ultimatums."

Gideon sighed and relaxed a bit, but those blue eyes of his were penetrating. They said, "Don't stop me."

"Uncle Lazar, I love you. I don't want you to have to get mixed up with this. It's better if I just go."

"What's going on? I'm no longer your guardian? I'm a bum off the streets?"

"Cripes. Look, you and Aunt Simone have been wonderful to me, better than anybody in my life, except Molly. I know if you sign for me, my dad and mom are going to raise blue hell. Why don't you let me make it easy for you by just slipping out?"

"From Nathan Zadok and Leah, I don't exactly tremble with fear. Can we talk, son?"

His eyes flitted about, now avoiding mine. He was very jumpy and jittery. He wanted out, to hit the road. His mind was closed. "You owe me twenty minutes' conversation, for God's sake," I said.

Gideon jumped on the bed, rested his shoulders against the headboard, and nodded to me, daring me to talk him out of it.

"Why the Marines?" I asked.

"That's funny coming from you."

"I joined the Navy, they attached me to the Marines. I was also a grown man. I have my reasons. They're not the same as yours."

"I've always wanted to go into the Marines when I could get rid of that Communist crap. I've seen them at the Fireman-Quantico Marine game, walking out of the stadium in their dress blues with a girl on each arm. I'd look at your picture with the *fourragère* around your left shoulder. I don't really know, Uncle Lazar."

"Then think of reasons."

"I'm not happy here. It's not you. It's not Molly. I'm flunking in school again. I'm not doing what's right with my life. I've got to get out there and find out about it. Maybe the war just makes it a good excuse, I don't know."

"Come on, you can do better than that," I said.

"My Uncle Matti was a hero during the Arab riots in Palestine. You were a hero at Belleau Wood. Miss Abigail was a heroine."

"So you need a war of your own, is that it?"

"I want to be wanted," the boy cried. "I know how much you and Molly love me, but you have your own people to love. I want to belong. I want to be needed. I have to be a writer and I have nothing to write about but sadness and despair."

"So go down to the burlesque show and copy their jokes."

"All right," he cried, "I have to go! I've got to fill my coffers with whores and buddies and feel good about living. I want to look sharp in a uniform. I want to be tough and drink like Hemingway and have mates like the Mexicans in *Tortilla Flat*. With my mom and dad, it's all hate. It's hate. We've all got our time, Uncle Lazar. My time is here. I have to answer."

"That's quite a mouthful, son." I brought the hardback chair up close to the bed, so we were very near to one another.

"I want to fight my own Belleau Wood," he whispered. "I want to be a man, a writer. Every day in the Marine Corps will be a new chapter."

"You know how many would-be writers are under the ground in France?"

"Do you know how many writers were born in war?" he answered.

I sighed because it hurt. All I went through was in vain. Look at his eager face. He couldn't wait to get at the world. There would be no stopping him now. What was that goddam tattoo some of the guys wore on their arm . . . "victory or death" or some shit like that.

"I never spoke much about Belleau Wood," I said. "I never talked about it to Aunt Simone. Writers make this shit glamorous, high adventure, spellbinding romance. So, let's talk about Belleau Wood. Yes, son, it is true I went into the Navy to free myself from Moses Balaban, a father I hated. I wanted to be free of the red-necked bigotry that took my brother, Saul, may his soul rest in peace. I wanted freedom from the Balaban women. . . . I'll tell you about Belleau Wood. . . .

When America entered the war in 1917, a brigade was made up of the Fifth and Sixth Marines and rushed to France to show the flag in the vanguard of the American Expeditionary Force. I was made a Chief Pharmacist's Mate because my special skills were badly needed. My unit, a naval unit, was assigned to the Marine Corps as their medical support group. That's how I got to wear a Marine uniform and won my decorations.

By mid-1917 we had crossed on the troop ship Henderson *and landed at St.-Nazaire filled with hatred of the Hun, looking for French poon and to make the world safe for democracy . . . that was the big slogan. They always have to sell you some kind of shit, so we were convinced the Krauts ate little babies for breakfast. We landed and the French pelted us with flowers as we marched through the villages.*

There were so many stars in our eyes, we didn't see Europe was soaked with the blood of millions of casualties, ravaged landscapes, hunger, disease, mud . . . always mud . . . mud is part of the uniform.

On the Western Front, the British and French faced the Germans on a static line. No one had been able to really dislodge the other for three brutal years. It was a stagnant, filthy line of trenches, a line of horror, set in eternal palls of smoke, poison gas, and barbed wire, and the forests and fields were destroyed with deep craters and muck. Men lived in corrugated tin and sandbag underground cities sharing their lot with millions of rats and billions of lice.

The battles were ferocious. Take one day at the Somme. The British had sixty thousand casualties. Twenty thousand of these men were killed . . . in one day. By the time the Yanks had gotten there, the toll was over ten million dead on both sides and twice that number wounded.

Well, the German staff and their commander, Ludendorff, didn't evaluate the Yanks too highly. When they were able to transfer divisions away from the Eastern Front after Russia sued for a separate peace, they massed a decisive edge in guns and troops. Their aim was to first knock the British out of the war, then break through to Paris.

To punch a hole in the French lines, they organized forty-two divisions of infantry and ten thousand pieces of artillery. No man who has ever been through a bombardment ever forgot it. Well . . . Ludendorff got his hole against the French Sixth Army at a place called Château-Thierry, a little town on the Marne River.

The French Sixth had been torn to shreds and was in full retreat. This opened the gates to Paris. German patrols could actually see the Eiffel Tower through their field glasses.

In order to avoid crossing the Marne River, the Germans decided to bypass it west of Château-Thierry where it took a big bend.

After three days of confusion and conflicting orders, the Marine Brigade drove part of the way and marched part of the way and we reached our destination without having slept for almost three days. It seemed like all of France was fleeing in the opposite direction, women hitched up to carts, old people, cattle filling the road. And the fucking mud.

We reached the line on May 30, 1918, and let the French Sixth Army pass through us and continue their retreat. It was a lovely spring day. The Marne Valley was magnificent. Rolling fields of wheat swayed like sensual women, dancing in rhythm to the kisses of the winds. The wheat was young and still green and the fields were speckled with thousands of blood-red poppies.

The countryside was interspersed by a number of small woods of silver-barked birch and second-growth scrub and thickets. One of these stands of trees was Belleau Wood. It lay on a hillock west of Château-Thierry. The wood was about a mile in length and several hundred yards deep, flanked by five lovely little farming villages. Before the war, Belleau Wood had been the private hunting preserve of a wealthy Frenchman.

The German offensive had swept forward so rapidly it had outrun its artillery and supplies and had to stop to consolidate in Belleau Wood.

To outflank the Marne River, the Germans had to strike right through the middle of a thin line held by the 5th and 6th Marines. We were green, untested troops, but we had been trained well and we were not war-weary as the French were.

My unit set up in a field hospital in the cellar of the church of one of the villages, Lucy de Bocage, just a few hundred yards to the rear of the front lines.

When the artillery fire opened, we had never experienced anything like it and the rest of the battle seemed like a surrealistic play, seen through a gauze . . . a haze . . . exhaustion . . . smoke . . . and we listened to voices and gunfire like they were distant echoes. We were there and functioning, but we were not there, if you know what I mean.

During the course of the war, the snipers from all of the armies had eventually been killed or crippled. The emphasis was now on massive fire, mostly by machine gun. The Germans did not realize that the Marines were the best rifle shots in the world. When they came out of Belleau Wood, our men started picking them off at distances of six hundred yards. We shot them down, accurately, as fast as we could load and fire. Hell, the Krauts never knew what hit them, but on they came, pouring out of the wood into the wheat field. They came all day long and continued through the night. We kept chopping them down, our rifles so hot we could hardly work the bolts. By the end of the second day, they had still not been able to reach our lines. On the third day, they threw everything at us—maybe five or six hundred artillery pieces. They threw out a solid curtain of machine-gun fire and they came again in droves, in hordes. By night, they had to leave the wheat field and retreat into the wood, leaving hundreds, maybe thousands, of their dead on the field.

The instant they stopped to regroup, the 5th and 6th Marines went on to the offensive. I watched them run at high port in line after line and disappear over the ridge.

Inside Belleau Wood . . . that tiny space was honeycombed with a hundred or more German machine-gun nests, dug in behind boulders, hidden in jungle-like thickets. Our job was to flush them out, nest by nest, with grenades and bayonets.

I was on a four-day cycle.

Day one, I drove casualties back to a base hospital about ten miles away and returned with supplies.

Day two, I worked in the field hospital treating the wounded and assisting in surgery.

Day three, I did battlefield duty, finding the wounded, treating them, and taking them back by stretcher.

Day four was my "rest" day. I was given four hours' straight sleep, checked the inventory, and caught up with the reports. One, two, three, four, around the clock without respite.

The worst of it was the field hospital. The wounded were coming off the field so fast we couldn't get to half of them in time. Gangrene set in quickly and some of the arms and legs turned slimy and green and scarlet and lots of bare bones were sticking out. Our medication was primitive. Fever, give them castor oil. Iodine on open wounds, or peroxide. The smell of gangrene . . . ugh . . . I can still smell it. Infection, aspirin. Mustard gas wounds, we just washed them with water. Lot of screaming, moaning, dying. Thank God we had morphine and codeine.

In the operating theaters the floor always had a half inch of blood and the surgeons and assistants like myself slipped and fell and were drenched in blood a half-dozen times a day.

In those days, we didn't know how to type a man's blood. If he needed blood, one of us would volunteer, and as often as not, the Marine died on the spot because we were different blood types. I gave blood twice during the battle.

Our offensive went on day after day. Our gains through Belleau Wood could be counted in yards. Most of the European armies rotated their troops off the front every five or six days, but we didn't have the experience and we didn't have the replacements. The Marines went on, day and night, for fifteen straight days until an American Army unit came in and relieved us.

They generally sent the troops back about six or seven miles behind the lines, out of German artillery range. The first thing was to get deloused. They'd boil their clothing in acid and shave their hair off and give them a sheep dip. Then they'd usually sleep for twenty to thirty straight hours. After that, they'd get their one hot meal and march back to the lines and rotate again.

As I said, we didn't get relieved till two weeks into the battle. We were

*in back of the lines for only five hours. Five stinking hours, after fourteen
days of constant battle. The unit that replaced us were green and it began
losing all the ground we had gained, so . . . after five hours we had to
march back to Belleau Wood and continue the fight.*

Baltimore

WHEN I HAd finished, I couldn't tell whether Gideon was entranced
or horrified. I did something then I had never done before. I always
wore a high-necked undershirt to hide my wound, even when I went
swimming. No one had ever seen it but Simone and my doctor. I took
my shirt and undertop off and showed it to him. It was a hideous scar
filled with little black specks.

"The black specks are part of a German officer's face. He was blown
up right in front of me. They'll never come out."

We sat looking at one another for an infinity of time, holding hands,
like Simone and I do.

It was twenty minutes before we spoke. It seemed an eternity. Had I
talked him out of it?

"You understand that I have to go," Gideon said. "Don't you, Uncle
Lazar?"

"Yes, I know," I said. "We've all got to carry the burden of our times,
fight our own wars, both inside us and out there on the battlefield. It's
the way men have always done things. Don't try to be a hero. Do your
job, and part of your job is coming through alive."

I scratched my signature on the document, giving him permission to
join the Corps. I took off my Marine ring and put it into the palm of his
hand and closed his fist around it. "Take it. This little sucker got me
through. You'll need all the luck you can get."

PART FIVE

JUST BEFORE THE BATTLE, MOTHER

MITLA PASS

October 31, 1956

1100 HOURS, D DAY PLUS TWO

Southern Command to Lions STOP Enemy convoy spotted from air moving on west side of Mitla heading for the Pass STOP We have diverted our air cover from Para 202 to attack convoy STOP We are out of communication with Para 202 STOP Do you know their location SIGNED Ram.

Lions to Southern Command—1130 Hours STOP Negative STOP we are not in contact with Para 202 SIGNED Ben Asher.

Southern Command to Lions STOP Our two northern columns have been slowed at Gaza and Jebel Livni STOP We have not made sufficient penetration for you to try evacuation by land STOP Attempt to clear your runway to length of twenty-five hundred feet by forty feet in order to accommodate Dakotas for possible air evacuation SIGNED Ram

Lions to Southern Command STOP Impossible to clear field by hand STOP Large rocks and boulders can't be moved STOP Advise SIGNED Ben Asher

Southern Command to Lions STOP Will attempt to parachute two bulldozers STOP SIGNED Ram

High Noon

Lions to Southern Command High Noon STOP One bulldozer received in operating condition STOP Estimate airstrip can be cleared by 1600 Hours SIGNED Ben Asher

Southern Command to Lions STOP Air strike against enemy convoy west of Mitla Pass successful STOP New intelligence directly from Cairo sources indicate that only two Egyptian companies are inside Pass STOP Included in enemy force are two mortar and two machine-gun platoons STOP Air Recon reports no activity now on western side of Mitla SIGNED Ram

The sun this day was another brutal bone bleacher. Lethargy had all but consumed the Lions. They shifted about lazily to conserve every molecule of energy. Soft voices were heard from the command post and hospital tent. The bulldozer inched forward, backward, forward, backward, shoving the larger rocks and boulders aside and filling in the pockets they left. Now and again, an Egyptian mortar from high up in the Pass tried to reach the airstrip, without success.

This indicated to Major Ben Asher that the Egyptians didn't have any larger artillery with them, or they would have certainly been using it. He was encouraged by the latest intelligence. The report had come from Cairo. An Israeli spy was apparently inside the Egyptian high command and in a position to know the size and whereabouts of the enemy deployments.

Two companies inside? Not too bad. A few hundred men, more or less. It also appeared that the Israeli Air Force owned the skies and had the western side of the Pass under constant scrutiny.

Gideon's leg seemed miraculously better. The blood had drained away from the enormous swelling in his hip, reducing it to nearly normal size. It was still tender and bruised, but he had gained back nearly full use of the leg.

"Come on, Zechariah, where the fuck are you!" someone shouted every five or ten minutes.

Their eyes were all reddened from constantly straining in the sun for a sign of Para 202. Earlier they thought they had spotted dust rising and sent out a patrol jeep to lead Zechariah's men in. It turned out to be a false alarm. The dust had originated from a sudden lurch of wind winding through a narrow opening in some rocky cliffs.

Ration time. To hell with it, Gideon thought.

"Eat or you'll get weak," Shlomo said. "Eat, this sun sucks the starch out of you."

"You sound like my stepmother, Lena. Did you ever know anybody who got their sex kicks out of stuffing people with food?"

"Yeah," Shlomo answered, "half the women in Israel."

Gideon ran his hand over his face. The stubble was getting prickly. He hated wearing a beard. It itched constantly. Penelope and Roxy had made him grow one once, a long one, because some of their girlfriends' daddies were growing them.

"Suppose you were in a nice comfortable sheik's tent," Shlomo ventured between vocal bites of food, "and you had a choice between Val and Natasha?"

"Who am I? King Solomon?" Gideon answered. "They come from two different planets. On the one hand, peace, comfort, steadiness, softness, fidelity, trust. On the other hand, it's wild fantasy, sensuality, the fine cutting line between love and rage."

"They both sound pretty good to me," Shlomo said.

"Sometimes you need one, sometimes you need the other. Too bad they don't come in the same package."

"What makes a woman like Natasha tick?"

"All women have a labyrinth inside their heads. Emotion is a woman's first priority. When a woman gets devious, I'm screwed. I went through every crooked move as a kid, in Hollywood, in my marriage. But I couldn't be as devious as the simplest woman. Anyhow, I'm pretty up front now. After Val went on her little binge and tore my office to pieces, I didn't want to shelter lies anymore. Even the most honest of women have crooked minds, and being a concentration camp survivor, Natasha is even more complicated."

"How many concentration camp survivors do you suppose we have interviewed?" Shlomo asked, rummaging through his pack. The fruit had gone soft and squishy. He tossed it, grudgingly, and out of nowhere little ants started appearing and feasted.

"I count between fifty and sixty," Gideon said. "Besides that, I've read maybe three hundred case histories. I'd read more than a hundred in St. Barths before I got to Israel."

"Every one different?"

"Every one different, but certain similarities in all of them. Every person who got through the camps left behind twenty, thirty members

of their families dead. I found that everyone who survived had to use
their wits. But every person who walked out of a concentration camp
alive had run into a piece of golden luck at the right moment. Sometimes four or five pieces of luck. This kind of luck produces guilt."

"My father died, my brothers died, but I got through because I had
luck at the right moment and they didn't. That what you mean?"
Shlomo asked.

"That's right," Gideon said. "I've never met a survivor who didn't
carry the cross of guilt on his shoulder because his being alive represented twenty who were sent to the gas chamber. Why did I, who was
no more worthy than the next guy, get through? Why am I alive? I'm
guilty for being alive."

"What's the toll on Natasha's family?"

"All of them. A big family . . . all of them . . . not only mother,
father, brothers, but uncles, cousins, the works. Natasha's guilt is compounded because she hated her father before the war. He was a professional, respected, important member of the community. Apparently he
was a cold number, very strict. He didn't abuse her physically, but she
was frightened of him and he brought a great deal of pain, sexually, to
his wife. She loved her mother dearly. And . . . she's got more than
ordinary, garden-variety guilt about her father's death. She felt responsible for his death because she hated him."

"So she looks for her father through lovers?"

"I read it this way," Gideon said. "She finds an attractive man and
gets him to fall for her. No trick, she oozes sex from every pore. She
loves him with a fury he didn't know existed. And she drinks him dry.
When he is completely exhausted, she has the symbol she is looking for.
She's killed her daddy again. So, she discards him like a dishrag, but she
always has a sentimental feeling for him. Poor dog, just couldn't cut it.
But her drive to find another man, and another and another, is insatiable. She can't control herself from playing it out, over and over."

"And you, my little friend?"

"I've got her stumped, Shlomo. Europeans, Czechs, Hungarians, Ro-
manians, people who live by their wits and guile are her meat. I'm
nobody's sweetheart, but my mind can only get so crooked. I'm not up
to games. What you see is what you get. I've done all the mean shit
before, and it's out of my system. Natasha has a hard time dealing with
that. She knows I'm on to her game, her reasons, and that I can handle
her sexually. Then, she made the cardinal error of falling in love with an
intended victim. She loves me. I love her in a way. Real messy. It drives
her nuts, but she can't put the sword through the bull's neck."

"Fucking to the death. It sounds like a great sport," Shlomo said.

The officers broke up a meeting with the major and commanded the troops to pack up and prepare to go down to the airstrip for evacuation.

"Isn't he early?" Gideon asked.

"No, it's almost time. The first Dakota is due in about twenty-five minutes."

The bulldozer had just finished the job and hand crews were filling in the potholes.

"God-damned, shit, piss, and corruption," Gideon blurted angrily. "Jesus, this has been like washing your feet with your socks on."

"Win some, lose some," Shlomo said. "Let's hope to hell the Dakotas are able to land."

At that instant, a jeep out on the perimeter raced toward the command post. The officer shouted at the top of his lungs, "I see Para 202! Zechariah is here!"

October 31, 1956
1700 HOURS, D DAY PLUS TWO

> *Lions to Southern Command 1700 Hours STOP Para 202 has linked up with us STOP Cancel Dakota air evacuation STOP We will radio list of most urgently needed supplies and equipment within the hour SIGNED Ben Asher*

> *Central Command Tel Aviv to all Southern Command Air Units 1720 Hours STOP Anglo-French squadrons have commenced bombing Egyptian airfields STOP Stay clear of eastern side of Canal and Gulf of Suez SIGNED Hod, Air Chief, more follows, more follows, more follows, more follows Central Command to all Ground Units STOP Anglo-French Expeditionary Force has launched an attack on Port Said area with objective of seizing Canal STOP Israel has agreed to ultimatum to halt our forces eight miles from Canal STOP Confirm and comply SIGNED Dayan, Chief of Staff*

Just before nightfall an air drop replenished the diminished inventory of Para 202, and a full assessment of the brigade's battle-ready condition was under way. A hundred and fifty miles of cruel desert had savaged men, vehicles, and arms.

Zechariah's paras were grungy and exhausted and craved sleep, like men in battle since ancient times. Most of them had been getting by on catnaps since the mobilization over a week earlier. They were punch-drunk, thick of tongue, and their mouths were too tired to chew food.

In the command tent, Colonel Zechariah studied the map with Major Ben Asher. The famed Colonel Z was both large and well-muscled, with a shining black beard that gave him a look of madness, like an ancient prophet in a rage. It seemed as though half the desert was caked on his face, his eyelids, his beard, and his baked, cracked lips. His clothing was torn in several places, sticky with sweat. He took no time for the luxury of a cleanup until plans were settled for tomorrow. Outside the tent, men were in deep sleep on the ground.

His aide, Captain Kofsky, entered with Dr. Schwartz.

"What's the story?" Zechariah asked.

"There is no way you can push this unit out tomorrow," Dr. Schwartz said. "They are beyond exhaustion and they will not perform. If you try to go tomorrow, you're going to lose half of them. They're just going to fold, collapse." The doctor was pointed in his opening remark because he knew Zechariah would drive them before they were ready, unless he made a stand.

"They'll rest at the end," Zechariah said. "I'll give them all a week to sleep after we take Sharm al-Sheikh."

"It's a hundred and seventy miles down the Gulf of Suez," the doctor retorted. "They need two days' rest and regrouping before they can go."

"Not before November third! Yoffe's Brigade is moving down the other side. He'll beat me to Sharm al-Sheikh! Half of his men are reservists. I will not let Yoffe beat the paratroops! I must get there first. I want to have a welcoming committee for Yoffe when he arrives!"

Captain Kofsky, the doctor, and Major Ben Asher held their tongues while Colonel Zechariah fumed. He peered out of the tent. It looked like a battlefield full of dead men.

"Why don't we wait till morning, see what shape the equipment is in, let the men have a night's sleep, and we'll also be in better shape to make a decision," Ben Asher said.

Wait! Zechariah did not like waiting! He did not like assessing! He did not like delaying decisions! Bang on through, that's the way! Damned! Damned! What if Yoffe actually got there first?

He dismissed Kofsky and the doctor with a wave of the hand, then turned to Ben Asher.

"We can't just screw up a day sleeping here while the whole Sinai is in flames. Ben Asher, your Lions have been sitting on their asses for two days now. They should be ready to do a little work tomorrow."

"What do you have in mind?" the major asked.

"Before we swing south, I want Mitla Pass secured. We go in with your battalion and take it tomorrow at dawn."

"Sorry, Zech, I've got specific orders from Dayan that we are not to enter Mitla under any circumstances."

"Since when can't the commander in the field change orders?"

"That's up to you, but you'll have to relieve me of my command first. I won't take them into the Pass until Central changes my orders."

"Come on now, Ben Asher. For Christ sake. You want me to move the brigade south and leave Mitla Pass wide open and our backs exposed?"

"I've had a chance to examine every piece of intelligence for two days. True, the Egyptians don't have a large force in the Pass. They are in there to try to prevent us from reaching the Canal. Okay? Purely defensive. But God dammit, Zech, even a few hundred Egyptians dug in in those cliffs and defiles could really mess us up. Besides, we are complying with the ultimatum to stop eight miles before the Canal. If we go in and take the Pass, we'd be in violation."

"Don't give me any political shit. I'm not going to let the Egyptians jump me in the back."

"Zech, there's no way on God's earth that Egypt can mount an offensive. Israel is winning on four fronts. The French and the British have jumped Egypt. Mitla Pass isn't worth a pound of camel shit. And we may get slaughtered if we go in."

"I gave you an order, Ben Asher. Yes or no?"

"No. I will not commit my troops to you without orders directly from Central."

"Your troops! Since when have the Lions been your troops? I created the paratroops. I put you in this command. Now get this, very clearly. At zero five three zero tomorrow, either you will lead the Lions into the Pass or the new commander will."

"No, not unless I get an order from Central," Ben Asher repeated softly.

It was concrete facing off against granite. Zechariah snarled over the map, took a message pad from his kit, and scribbled out a communication.

"Runner!" Zechariah yelled. A para spilled into the tent.

Para 202 to Central Command STOP 1800 Hours STOP Urgent STOP Most secret STOP It is my considered opinion as the commander in the field and on the scene that Mitla Pass poses a threat to our rear STOP Request permission to remove Ben Asher from his command and use Lions to take the Pass SIGNED Colonel Z.

Zechariah settled in on a canvas field chair, propped his boots up on the map table and tilted back and forth and sipped from his canteen, waiting for the return message.

Central Command to Para 202 STOP 1820 Hours STOP Permission to relieve Ben Asher denied STOP Permission to capture Mitla Pass denied STOP REPEAT denied STOP Late intelligence via Cairo now indicates full infantry battalion inside Pass with one dozen medium machine guns STOP One dozen 57MM anti-tank guns and forty Czech recoilless rifles STOP Enemy dug in at Heitan Defile STOP Egyptian posture is entirely defensive to block a move against Canal STOP They pose no offensive threat to our forces in the Sinai STOP We consider it extremely dangerous to try to dislodge them. CONFIRM, SIGNED Dayan, Chief of Staff

Zechariah was a man known for his power to bulldoze his way through anything, circumvent orders he did not care to read, run his own show. He almost always won his battles, so opposition usually melted before his wrath. Not so this time. Everyone at Central was aware. The Lions' commander was aware. It was no go into Mitla Pass. He wrote out another communication and handed it to the major.

"I hope you'll see my point, Ben Asher."

"All right, I'll agree to this," the major answered.

"Let's shake hands and forget the threats and harsh words."

"Of course, heat of the battle."

The two men shook hands like two pieces of steel clanging and embraced with rib-breaking slaps of affection.

Para 202 to Central Command STOP 1830 Hours STOP Confirming orders not to capture Mitla Pass STOP Nevertheless our defensive position around the airstrip and Parker Monument is extremely exposed to both artillery and air STOP Ben Asher is in agreement with me that we should probe into the Pass with a patrol to see if we can find a better defensive position STOP We will stop short of the Egyptian defensive position at the Heitan Defile STOP We will withdraw patrol as soon as it meets enemy opposition STOP With our new defensive position inside the Pass I will feel safe to swing south STOP Will try to find a position inside Pass that can be held by no more than two infantry companies STOP Brigade plans to move south along Gulf of Suez at 0600 November 3 STOP Confirm SIGNED Colonel Z.

Central Command to Para 202 STOP 1900 Hours STOP Permission granted to use Lions for a limited patrol into Pass stopping short of the Heitan Defile STOP Withdraw immediately if opposition is encountered. SIGNED Dayan, Chief of Staff

"Put the Lions on alert to jump off at zero five three zero."

"What do we need the entire battalion for? This is only a limited patrol," the major said suspiciously.

"Calm down, Ben Asher. I'm not going to use the full battalion. I'm too damned tired to make out a plan now. Just have them at the ready; I'll only use a part of them. I can't think straight at the moment."

Ben Asher gave a reluctant "Very well."

Shlomo and Gideon caught up with Colonel Z. at the water tanker, stark naked and chipping away at his grime.

"Ah, there's my writer," Zechariah said. "I heard you got a few bumps on the parachute drop."

"I'm okay."

"Well, are we as good as the Marines or not?"

"Pretty close, I'd say."

He dried himself and put on the same uniform he had been wearing for over a week. "Airplane hit the truck with the extra clothing. Everything went up in smoke . . . *pssst.* The Egyptians will probably run when they smell us."

"You in a good mood?" Gideon asked.

"Why not? I'll still beat Yoffe's Brigade to Sharm."

"I want permission to go into the Pass on the patrol."

Zechariah dug his fingers into his beard and thought as he scratched. "Sure," he said at last, "you ride in the command vehicle with Ben Asher."

"That includes me," Shlomo said.

"Fine. You two can handle the machine gun in the command car. You want a game of chess later, writer?"

"I think I'd better get some sleep," Gideon said.

GIDEON HUMMED a tune as he checked his gear for the morning patrol.

Shlomo was very pensive. He didn't like the idea that the entire Lion's Battalion was on standby. Colonel Z. had also ordered half-tracks and the three operating tanks to be ready. He wouldn't back away from a fight, no matter what the orders were. Zechariah had punched through the Egyptian position at Thamad like a battering ram. That one was vintage Colonel Z.

Gideon sang his song louder and louder. . . .

"What the hell's the name of that song? You sing it all the time."

"It's an old American Civil War tune, 'Just Before the Battle, Mother.' We sang it in school when we were kids."

"Sounds like you're hoping for a fight," Shlomo said.

Gideon became serious. "Maybe that's why I'm out here. To see how Jews fight in rocky places. Shlomo, I meant to tell you, this patrol is not a Foreign Office assignment. I really don't think you ought to come. It's not really your business, but it is mine."

"I've got nothing else to do tomorrow," he answered.

"You sure?" Gideon asked.

"I'm sure."

Gideon rolled up in his blanket fairly close to his mate. "I think I'm too damned excited to sleep," he said.

"Who is Pedro?" Shlomo asked abruptly.

"Why did you ask that?"

"You've called me Pedro a half-dozen times since we've been here."

"Freudian slip, I guess."

"So, who is he?"

"Just a buddy in the Marines."

"What happened to him?"

"Let's get some sleep," Gideon answered.

"I thought you said you couldn't sleep. What happened to Pedro?"

"I didn't get to him fast enough."

"What do you mean?"

"I hesitated. He was killed."

Shlomo heard Gideon's hard, nervous breathing. Just before the battle, Mother, he thought. Oh boy, Gideon had come home. "Don't do anything foolish tomorrow," he said.

November 1, 1956
0515 HOURS D DAY PLUS THREE

ORDERS OF THE DAY 11/1/56 The following units will fall in
at 0530 in full combat gear:

Company A Lion's Battalion
Company B Lion's Battalion
Company C Lion's Battalion
Recon Unit—Para 202—with full rock-climbing gear
Tank Squadron B—remaining three tanks
Heavy Mortar Platoons—Para 202

Companies A and B will proceed into Mitla Pass in half-tracks.

Company C will be in ready reserve west of Parker Monument.

Medical and Command Post units will follow into Pass and establish communications center in secure area around map coordinate
A-16

Recon unit will enter by heavy truck to map coordinate C-17 and
then proceed by foot to climb to the top of cliffs and attack
enemy from above.

All messages by voice in Hebrew.

OBJECTIVE: To secure and maintain defensive positions inside
Mitla Pass to prevent an Egyptian breakout into Sinai proper.

Major Ben Asher in command.

SIGNED: Colonel Amos Zechariah, Commander Para 202.

Ben Asher marched briskly, at a half trot, into the command tent,
ordering his officers to wait outside.
"Good morning, Ben Asher," Colonel Zechariah said, "I've been expecting you. Have the units formed?"

"They are forming now, Colonel, but I think we'd better talk about this so-called patrol."

"As I said, I was expecting you."

"Last night you and I and Command Central agreed to send in a patrol to probe for better defensive positions. This is not a patrol you've ordered. This a full combat team. I think you have deceived us, and I believe you are planning to capture the Pass."

Zechariah remained calm to belie his reputation. "Read this," he said. "I was making up an order during the night, when this message arrived." He handed the message to Ben Asher.

Command Central to all ground, air, and naval units STOP 0330 Hours URGENT URGENT URGENT Anglo-French Expeditionary Force has been forced to cease all operations due to pressures from Washington and Moscow STOP We will continue operations on all fronts until objectives have been reached SIGNED D. Ben-Gurion, Prime Minister SIGNED Dayan, Chief of Staff

"Jesus Christ," Ben Asher mumbled. He read the communiqué again, dropped it on the map table, and stared at it.

"We're all alone now," Zechariah said. "Jordan may take a crack at entering the war. So might Syria."

"Can our units reach their objectives before America and Russia force us into a cease-fire?"

Zechariah shrugged. "We have to move very fast. On the Northern Axis, the Seventh Armored has probably reached El Arish. They'll get a fight there. They'll have to go like hell to reach the Canal. Central Axis . . . we've broken through at Jebel Livini and are probably now facing opposition at Kfar Gafafa. We are here at Mitla. Yoffe's Ninth Brigade is just kicking off. They'll reach Taba by tonight and then their fun begins. They've got close to a hundred and fifty miles of mountainous, untracked desert before they reach Sharm al-Sheikh. How do you say it . . . there's good news and bad news. Every column has to perform perfectly from here on out to avert a disaster."

"How long have we got?"

"The way I figure it, if our two northern columns haven't reached the Canal by tomorrow night and if we haven't captured Sharm al-Sheikh by the fourth, we're fucked."

"Why don't I take our combat team and head south now?" Ben Asher asked. "You can start with the rest of the brigade tomorrow morning and we can leapfrog down to Sharm."

"With France and England out of it, the Egyptians may get bold and release their reserves. I don't want to get pinned down here at the Pass."

Ben Asher nodded that he understood. The two were in accord for the first time. "What do you want me to do, Zech?"

"Capture Mitla Pass."

"We're going to get our asses fried."

"So, we'll get our asses fried. Dayan did the same kind of thing during the War of Independence. He broke orders so he could take Lydda. We still have the basic rule of war: that the commander in the field can make the ultimate decision. You being in agreement is all the support I need."

"Let's talk about this plan," the major said. "I don't like taking our armor, men, and vehicles right through the middle of the wadi bed. The Egyptians will be entrenched over the top of us, shooting down."

"There is no easy way. We have no room for tactical finesse. As soon as we encounter fire, disperse for the best cover and keep the Egyptians pinned down. That will give the Recon unit the opportunity to climb the cliffs near the Egyptian positions and get above them at the Heitan Defile. It's going to be a dirty day, Major, a very dirty day."

Captain Kofsky entered. "The troops are formed, Zech," he said.

"I'll give them a little pep talk," Colonel Z. said.

THE TAUNTING MYSTERY of Mitla Pass was about to be answered. That silent conglomerate of massed pale red rock loomed large as the Lions moved forward into its ominous but alluring jaws.

As they entered the wadi bed and the Pass itself, Gideon and Shlomo lifted a fifty-caliber air-cooled machine gun onto a stationary pole attached to the command truck. The gun was set down on its swivel, and Gideon whistled lightly through his teeth as he swung it around in an arc to set up his field of fire. In a moment they were inside, beneath hundreds of feet of sheer cliffs filled with fissures and caves. Where was the enemy? They could be there, there, there, or there. Anywhere? Holy shit. A platoon of Marines could hold this pass forever.

Scared, Gideon whistled "Just Before the Battle, Mother" beneath his breath. It was like the landing at Tarawa . . . jumping out into chest-high water with the Japs pouring fire at them.

Gideon signaled to Shlomo to feed a belt of ammunition to him. He cracked the bolt twice as Shlomo tidied it to feed it in straight, so it wouldn't jam. They were ready.

"Forward to Ben Asher, do you read me?"

"Ben Asher to Forward, loud and clear."

"Forward to Ben Asher, no sight of enemy."

"Ben Asher to Forward, how far in are you?"

"Forward to Ben Asher, one mile."

"Ben Asher to Forward, slow your movement. Look for cover if you are attacked. Ben Asher to all units, look around you for cover."

The tanks crunched the rock, and the heavy trucks tossed their human cargo around, as the mass of rock in the wadi bed grew larger from slides. Up and down the canyon walls a discordant cantata of half-track engines roaring and barfing exhaust.

"Forward to Ben Asher, Heitan Defile dead ahead."

"Ben Asher to Recon, hide your vehicles and commence climbing out of enemy sight. Work your way over the top of Defile."

"Recon to Ben Asher, order received."

"Ben Asher to Recon, can you estimate length of time needed to scale Defile?"

"Recon to Ben Asher, rough estimate, three or four hours."

"Shit," Ben Asher mumbled. "Okay, we'd better prepare for a messy day. Ben Asher to all units. Start seeking cover immediately outside of wadi bed. Dig in, cover Recon unit. Hit anything that moves. Keep enemy pinned."

The instant the Recon unit began their climb, a smoke shell from the caves in the Defile arched out and down to the wadi bed, exploded, and signaled the Egyptians to open fire. In what seemed a single blast, Mitla Pass erupted with cannon, mortar, machine-gun, and small arms fire.

"Scatter!"

The paras leaped from their vehicles and hugged the canyon walls, seeking crevices and boulders for cover.

Whoooomph! The fuel truck took a direct hit and sent a column of flames leaping two hundred feet up the canyon wall.

Gunfire came not only from the Defile, but from almost a full circle of positions in front, alongside, and behind the para column.

"God dammit!" Ben Asher roared. "They slipped back into other positions during the night! Driver! Pull into that draw over there." It gave barely enough cover to hold the command car and the ambulance. They set up a first-aid station and message center. Ben Asher's view was not far enough into the Pass. He looked about. A ledge above him showed more promise. He climbed to it with the radio man, the driver, and a half-dozen command post personnel. Yes, it was much better . . . a good look down the wadi bed, clear to the Defile. Gideon and Shlomo hid the command car and carried the machine gun to the command post ledge and manned it.

The fire fight intensified as the paras first dug in, answered fire, then sent out squads to pick off the Egyptian nests, one by one, with bayonets and grenades.

A half-track in the wadi bed exploded and then ten thousand rocks shook loose as the ammunition truck blew to kingdom come . . . then the ambulance went . . . another half-track and another . . .

"Ben Asher to Colonel Z., can you read me?"

"Z. to Asher, you're coming in about three and three, very low. I can barely make you out, over."

"Ben Asher to Z., we have lost our ambulance and ammo truck. We are completely surrounded. All troops well deployed, but we're having to take positions one at a time."

"Z. to Asher, ammo truck and ambulance on the way."

"Asher to Z., you're going to have to have the reserve company lead them in. We're blocked. C Company has to open a hole and keep a lane, so we can move in and out around map coordinate A-12."

"MiGs! Hit the dirt!"

Flying in a line, six MiGs came in from twelve o'clock high, strafing the middle of the wadi bed. More vehicles were torched.

"Medic! Medic!"

A dozen wounded were pulled, dragged, carried back to the aid station a few feet from Ben Asher's ledge. Israeli tanks and mortars had established cover and were firing at the Egyptian positions, but the fire seemed ineffective. Runners and radios crackled with messages . . . Hallelujah, two Egyptian machine guns had been reached and taken!

Ben Asher gained control of the battle, directing the movements of his units until the Egyptians spotted the command post and plastered it with mortar fire.

"We've got to get them out of there!" the major yelled. "Dammit, we've got to give better firing directions."

Gideon spotted a fissure some twenty feet above them. It appeared to afford a better view down the wadi. He tapped the commander on the shoulder and pointed up.

"Good," Ben Asher said and looked for people to run up a phone line. "Shit, where is everyone?"

"Comm truck was hit. We're short of radio and telephone men—I'll run it up," Shlomo volunteered. Gideon grabbed the second handle on the phone reel. "You'll never get up there with your leg," Shlomo said.

"Want to bet!"

Ben Asher handed Gideon his binoculars, and Gideon and Shlomo struggled up with the wire moving hand over hand up a sheer wall to the fissure. He pulled Gideon in. Gideon scanned with the field glasses. "It's a beauty! We can see everything! Hey! There's Recon. They're going up the cliffs like mountain goats!"

"Ben Asher," Shlomo shouted down, "we can direct the tank and mortar fire from here! Send up a map!"

The map was hurled up tied to a rock as Gideon spliced on a field phone.

"Stay here with the phone," Gideon said. "I'm going up a few more yards. I'll call the numbers down to you."

Shlomo looked at the place Gideon intended to crawl to. It was terribly exposed. "No, better let me go, you phone down."

"I can't speak Hebrew. You'll have to man the phone," Gideon said. "Don't look so worried. I spotted for artillery on Tarawa." And he was gone. Ten yards away and out on a ledge he lay on his belly and with his binoculars brought the battle into focus: Three tanks hidden behind large boulders; the infantry working their way toward machine-gun nests; and the Recon unit scaling the sheer rock wall of the Defile.

"Oh boy! Hot damned! I'll whack the living shit out of them!" Gideon cried. In a moment he settled down. Fear diminished and hard work began.

Shlomo called up the numbers of the three tanks.

"Shlomo! Have Tank J move forward about twenty yards!"

"I've got it!"

"Tank H, raise elevation two feet!"

"Got it!"

An Egyptian squad across the wadi spotted Gideon and fired. Shlomo didn't like it, but instructions were coming down so fast, he didn't protest.

"Whammo! Tank H is right on target. They're hitting the line of caves in the Defile. Keep firing and move fire fifteen yards left after each shot!"

"Got it!"

The noise was now eardrum-breaking. The sound of every shot, rifle, pistol, gun, grenade, mortar, artillery was magnified a half-dozen times by the narrow walls. The roar became gigantic. Cotton and ear plugs helped slightly, but it was almost impossible to hear and Gideon's shouts had to be repeated a half-dozen times on each order.

"Where the fuck's our air support!" Ben Asher demanded. "Shlomo! Where the fuck's our air support!"

"Gideon! Can you see our air? We need their support! The canyon walls are fouling our transmissions."

"Too tight to send them down here!" Gideon shouted. "Suggest you radio back to Colonel Z. to speak to them. Suggest you have them circle above the Defile and keep the Egyptian planes off our asses. That's the best they can do!"

After three repeats the message got to Shlomo, who phoned it down to Ben Asher.

"Shlomo! Tell Tank K he's firing way too high! Lower elevation at least ten degrees!"

"Got it!"

In a few moments sight of the Israeli Ouragans hovering above the scene caused an eruption of cheers, but they could no longer be heard over the din.

For two murderous hours gunfire continued to pour from the muzzles of both sides. The canyon shook and spewed rocks, as Company C fought its way in with more ammo and medical supplies.

The Recon squad continued up the face of the Defile like a group of alpine rock climbers. It was slow, torturous going. Gideon was able to direct them from his vantage point to avoid Egyptian fire.

"Ben Asher to Z. Casualties heavy! I need trucks to carry them out!"

"Medic! Medic! Medic!"

"Command to Z. Major Ben Asher has been hit! Captain Masada is taking command."

"Z. to Masada. How badly is Ben Asher hurt?"

"Masada to Z. He's dead."

Another hour passed and another. The Egyptians, realizing the gunfire spotter was causing major damage, opened a mortar barrage on the semi-exposed ledge. Gideon cringed as the impact of their shells smashed his face against the rock, shattered his binoculars, and flipped him over like a pancake.

All around the canyon wall, small units of paras knocked out one enemy position after another. At last they destroyed the Egyptian mortar nest which had zeroed in on the spotter.

Para toeholds in the high ground rolled up the solid line of the Egyptian infrastructure. The paras had squeezed out some breathing and maneuvering room and continued methodically to wipe out the nests.

"Recon to Masada! We have reached the top of Heitan Defile! Casualties heavy! We should be above the main Egyptian defenses in another hour!"

Gideon's binoculars were gone, Shlomo's line was cut, and the tanks and mortar squads ran out of ammunition at the same moment. "Come on down, Gideon. Let's get the fuck out of here!" Shlomo yelled.

"Good! I can't direct any more fire. Look!"

Shlomo saw the tanks retreating and became fascinated watching the Recon men lowering each other down a sheer wall on ropes and tossing grenades into the Egyptian caves.

"Masada!" Shlomo shouted down. "We're securing our position! Tanks are withdrawing and none of the mortars are in operation!"

"Get your asses down here quick!" Masada called up.

Stray bullets had been ricocheting off the walls all day. As Shlomo raised himself to assist Gideon coming down, he caught a bullet in the stomach and slid, rolled, bounced, and hurtled off the ledge into the command post. Gideon, his injured leg all but inoperable, limped; then he leaped to the ground and crawled to Shlomo.

"Hey, baby! Hey, baby! Talk to me, Pedro! Pedro! Talk to me, man! God dammit, talk to me . . . Shlomo! Pedro! Shlomo! Pedro!"

Central to Para 202 STOP Our forces have broken through on northern and central axis STOP They will reach Canal by tonight STOP Yoffe's Brigade ahead of schedule STOP At dawn tomorrow move Para 202 down Gulf of Suez to assist in capture of Sharm al-Sheikh. SIGNED Dayan, Chief of Staff

Para 202 to Central STOP 1430 Hours. Inquiry STOP Should I leave a defensive force inside Mitla Pass SIGNED Colonel Z.

Central to Para 202 STOP 1435 Hours STOP Negative to your inquiry STOP Abandon Mitla Pass STOP It has no military value SIGNED Dayan, Chief of Staff.

Gideon sat on a tiny knoll at the edge of the airstrip and looked down at the row of corpses, now sacked in plastic bags, waiting to be taken back to Israel. The wounded had already been evacuated. This would be the last flight.

Gideon felt a presence and looked up. Zechariah towered above him, then sat beside him and also stared at the dead.

"Hello, writer. I heard you had a big day directing tank and mortar fire."

"I don't speak Hebrew," Gideon said in an angry whisper. "Shlomo did all the work."

"You're too modest. You were very courageous, both of you. You stayed out there in an exposed position for hours."

"It was the only place we could find with a clear view."

There was a long silence; bitter nothings passed between them unsaid.

"Do you have a clear view now?" Zechariah asked. "Did we stage for you the battle you craved? Can you now march forward into immortality?"

Gideon closed his eyes and shed a tear. "Shut up, Colonel," he said.

"Oh, I see. The writer thinks it got too untidy in there. The writer is now passing great judgments. Mitla Pass did not have to be taken. Zechariah is a butcher."

"You're reading my thoughts exactly," Gideon said.

"What the hell did you think you were going to find out there? Supermen? Ancient Hebrews scaling sheer walls with God's angels circling around them and turning enemy bullets into rose petals?"

Gideon started to move away, but Zechariah grabbed his arm. "Do you think I am without tears, writer?"

"You? Don't be ridiculous."

"My kid brother was killed today at El Arish. He was . . . he was . . . my kid brother. . . ."

"I'm sorry."

"Fifty of my boys lie dead down there. I had to learn at an early age to cry inside and only when I'm alone."

"But this was such an act of futility!" Gideon said clenching his fists.

"All wars are acts of futility, writer. So, Zechariah maybe made a bad judgment in battle. Maybe not. History and the Lord alone will pass on that. We wanted a state. From the time I was twelve years old, I have done nothing but serve that state. Zechariah, Bedouins are marauding a village; Zechariah, give us a paratroop brigade; Zechariah, cross the border and give the Syrians a lesson. Make those boys hard, Zechariah, make them invincible, make them scale cliffs under enemy fire. Ah yes, but Jews are not supposed to die in battle. Jewish generals are supposed to get their wisdom directly from the Almighty. Well, writer, we have been under arms from birth, all of us, and twice in less than a decade we have been called to all-out war. Win it fast, Zechariah! We don't have the time and resources for a long war! Get it done any way you can! Do you think this is the last time Israel will have to come through Mitla Pass?"

Gideon stared into the troubled face of the colonel.

"But we are a democracy. We will talk and talk and talk. Jews are liberal, peaceful. Warriors are fascists. So, there will be a commission of inquiry filled with intellectuals and our free press will roast me alive. And then all those great thinkers and great statesmen will go and fuck everything up and lead us to the brink of another war. And they'll come to me and say, There's a mess out there, Zechariah. Go clean it up for us. They do the talking. Zechariah does the dirty work. And maybe, mistakes will be made in battle and there will be another commission of inquiry. Perhaps someday we will find that flawless general who can lead us into bloodless victories. Or have you forgotten how many times your glorious Marine generals fucked up in battle?"

Captain Kofsky approached them. "Dakota is in radio contact. It will be landing anytime now, Zech. The brigade is forming up to bid them farewell."

Zechariah came to his feet. "We're heading south tomorrow, writer. I've got to beat Yoffe to Sharm al-Sheikh. You want to ride with us? Come on, I'll take you in my own jeep."

Gideon pulled himself to his feet and massaged his gimpy leg. "I want to take Shlomo home," he said.

"You're a good man, Zadok. Write us a hell of a book, will you?"

The three of them stood transfixed as the Dakota appeared on the horizon. The desert air stirred a bit and the plane wigwagged down to hit the narrow runway like a child's paper toy, screeched, spat up dirt from its wheels, and sputtered to a stop. Voices of the officers called Para 202 to attention. The bugler sounded taps as Zechariah and Captain Kofsky walked briskly toward them and Gideon limped, a few steps behind.

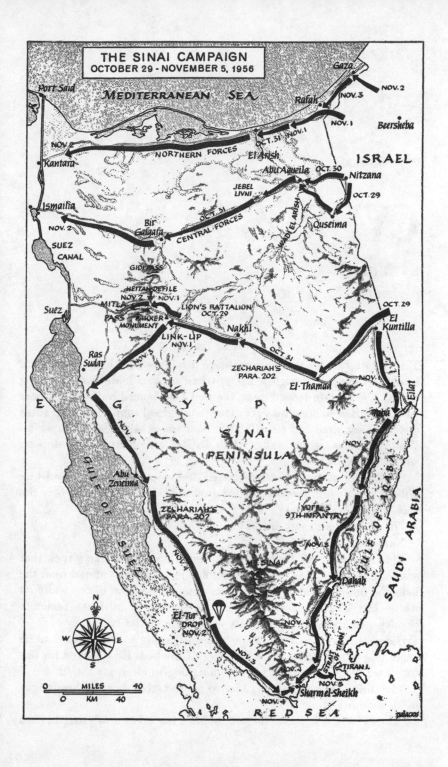

CYPRUS

KYRENIA
November 12, 1956

THE BREEZE OFF the sea was sharp; it billowed the long lace curtain into the room, as though a big sail had broken loose from a racing yacht. The curtain leaped upon the bed and danced on Gideon's bare back. He tried to open his eyes. They were glued shut. He forced them open and squinted and teared. The room was a bright white on white. White curtains, white walls, white wicker armchairs, white dresser, white, white white.

"Shithouse mouse," Gideon blurted, his voice drowned in the white pillows and a white sheet entangled around his naked body. "Where the fuck am I?"

"Right here with me, *habibi.*"

Natasha's voice.

Gideon tried to lift his head from the pillow. It was like a rock that someone was pounding with a sledgehammer. Natasha entered from the balcony, flowing. Natasha! Red hair, a joyous invasion of the white on white. Her long, slender neck bore an expanse of intricate Yemenite jewelry and a smashing green silk robe clung to her body.

Gideon inched up like a fighter using the ropes to climb up, until he came to a sitting position on the edge of the bed. He smacked his lips together. They were dry. "I need something to clean my mouth out."

"Try this," she said, pulling him to his feet, then burying her tongue in his mouth.

"Honey, don't, I stink," he said, holding her off at arm's length, then kissed her. "I lost my head for a minute. I forgot how much you like sweaty, stinking workmen, and perfumed barons, and wop race car drivers, and big black stevedores, and roughnecks with tattoos."

"Yes, darling, and you played every single part to perfection. But most of all, I love mean little five-foot-eight, Jew, cowboy, writers."

"It's so white here. Where are we? Morocco?"

"Cyprus."

"Cyprus? Really? I'll be go-to-hell. Tell me about it."

"I met you when you landed at Beersheba. We took Shlomo back to his kibbutz and saw his wife and children," she said.

Gideon leaned against the wall and bit his lip. "God, he's dead." He rubbed his hand over his stomach. "He caught one right in the belly. We were standing this close together. It could have just as well been me."

"I know, darling, you've told me about it over and over."

Gideon couldn't stand the foul taste in his mouth. He wobbled into the bathroom and spotted her Swedish mouthwash, the brand that could blow a hole in a tank, and drank it straight without mixing it in water.

"Yow!" He opened both faucets and splashed water into his mouth handful after handful. He found his bathrobe on the door hook, put it on, and sauntered out to the balcony, shading his eyes from a blast of sunlight. He was on the third story. A block or two away and below him lay a tiny circular jewel-like little harbor.

"Hey, did Yoffe ever reach Sharm al-Sheikh?"

"Yes, and he beat Zechariah by a half day."

"Good. Cyprus, huh. Where?"

"Kyrenia."

"Any idea how we got here?"

"A friendly driver brought us from Famagusta. He is with relatives across town."

"Jeeze, that's interesting."

"We landed on Cyprus three days ago. You were blotto, oblivious. I have learned every Marine Corps song from the American Revolution on. Anyhow, we cruised out from Nicosia and wound up in the Turkish Quarter of Famagusta yesterday and ran into this nice gentleman, whom we hired as a driver. He introduced us to the delights of opium. Seeing that neither of us had ever tried it before and seeing that mere alcohol was not going to do away with your blues and blahs, and seeing that you declared with bravado that every real writer had to try everything at least once, we did, and here we are."

"I said all that, huh?"

"And much, much more. You wanted to send Shlomo off in grand style. You did him proud."

"You know something, my goddam stomach feels like a sewer is running through it, and my head is about to explode."

Natasha went inside and fixed a potion in a glass, fished for a pair of aspirins in her purse, and drew a glass of water. "Here, just close your eyes and drink this first."

"What is it?"

"Cognac and bitters, an old Hungarian cure-all."

"That's not Israeli cognac, is it?"

"Of course not. You lectured me about that for a full hour in Jaffa."

"I did, huh." He drank, winced, and then downed the aspirins.

"Catch some air out here; it will do you good. I'll order up some lunch."

"I, uh, really don't think I want anything to eat."

"You haven't had anything but booze and opium in your stomach for forty-eight hours."

"All right, but nothing too . . . you know, greasy."

When Natasha returned to the balcony, she found Gideon entranced with the beauty of the harbor. On the far side was an ancient fortress, probably Venetian.

"That harbor is one of the most beautiful things I've ever seen," he said. "What's the name of this hotel we're in?"

"The Dome. It's veddy veddy British, middle-ranking civil-servant type holiday place."

Gideon scratched his stubbly face, then held his hands out, making a square as though it were a camera view finder, putting the quay into focus. "Dome Hotel, Kyrenia, Cyprus," he said, like a "voice-over" of the scene in a screenplay. "I just might start my novel here. That would be wild! We'll have to go down there and take a good look later."

Gideon turned around and, seeing her radiant in her colors, hair now flowing with the breeze, her robe a violent verdant with the sun shimmering off it. He brought her to him, untied the front of her gown. The knot disappeared easily, and he reached inside around her waist and brought all that white softness to him, then lifted her in his arms and took her through the French doors to the big fluffy down featherbed where he buried himself in her.

It took no more than a touch from either of them to set them off again yet one more time, only to be halted by the arrival of the food.

"Good," he said, "I think our tanks are trying to run on empty."

Fortunately the British chef, a former hard-assed cook in the Navy, was on vacation, and his Greek assistant had made up the sumptuous platter of seafood, lobster, squid, dainty little eels, shrimps, chips, veggies, and vino . . . retsina and ouzo. They tried the ouzo. It blended well, not agitating his hangover.

They recounted the past week or so, much of which was very hazy.

"You said to me, I wanna go get fucked up," she swaggered, imitating an American accent. "So, what girl could refuse such a charming invitation?"

The first stop was the King David Hotel. "We barely made it inside our room. Some people in the hall were quite shocked. You stood in the doorway and started to unzip your pants before a group of Hadassah ladies."

"Oh shit, real kid stuff," Gideon chastised himself.

"Then you turned around and mooned them, much to their delight."

"Gimme some more ouzo. This stuff is really straightening me out."

"Closing the door and locking it behind you, you threw the key over the balcony and declared, Ever see turtles fuck? They sit on top of the water in the sun, humping each other with the only movement, the rolling of the waves, and they don't quit till one dies. Well, you weren't exactly a turtle, *habibi*, because every hour or so you would dismount, go out on the balcony, and look across no-man's-land to the Old City walls, and shake your fist and deliver your sermon from the balcony.

"From there the party went to Jaffa . . . for atmosphere, you know. You were determined to find the sleaziest Arab hotel in the Middle East. We came very, very close . . . then Tel Aviv, that part of the city where the gangsters hang out, near the beachfront, and then to Herzlia to the Accadia, where you read me twenty-two letters from your father. My, my, my, Nathan is quite a chap."

Gideon now remembered. He tried to take Natasha to his home, but she had refused to enter, much less make love in Val's bed. From then on, things became fuzzy in his memory.

"So, here we are on good old Cyprus, the next jewel to fall out of the king's crown," Gideon said.

Suddenly the battle for Mitla Pass took over. Shlomo took over. Major Ben Asher and Zechariah and Val and his daughters, now waiting in Rome, took over. And there was the woman across from him, her emerald eyes glowing and singing with love for her wayward cowboy.

They made love again. This time it was sober and hungry and deep. No more little "chicken" contests of who would give up first and have an orgasm, stretching their powers for three, four, five hours before one of them had to quit and explode. No fantasies, no toys, no costumes, no ropes, chains, cuffs, no drugs, no mock wrestling matches, no slaps, no mirrors, no belly dancers in Nicosia's fleshpots, no more pickups in dark cobblestone alleyways, no more sex in the elevator between the first and fourth floors, no more rolling in the fields off the Jerusalem highway, in sight of the Christian Brothers Monastery, no more flashing exhibitions, no more watching paid performances, no more getting it on in the lavatory of the airplanes, no more fingering each other under the tables in restaurants, no more oils, wigs, backs of taxicabs.

They'd done all that. Now it was just plain, raw, naked, screaming sex.

And they collapsed in each other's willing arms, weeping from the continued magic of it, all day, late into the evening.

They went down to the harbor and climbed the steps to the parapets of the old fort. She became entranced watching Gideon's movements; he was like a lion stalking forward, speaking under his breath as his mind whipped the fort and harbor into chapters of a story.

They returned to the Dome Hotel, thought it best to round up their driver and get to the airport at Nicosia, but as they packed they went after each other again and made love and fell asleep, clinging to each other. And darkness came.

Natasha woke up with a start! Gideon was not beside her. She flung off the sheet and leaped from the bed, heart pounding. No! It was all right. He was outside, feet up on the railing looking out to the sea, off again on one of his mystical journeys in that strange world of his own making.

"Hi, cowboy."

"Hello, sweetheart. Jesus, I've got a super first chapter."

She pulled up a chair alongside him and only then saw how troubled he was.

"What's going on inside there?" she asked.

Natasha had caught him cold. He couldn't speak.

"Well, out with it."

He shook his head for her to leave him alone.

"Shlomo?"

"I suppose . . . he didn't have to go into the Pass . . . nobody did."

"You've already said that a hundred times in the past week."

"So I did. At least . . . at least . . ."

"What?" she pressed.

"Nothing," he answered sharply.

"Something's choking you, Gideon. There's a lump in there. I knew it

the first time we met. I've known it every time we've made love. I think
it's time you let it go."

It was quite chilly, but perspiration broke out on his face.

"Gideon, I've learned so much from you. You were the first man to
understand the pain I was in. You were the first man who knew I hated
my father and taught me to stop trying to kill him through other men.
Pussy power is an awesome thing, you said. Don't kill with it. Find a
man you can love in a precious way . . . wild as you want it . . . but
let him live. You held my shoulders and shook me and made me shout
aloud to stop destroying . . . myself . . . and my lovers."

Gideon grunted.

"What is it, man!"

"At least," he cried with a sudden sound that was not his voice, "I
didn't disgrace myself! At least I didn't let Shlomo down!"

"So, that's it. Just let it happen. Natasha is here!"

"I can't," he said shivering.

"Who was Pedro?"

Gideon reacted as though he had been shot. He spun from his chair,
jammed his hands in his pockets, and shook. "It's . . . c . . . c . . .
cold out here. I'm going inside." She came after him. "Don't turn on
the lights," he ordered.

Natasha found a match and lit the candle on the dresser. The breeze
caught the flame and hurled a wild shadow off the white walls and
ceiling. Gideon was silhouetted, sitting on the edge of the bed, his shoulders slumped in grief, his hair falling into his eyes, a Hamlet of Cyprus.

"Pedro was my buddy-buddy," he moaned like a ghost. "I loved him
like a brother. We were in it together from the start, boot camp, radio
school, and then the 6th Marines . . . I was so proud to go into the
6th . . . that was my Uncle Lazar's regiment in the First World War
. . . Belleau Wood . . . I got to wear a *fourragère* around my left
shoulder . . . but he was the one who won it. Pedro and I . . . we
were something else . . . he was just a Mexican kid from San Antonio,
but he had one of those voices only Mexicans have . . . it was like a
nightingale . . . La Paloma . . . Cookoo Rookoo Coo . . . he could
melt the heart of an iron maiden when he sang . . . hell, we'd have
broads waiting for us at the Wellington train station, and they'd just
grab us by the stacking swivels and march us off to bed. I was seventeen, Pedro was nineteen. Can you imagine our chutzpah? Pedro and I
and two other guys rented the God-damned Wellington Opera House
and then conned the commanding general of the division into letting us
put on a review . . . I wrote a good part of it . . . funnier than hell

... but the moment of the night was when Pedro came out in front of the curtain with just a spotlight on his face ... and his guitar ... and he sang. ..."

Gideon sang the song to the tune of "Road to Mandalay" in not much more than a whisper. ...

"on the road to Gizo Bay, ...
where the Jap flotillas lay, ...
and the dawn comes up like thunder, ...
out of Burma cross the way. ...

"ship me somewhere east of Lunga, ...
where the best ain't like the worst, ...
where there ain't no Doug MacArthur, ...
a gyrene can drown his thirst, ...
oh, the Army takes the medals, ...
and the Navy takes the queens, ...
but the guys that take the fucking, ...
are United States Marines. ..."

"He'd made buck sergeant by the time we hit Tarawa. Me? I was a PFC, one rank lower than Hitler. Oh, I got to corporal twice and got busted back to PFC twice. I was always in some kind of mischief. Nothing big ... AWOL a few hours here and there, ducking mess duty, that kind of stuff."

The silence was awful as he tried to force more words up. His chin dropped to his chest.

"... he was in a clearing. He had to expose himself because the fucking radios were some kind of asshole models unfit for combat ... the Marines always got shit gear. So he had to find a clearing to the water, and he was transmitting a message, a very important one. A landing boat bringing us ammo was heading into Jap lines. Pedro was steering them into us. I was on the generator. The Japs opened fire. He kept on transmitting. I kept on winding the generator. Not until he got the message to them did he quit. I started to break down the generator to shag ass, when Pedro toppled over ... maybe twenty yards from me ... I stood there and gaped ... gaped ... I was frozen. Before I could move Captain Farney and Corporal Burns dashed out from cover, passed me, and reached him. They got hit too. All three of them dead."

Gideon suddenly stopped speaking. He stood up and screamed in anguish. "I didn't get to him! I let my buddy down!"

He fell on the bed, rolled onto his stomach, and babbled. "They sent the division to Hawaii to recuperate. I didn't want to go on anymore. I wanted to quit and go home. I had a bad case of dengue fever on Tarawa . . . it's a kind of shit disease where all your joints, elbows, knees, knuckles, all swell up and you've got this crazy fever . . . I wasn't any good to anyone, anymore. Then my asthma came back from the volcanic dust in our camp. So they sent me home. My outfit went on to the invasion of Saipan, and all my buddies got slaughtered on the beach. The guy carrying my radio got his guts blown out. And there I was, safe in the hospital in Oakland, putting on another fucking play!"

He felt her loving hand.

"Don't touch me! I'm no good! I'm a fucking fake! I've faked my way through everything!"

"Don't you know that all soldiers want to go home?" Natasha said. "From the beginning of time, all soldiers want to go home."

"But I . . ."

"What?"

"I was a coward! I was a Jew coward!"

"Shut up, Gideon! Sit up and look at me! I said look at me, God damn you, look at me!"

He rolled over slowly and stared up at her. Natasha's face was wild, and the light and shadows whirling around her were wild.

"What happened to Pedro! He was killed, right!"

"He was killed!"

"How many bullet holes?"

"Just one."

"So he was already dead when Captain Farney and Corporal Burns reached him, wasn't he?"

"He'd been shot through the head."

"And if you had gone out to get him, you would have been killed, just like Farney and Burns, isn't that right? Well, tell me, isn't that right?"

"I don't know . . . maybe I could've . . . maybe if I had acted faster . . . maybe . . ."

"But you stayed on the generator until the message got through. You didn't run. They were shooting at you too."

"We had to save the ammo boat."

"So you stuck in until your job was done. Pedro was dead and the men who went after him got killed. And you've let yourself be filled with guilt because you survived. Darling, remember when you said to me . . . Natasha . . . you can't be guilty because you lost everyone in the gas chambers. You told me that. All survivors have a guilt syndrome. I have it from Auschwitz, you have it from Tarawa. It has nothing to do with you being a Jew. All your life, that's been pounded into you. I'm a Jew, so I'm a coward. So, to absolve yourself of your guilt, you had to write a book, a great book, to redeem yourself in your own eyes and win the respect of your fellow Marines. And then you had to come to Israel and go to Mitla Pass to redeem yourself as a Jew and win the respect of the Jewish people. Why can't you see that, man!"

"Oh, Natasha," he cried, "hold me, hold me, hold me."

Natasha rocked him in her arms, and after a long time Gideon fell into a dead sleep. A knock on the door and she opened it a crack.

"Waiter, ma'am. You asked for the dinner menu."

"Just a moment, please," Natasha said and looked about for a bill to tip him. She went to the armoir, reached inside Gideon's jacket pocket, and took out his wallet. His airline ticket fell to the floor.

She tipped the waiter. "I'll call down when we are ready to order."

"Thank you," he said and closed the door behind him. Natasha returned to the armoir and picked up his ticket, then became curiously entranced by it. As she read it, she paled.

Gideon reached for her on the bed and, feeling nothing, opened his eyes, got his bearings, sat up, and yawned. Natasha advanced toward him ever so slowly.

"Hi, honey," he said. "Must have conked out."

"Bastard!" she said and flung the ticket in his face. Gideon avoided her eyes.

"You were going to take me back to Israel, then head for Rome alone, if I read your ticket right."

"You read it right."

"I was under the illusion that we were on our way to St. Barths to write a book."

"Somewhere along the line during this binge, I had a few moments of clarity," he said. "Natasha, you are every fantasy I ever imagined. But you and I are going to kill each other."

"Why, *habibi*, what makes you say something like that? You know Natasha like a book."

"That's the problem. We seem to have death wishes, you against your father, me against my mother. We can't control them. You're too tough for me and I'm too tough for you. Let's call it a draw."

"You think that little cock of yours is a lethal weapon!"

"We're a shit pair, Natasha."

"You fucking cowboy bastard! You son of a bitch!"

"Don't curse in Hungarian and don't start throwing things."

"Huh! Me! So, go back to your lily-white puritan Protestant wife. You'll come back to me, always! You'll come back to me crawling and I'll make you bark like a dog! They all did!"

"It's a blood sport with us, honey. Sorry to deny you the kill. I guess we'd better round up that driver and get back to Nicosia."

"What's the hurry, cowboy? Let's you and me have one for the road."

ROME

November 15, 1956

"THERE HE IS!"
"Where?"
"Over there!"
"Look, Mommy, he's got Grover Vandover with him!"
"Daddy!"
"Gideon! Here we are!"
"Daddy!"
"Val! Penny! Roxy!"

VAL'S HAND SHOOK SO, she couldn't turn the key. Their room in the Excelsior Hotel was large and splendid and overlooked the elegant Via Veneto thoroughfare. The girls had a smaller connecting room.

"Pretty fancy for poor folks," Gideon said.

"Mother sent me the money," Val said. "And our fare to get home. She's very anxious to support us while you're writing. She really wants to help."

"That's nice, but I'll pick up some screen work. How is your mother?"

"She is in good shape. We'll talk about it later," Val said.

"We've been going to the American school here, Daddy."

"Oh, Rome is so much fun, Daddy. . . ."

There were presents and a big pillow fight and a wrestle on the bed,

Mother, Dad, dog, and daughters, all mixed up together, until they were gasping for breath, and they jabbered, overlapping each other. After a long time, the girls were worn out and slept a lovely sleep with their dog, a sleep of peace they had not known in so long.

Gideon closed their door and smiled. And now he and Val were alone.

"I'm so terribly sorry about Shlomo and all the others," she said.

"Yeah, it was a nasty little war."

"Say, I've got an idea," Val said. "We've got a tub big enough to float a cruiser in. How about you and me sudsing up a tub and getting in and popping the cork on some bubbly?"

"Deal."

After they had luxuriated and fooled around in the bath, as a prelude of sweeter things to come, they wrapped themselves in big terry robes which had been warmed on special heating pipes. Val's hair was still wet from the shampoo. Even under the thickness of her robe, the beautiful lines of her body could be discerned.

"You look terrific, Val," he said.

"You look like you could use a lot of T.L.C.," she said.

There was a stack of mail on the desk. "Anything urgent?"

"Let's see. Sal Sensibar has a couple of screenplays for you to look at. He says he can get you thirty-five thousand on a flat deal, for twelve weeks' work."

"That's real good. Three months. It won't hold the novel up too badly. Should be enough bread to see us through."

"I've booked passages home on an Italian liner. We're so damned broke, I thought it would be a good idea to have Christmas and New Year's at sea."

"Fabulous idea," he said.

"I had to bargain like hell, and we've got two first-class staterooms, and they'll let the girls keep Grover in their cabin. Let's see, stack of letters from your dad. Why don't we let that go till tomorrow."

"Brilliant idea."

"And I'm dying to show you Rome," she said.

"All yours, baby."

"How's the book coming along in your head?"

"It's going to be real good, Val. I mean, real good. I've got a lot of things solved."

"Any new ideas for the title?"

She filled their champagne glasses again.

"I'm thinking *Galilee*. Anyhow, that's good enough for a temporary title. Let's see how it wears."

"Galilee. It's beautiful, Gideon."

They clinked glasses again and sipped. Val turned her back, took a deep breath, and braced herself. "Is Natasha over and done with?" she said, unevenly.

He turned her around and lifted her chin so he could see into her eyes. "I think so, with all my heart. I don't ever intend to see her again. Val, I need your forgiveness for her and for a lot of others."

"I've always forgiven you," she said.

"I don't ever expect you to forget. I'll try to know when you are hurting and I'll comfort you. But I promise . . ."

"No promises," she interrupted, "just do your best and remember, we're very touchy and we've got to learn how to manage our own pain and to help each other."

"Val."

"Yes, dear."

"I forgive you for your little deal, too."

"Thanks, pal," she said, "I've really needed that."

They held each other softly. The song over the American Armed Forces radio station played . . .

"Dance, ma'am?"

"Love to, Marine."

I saw you last night,
And got that old feeling,
When you came in sight,
I got that old feeling.
The moment that you passed by,
I felt a thrill,
And when you caught my eye,
My heart stood still.
Once again I seemed to get,
That old yearning,
And I knew the spark of love
Was still burning.
There'll be no new romance for me,
It's foolish to start,
For that old feeling
Is still in my heart. . . .

"Hey, Marine."

"Yes, ma'am."

"You've got a lousy voice."

"Singing is not my long suit. I'm going to be a great writer someday. Hey, why don't you come over to the hospital tomorrow night? I'm putting on a play."

"Really?"

"Yep. Wrote it, directed it, produced it, and I'm starring in it."

"Cocky, aren't you?"

"You bet. Stick with me, honey, and I'll take you over the rough spots."

The music stopped. "God, that bed looks good," he said.

She lay down and opened the top of her robe for him.

"I love your tits," he said, crawling alongside her and rubbing his face against a breast, gently, with sweet soft brushes of his lips.

"My tired little warrior. Shhhh. Shhhhh. The battle's over for now. The fighting's all done."

He was already half asleep. Tomorrow you go into battle again, Val thought. All of your strange breed seem to have this compulsion to take on the pain of the world. That's why you love John Steinbeck. What pain you must be in now. I have to understand it better and help you. My Gideon, the soul of a poet, the rage of a lion.

They had never felt so good to each other. His head was now buried in her bosom as she ran her fingers through his hair. She and Gideon had inflicted terrible damage on each other, and much of the bitterness was just below the surface. They'd get through this book together; then what? What war would her warrior seek next? Could he ever stop fighting?

Well, no use thinking about it now, Val thought. There was Rome, Christmas at sea, then the greatest time of all, *The Galilee* would be set down on paper.

"Sleep, baby . . ."

"Sleep . . . sleep . . ."

Just before the battle, mother,
I am thinking most of you,
While upon the field we're watching,
With the enemy in view,
Comrades brave are 'round me, lying . . .

Miss Abigail! Miss Abigail! Oh, look at the stars! It's so beautiful up here! Watch me! I'm going to step out of the plane! I'm not scared anymore! You'll be so proud of me! Look! Here I go! MISS ABIGAIL! MISS ABIGAIL! I'VE CAUGHT THE TAIL OF A COMET!

ABOUT THE AUTHOR

Leon Uris lives in Aspen, Colorado, with his wife, the photographer Jill Uris, and their two children. He has been an internationally acclaimed novelist for over thirty years, and his works include *Exodus, Trinity, Mila 18, QB VII,* and *Battle Cry* and, in collaboration with his wife, *Ireland: a Terrible Beauty* and *Jerusalem: Song of Songs.*